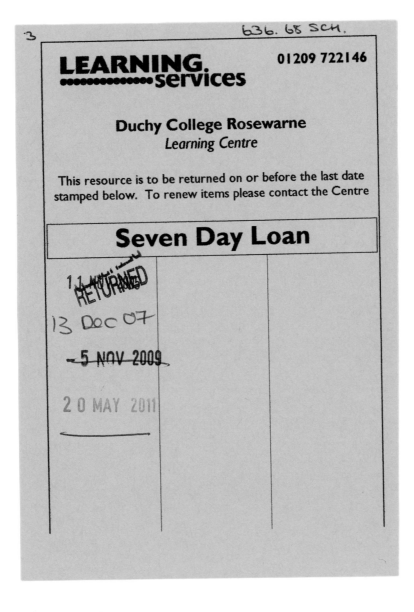

PATHOLOGY OF PET AND AVIARY BIRDS

PATHOLOGY OF PET AND AVIARY BIRDS

Robert E. Schmidt, DVM, PhD
Diplomate American College of Veterinary Pathologists
Zoo/Exotic Pathology Service

Drury R. Reavill, DVM
Diplomate American Board of Veterinary Practitioners
    (Avian Practice)
Diplomate American College of Veterinary Pathologists
Zoo/Exotic Pathology Service

David N. Phalen, DVM, PhD
Diplomate American Board of Veterinary Practitioners
    (Avian Practice)
Department of Large Animal Medicine and Surgery
College of Veterinary Medicine
Texas A&M University

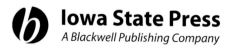

Iowa State Press
A Blackwell Publishing Company

Robert E. Schmidt, DVM, PhD, is a veterinary pathologist and consultant for Zoo/Exotic Pathology Service, Citrus Heights, California. He received his BS and DVM degrees from the University of California, Davis; his MS in veterinary pathology from Michigan State University; and his PhD in veterinary comparative pathology from Oklahoma State University. He is a Diplomate of the American College of Veterinary Pathologists and has been involved in diagnostic pathology of pet and exotic birds for more than 35 years. His professional affiliations include the Association of Avian Veterinarians, The American Association of Zoo Veterinarians, The American Veterinary Medical Association, and the American Association for the Advancement of Science.

Drury R. Reavill, DVM, is a 1986 graduate of the College of Veterinary Medicine, Colorado State University. She is a Diplomate of the American Board of Veterinary Practitioners in avian practice and Diplomate of the American College of Veterinary Pathologists. Dr. Reavill has more than 15 years of experience in avian and exotic animal clinical medicine, clinical laboratory diagnostics, and exotic animal pathology. She currently owns and operates Zoo/Exotic Pathology Service and is a consultant for Veterinary Information Network. Her professional affiliations include the Association of Avian Veterinarians, The American Association of Zoo Veterinarians, The American Veterinary Medical Association, and the International Association for Aquatic Animal Medicine.

David N. Phalen, DVM, PhD, earned his BA at the University of Chicago, his DVM from Cornell University, and his PhD from Texas A&M University. He has been an avian practitioner for 20 years and is a Diplomat of the American Board of Veterinary Practitioners in avian practice. Dr. Phalen has spent the last 10 years studying the epizootiology, diagnosis, and control of infectious diseases of aviary, companion, and wild birds and has published extensively in this field. He is currently an Associate Professor of zoological medicine at Texas A&M University, is included in the Veterinary Honor Roll of the Morris Animal Foundation, is a member of Gamma Sigma Delta, and has received the Excellence in Avian Research Award from the American Veterinary Medical Foundation.

© 2003 Iowa State Press
A Blackwell Publishing Company
All rights reserved

Iowa State Press
2121 State Avenue, Ames, Iowa 50014

Orders:　1-800-862-6657
Office:　1-515-292-0140
Fax:　1-515-292-3348
Web site: www.iowastatepress.com

Authorization to photocopy items for internal or personal use, or the internal or personal use of specific clients, is granted by Iowa State Press, provided that the base fee of $.10 per copy is paid directly to the Copyright Clearance Center, 222 Rosewood Drive, Danvers, MA 01923. For those organizations that have been granted a photocopy license by CCC, a separate system of payments has been arranged. The fee code for users of the Transactional Reporting Service is 0–8138–0502–3/2003 $.10.

♾ Printed on acid-free paper in the United States of America

First edition, 2003

Library of Congress Cataloging-in-Publication Data

Schmidt, Robert E. (Robert Eugene), 1939–
　Pathology of pet and aviary birds/Robert E. Schmidt, Drury R. Reavill, David N. Phalen.—1st ed.
　　p. ; cm.
Includes bibliographical references and index.
　ISBN 0–8138–0502–3 (alk. paper)
　1. Birds—Diseases. 2. Veterinary clinical pathology.
　[DNLM: 1. Bird Diseases—pathology. SF 994 S353p 2003] I.
Reavill, Drury R. II. Phalen, David N. III. Title
　SF994. S36 2003
　636.6'8—dc21
　　　　　　　　　　　　　　　　　　2002013214

The last digit is the print number: 9 8 7 6 5 4 3 2 1

Contents

Previously Published Materials

The following images in this book are:

Reprinted with permission from R.E. Schmidt and G.B. Hubbard, *Atlas of Zoo Animal Pathology*, volume 2, 1987. Copyright CRC Press, Boca Raton, Florida.

Chapter 1—1.19, 1.20, 1.21, 1.30, 1.32, 1.35
Chapter 2—2.14, 2.15, 2.28, 2.31, 2.49, 2.50, 2.59, 2.60
Chapter 3—3.36, 3.47, 3.51, 3.52, 3.54
Chapter 4—4.2, 4.6, 4.25, 4.33, 4.44, 4.46, 4.47, 4.51, 4.70, 4.80
Chapter 5—5.10, 5.13, 5.34
Chapter 6—6.3, 6.13, 6.15, 6.24
Chapter 7—7.15, 7.19,
Chapter 8—8.19, 8.30
Chapter 9—9.1, 9.4, 9.7, 9.8, 9.10, 9.40

Chapter 10—10.9, 10.26, 10.27, 10.35
Chapter 11—11.12, 11.28, 11.29
Chapter 12—12.6, 12.13, 12.14, 12.16, 12.17, 12.23, 12.24, 12.27
Chapter 13—13.7, 13.8, 13.11, 13.15

Reprinted with permission from R.E. Schmidt, *Diseases of Cage and Aviary Birds*, 3rd edition, 1996. Copyright Lippincott Williams & Wilkins, Baltimore, Maryland.

Chapter 2—2.35
Chapter 3—3.44
Chapter 4—4.27, 4.52, 4.56
Chapter 11—11.1, 11.4, 11.15, 11.31
Chapter 12 —12.1

Preface

The number of birds in captivity, as pets and breeders, and in ornamental and zoological collections has increased dramatically in the past 30 years. In many cases, wild populations of some of these species are threatened or have disappeared entirely, leaving the survival of the species to captive-bird breeding programs. With the growth in the bird-owning public has come a commensurate growth in the number of veterinarians providing care for birds and an enormous increase in the knowledge of the husbandry and diseases of these birds, including several comprehensive textbooks of avian medicine and surgery. Since birds are now common mainstream pets, there is also a need for diagnostic veterinary pathologists to be familiar with the diseases of these species.

The necropsy and related diagnostic services are an integral part of avian medicine. Both private and public collections are often large and closely housed. The death of a bird may be the first indication of a serious infectious disease, nutritional disease, or other management-related problem. Avian veterinarians and bird owners depend on pathologists to make an accurate diagnosis and provide advice on the significance of their findings.

Diseases of pet and aviary birds differ significantly from those of poultry. They also differ from many of the common diseases seen in wild birds, even wild birds of the same species. Much of the literature on the diseases of pet and aviary birds is widely scattered in individual articles and in proceedings that most pathologists would not routinely review. Additionally, much information has never been published in any form. The goals of this book are to bring together in one volume a comprehensive review of the gross and histologic features of the diseases of pet and aviary birds and to provide a guide to ancillary diagnostics and a context in which to interpret the pathologic findings. While we feel this book will be of greatest value to veterinary pathologists, we also feel that it will be a valuable reference for practitioners and students of avian medicine, helping them to understand the pathogenesis of the clinical manifestations of disease.

We have organized this material in a systemic format, so that pathologists faced with a diagnostic challenge involving a particular organ can hopefully go to the appropriate chapter rather than having to search through extraneous listings under etiology or by bird species.

For the most part, this book deals with diseases of common, and a few uncommon, pet birds. However, the authors have also included material relating to other avian species that private practitioners and pathologists might occasionally be expected to encounter.

Acknowledgments

The authors thank the many veterinarians who have contributed the material that has led to this book. In particular, we thank Drs. Brian Speer, Alan Fudge, Irv Ingram, Douglas Mader, and Michael Murray for the contribution of photos of gross lesions. For his darkroom expertise, we thank Mr. Larry Wadsworth. Thanks also go to Drs. Roy Pool and Pat Wakenall for reviewing chapters 9 and 8, respectively.

PATHOLOGY OF PET
AND AVIARY BIRDS

1 Cardiovascular System

NORMAL STRUCTURE

The bird's heart sits squarely in the middle of the coelomic cavity just caudal to the thoracic inlet. The axis of a normal heart deviates only slightly from the midline. Enlargement of any of the chambers may result in a change in the heart axis. The cranial ventral surface of the heart is in contact with the sternum, and the liver lobes cover the apex of the ventral surface.

The thin-walled atria have a scalloped surface and margins and are symmetrically located at the base of the heart. The right atrium is somewhat larger than the left. The right atrioventricular (AV) valve is a single muscular flap and is not membranous. The right ventricular free wall wraps around the heart from the caudal right lateral aspect of the heart to the cranial ventral surface of the heart. The wall of the right ventricle is approximately one-third to one-half the thickness of the interventricular septum and the free wall of the ventrical.

The pulmonary and aortic values are essentially the same as those found in mammals. The left AV valve is membranous but is a continuous sheet and does not have clearly defined cusps. The valve is connected to papillary muscles by chordae tendineae. The brachiocephalic trunks immediately branch off the aorta as it leaves the heart. The first arteries to leave the brachiocephalic trunks are the carotids, which are relatively thin walled and narrow. The aorta arches to the right in the bird, as opposed to the left in mammals. Birds have a larger heart compared with body mass. Myocytes have a smaller diameter (approximately one-fifth to one-tenth) than in mammalian hearts and a more rapid depolarization leading to a faster heart rate and relatively greater cardiac output. Purkinje fibers of the conduction system are relatively large.

CONGENITAL ANOMALIES

Most of the literature on avian heart anomalies concerns chickens. Congenital lesions in pet birds are rarely described. Ventricular septal defects appear to be increasingly common in umbrella cockatoos. The defects

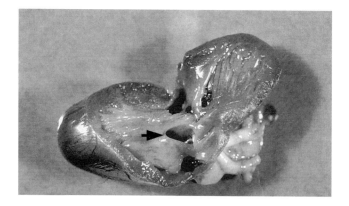

1.1. Interventricular septal defect (arrowhead).

between the ventricles are typically 1 to 3 mm in diameter and are located in the interventricular septum just below the pulmonary and aortic valves (Fig. 1.1). Right-sided and left-sided heart failure typically develops in these birds between 1 and 3 years of age. Dilation of both ventricles is common, and the pulmonary veins are markedly distended (Fig. 1.2). Perihepatic effusion and cirrhosis of the liver with dilation of the hepatic veins may be present secondary to right-heart failure.

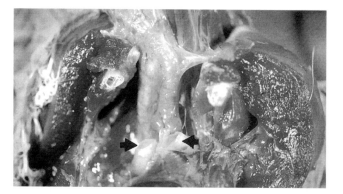

1.2. Marked distension of pulmonary veins (arrows) secondary to right-sided and left-sided failure in a bird with an interventricular septal defect.

3

Congenital aneurysms of the left ventricle are uncommon. One of us (D.N.P.) has seen several of these in cockatiels. All were small, typically 2 to 4 mm in diameter. A large left ventricular aneurysm (2 cm in diameter) was found in a mature blue and gold macaw. There was no other evidence of heart disease, and the lesion was not thought to impact the heart function.

An epicardial keratinaceous cyst presented as a yellow nodule containing caseous material. Histologically it was lined by stratified squamous epithelium, and the grossly noted material was laminated keratin. Based on the gross appearance, the differential diagnosis for this type of lesion would be an abscess. We have seen an African grey parrot with a focus of capillary proliferation in the myocardium (Fig. 1.3) that was considered to be congenital telangiectasis or possibly an example of a hamartoma.

In chickens, cardiac anomalies are thought to be associated with stress during organogenesis, including increased temperature and hypoxia. Vitamin deficiencies may also be responsible for these malformations in chickens. Aortic anomalies are reported in chickens and have been associated with excessively high or low humidity during incubation. Given that ventricular septal defects are seen most frequently in umbrella cockatoos, a genetic defect may be to blame for this anomaly in this species.

PERICARDIAL DISEASE

Pericardial lesions can be a manifestation of infectious, noninfectious, or neoplastic disease.

Infectious Disease

Infectious disease of the pericardium can be localized to the pericardium or may be just one manifestation of a systemic disease. A variety of organisms have been found to cause pericarditis, including numerous bacteria, such as *Mycobacteria* and *Chlamydiophila psittaci*, fungi and, occasionally, polyomavirus.

Grossly the pericardium is variably thickened and gray to yellow-white, with red foci seen occasionally. The pericardium may have a shaggy appearance. In less severe cases, multifocal plaques are seen. There may be adhesions to the epicardium. Pericardial fluid is increased, gray-yellow, and cloudy and may be flocculent. Histologically, bacterial and fungal infections cause edema, fibrin deposition, and an initial purulent response containing numerous heterophils and macrophages. Relatively more lymphocytes and plasma cells may be found in fungal infections. The pericardium may be adhered to the epicardium (Fig. 1.4).

With chronicity, there can be abscess formation. Macrophages and possibly giant cells as well as a more pleocellular response surround a central necrotic area. In both acute and chronic conditions, specificity depends on finding organisms that may be present.

Mycobacterial infections usually present grossly as large irregular masses that can mimic neoplasia. They are relatively firm, gray-white, and most often near the heart base. Early mycobacterial infections elicit a response of heterophils and macrophages. Organisms may be present infrequently. In advanced mycobacterial disease, the response will be primarily large macrophages with abundant light basophilic cytoplasm. Organisms can be seen within the cytoplasm with acid-fast stains.

Noninfectious Disease

The pericardium is a common site of visceral urate deposition (gout). Grossly the lesion can be similar to an infectious pericarditis, with a thickened membrane containing gray-white plaques. However, pericardial thickenings associated with gout are typically white, smooth, and shiny as opposed to the yellowish, roughened, and dull exudates seen in infectious conditions. Flocculent material, along with an excess of turbid fluid, may be present in the pericardial sac (Fig. 1.5).

Histologically, urates may be crystalline or amorphous and are lightly basophilic on hematoxylin-eosin stains.

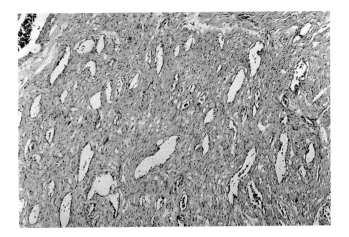

1.3.   Congenital myocardial lesion comprised of irregular, dilated vascular channels.

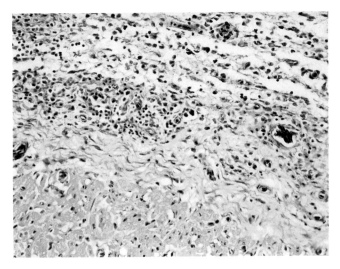

1.4.   Chronic pericarditis. Note the diffuse inflammatory reaction and adherence of the pericardial tissue to the epicardium.

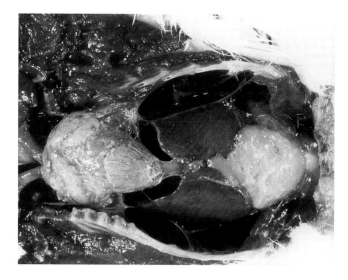

1.5.   Severe pericardial and epicardial urate deposition. The lesion must be differentiated from infection.

Although the crystals dissolve in formalin, the remaining characteristic needle-shaped spaces can be found in most cases. Alcohol fixation and special staining can be used if there is any doubt that the lesion is gout. Depending on the duration of the urate deposition, there will be an inflammatory response comprised primarily of heterophils. Focal necrosis may also be seen.

Neoplastic Disease
In mammals, sarcomas and mesothelioma have been reported in the pericardium. Primary pericardial tumors are not documented in pet birds, and we have not seen any examples of them.

Pericardial Effusion
Effusion may accompany primary heart and pericardial diseases, as already discussed, and may be a part of systemic problems, including anything leading to right-sided heart failure or hypoproteinemia. Effusions may be transudates, modified transudates, exudates, or hemorrhage. The gross appearance will depend on the composition of the fluid. Within several hours of death, high-protein effusions will often become gel-like.

HEART DISEASE
Diseases of the heart can be divided into inflammatory, noninflammatory, and neoplastic. Infectious disease can be further divided into viral, bacterial, mycobacterial, fungal, and protozoal infections. Most diseases of the heart are confined to the myocardium, but, less commonly, lesions can also be seen in the epicardium and endocardium.

Infectious Disease
Several viruses are known to cause myocardial lesions in pet birds. Polyomavirus is seen in a variety of psittacine birds and can also cause heart disease in finches. In

budgerigars, gross lesions include hydropericardium, cardiomegaly, and hemorrhage. The myocardium may have patchy pale areas. Histologically there is coagulative myofiber necrosis and variable nonsuppurative inflammation and hemorrhage. There may be karyomegaly of myocyte nuclei, with margination of chromatin and inclusion body formation. Polyomavirus inclusions are usually pale or almost clear, or granular and basophilic.

In nonbudgerigar psittacines, gross and histologic lesions are similar (Figs. 1.6 Figs. 1.7 Figs. 1.8 Figs. 1.9) to those of budgerigars, although hemorrhage and muscle pallor are more prominent. If there is an inflammatory reaction, it is primarily lymphoplasmacytic. In finches, necrosis, inflammation, and inclusion bodies have been reported.

Proventricular dilatation disease affects a wide variety of psittacine and nonpsittacine birds, and heart lesions are relatively common. Grossly there may be slight dilatation of the ventricles, and occasional pale foci and streaks are seen. Histologically, multifocal lymphoplasmacytic and histiocytic infiltrates are seen in nerve ganglia

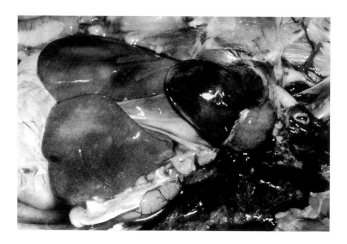

1.6.   Polyomavirus infection causing patchy epicardial and myocardial hemorrhage.

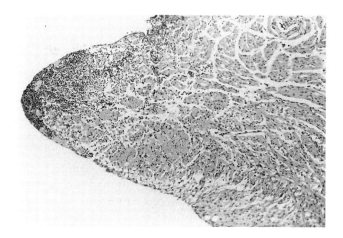

1.7.   Focus of epicardial and myocardial hemorrhage in a bird with polyomavirus infection.

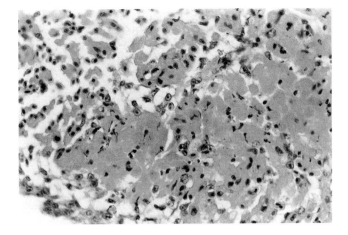

1.8.   Severe myocardial degeneration due to polyomavirus infection.

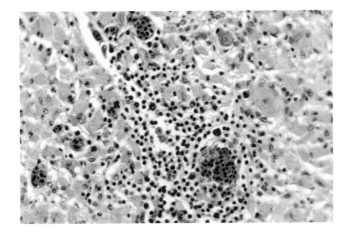

1.9.   Nonsuppurative myocarditis in a bird with polyomavirus infection. Inflammation is seen infrequently in the heart in this disease.

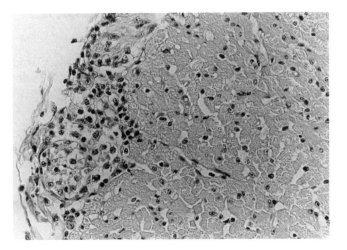

1.10.   Epicardial ganglioneuritis in a bird with proventricular dilatation disease. A lymphoplasmacytic infiltrate is visible.

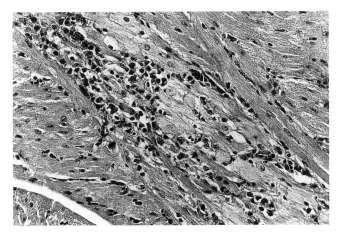

1.11.   Lymphoplasmacytic inflammation in cardiac conduction fibers in a bird with proventricular dilatation disease.

(Fig. 1.10) and in the epicardium and myocardium, particularly near cardiac conduction fibers (Fig. 1.11). The conduction system may be involved, and, when severe, these lesions may cause the bird to die suddenly. Myocyte necrosis and, less commonly, fibrosis are seen.

Togavirus (eastern equine encephalomyelitis or EEE) is thought to be the etiologic agent of a disease described as avian viral serositis. Heart lesions in this disease include a fibrinous gray-yellow epicarditis. There may also be excessive cloudy pericardial fluid. Histologic lesions include the infiltration of lymphocytes, plasma cells, and histiocytes. Inclusion bodies are not seen, but ultrastructurally viral nucleocapsids are noted near cytoplasmic and intracytoplasmic membranes.

There is one report of a parvoviral myocarditis in canaries. A nonsuppurative myocarditis and viral particles were seen on electron microscopy.

Myocardial necrosis is reported in systemic poxvirus infection. The diagnostic features of the disease involve other organ systems.

Bacterial infection of the heart can result in endocarditis, including valvular endocarditis, myocarditis, or epicarditis, although in most cases at least two areas are affected. Bacterial heart disease may be the result of hematogenous spread of infection or direct extension from air sacs or adjacent tissues.

Primary gross changes in myocarditis are multifocal to confluent yellow-white foci (Fig. 1.12) that extend into the myocardium when sectioned. In advanced cases, large yellow nodules may be seen and must be differentiated from other types of infectious disease and neoplasia. Endocarditis may involve the wall and/or valves. Lesions are usually friable and vary from red-gray to yellow. Lesions may be seen on the chordae tendineae. Valvular endocarditis is relatively rare, and, in our experience, the left AV valve is generally the only valve affected.

Histologically, bacterial infections vary with age. In early infections, there is acute necrosis and heterophilic

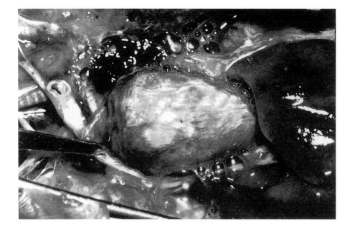

1.12. Severe bacterial myocarditis.

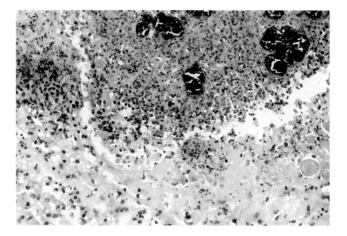

1.14. Severe valvular endocarditis. Large numbers of bacteria and a chronic-active inflammatory response are seen.

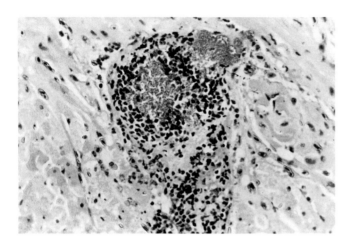

1.13. Bacterial myocarditis. Bacterial colonies are present in necrotic foci. A pleocellular inflammatory infiltrate is seen.

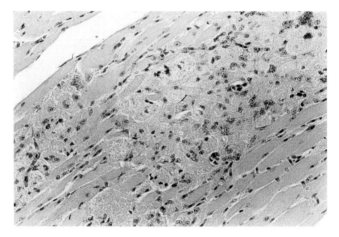

1.15. Mycobacterial infection of the myocardium. Numerous large macrophages are infiltrating the area. Granular material in the macrophage cytoplasm represents bacterial organisms.

reaction, and organisms may be seen (Fig. 1.13). As the lesion becomes more chronic, necrotic foci become surrounded by increasing numbers of macrophages, plasma cells, lymphocytes, and giant cells (Fig. 1.14). Organisms are usually seen in the center of these lesions. In endocardial lesions in particular, fibrosis may occur as mural thrombi are organized. In cases of endocarditis, septic emboli may form, leading to disseminated infection in any other organ.

Mycobacterial infections are usually secondary to hematogenous dissemination or extension from cervical or thoracic air sacs. They usually involve the aorta or pericardium at the base of the heart and have been previously described. If there is myocardial extension, the lesion is similar grossly and histologically to those seen in the pericardium (Fig. 1.15).

Mycotic infections of the heart are infrequent and usually the result of disease extension from air sacs. They usually involve the epicardium and superficial myocardium. Gross lesions are nodular or diffuse, gray-white, and friable. If the fungal infection extends from an adjacent air sac, the fungus will sometimes produce conidia, giving

the fungal plaque a green or black color. Histologically the lesions are similar to bacterial infections, with a pleocellular exudate whose character depends on chronicity. Fungal hyphae must be found for an exact diagnosis. Aspergillus is the most common organism involved, but a specific etiologic diagnosis requires that the organism be cultured.

Disseminated infection by *Aspergillus* sp., other mycelia fungi, and *Candida* sp. can develop in immunocompromised hosts, resulting in hematogenous dissemination to the heart. These lesions are grossly similar to bacterial infections of the heart, but fungal organisms are seen in necrotic foci. The inflammatory response is variable and involves both granulocytes and mononuclear cells.

Protozoal myocarditis is seen in some cases of systemic infection by *Sarcocystis* sp. *Sarcocystis falcatula* is a common cause due to the wide range of the definitive host, the Virginia opossum. The disease in most New World psittacine birds (macaws and conures) is usually subclinical, and the only evidence of infection is the incidental histologic finding of protozoal cysts in the myocardium at necropsy. Old World psittacine birds and some Amazon parrots have an acute disease with pneumonia and widespread dissemination of the organisms.

Gross myocardial lesions are often not seen, but small white foci and streaks may be present in severe cases. Histologically there is a spectrum of myofiber necrosis, hemorrhage, and an inflammatory response comprised of lymphocytes, plasma cells, and macrophages. Newly formed cysts may be found (Fig. 1.16).

Filarid nematodes are an occasional necropsy finding in wild-caught cockatoos. These 1.5-cm white worms may be found in the right heart. Histologically, adult nematodes may be found in hepatic and renal veins, and microfilaria are seen in capillaries throughout the body. In addition, focal endocardial hypertrophy and intimal hypertrophy of intramural vessels are noted. The intimal changes may be due to partial blood flow blockage by adults or a large number of microfilaria. Filarids are a common finding in the heart of some species of wild-caught African storks.

Noninfectious Disease

Inflammatory Disease. Deposition of urates in the epicardium or occasionally myocardium results in grossly noted white-gray foci or streaks. Similar material may be seen in the pericardial fluid. Histologically the urates can be crystalline or amorphous and may elicit an inflammatory reaction comprised primarily of heterophils, although urate deposition without inflammation is also seen.

Nonseptic valvular endocarditis with formation of nodules and accumulation of inflammatory cells and fibrin has been seen as a secondary condition in cases of severe frostbite.

Inflammatory Disease of Undetermined Etiology. Nonsuppurative myocarditis with no obvious cause occurs sporadically in birds. The possibility of autoimmune or immune-mediated disease should be considered in these cases even though not documented. It is known that certain peptides produced by *Chlamydia* mimic murine heart muscle-specific alpha-myosin heavy chains can lead to nonsuppurative perivascular inflammation of the heart of mice. Since pet birds have a moderate incidence of chlamydial infection, perhaps the same mechanism may be operational in birds.

Noninflammatory Disease

Serous Atrophy of Fat. In cachectic birds, fat in the coronary grooves and epicardium may appear clear and watery as well as being reduced in amount. Histologically adipocytes are small, and proteinaceous fluid may be present. Loss of heart fat is one of the first changes in birds experiencing a negative calorie balance, and it may even precede pectoral muscle atrophy.

Mineralization. Deposition of mineral may occur for several reasons, including dietary calcium/phosphorous imbalance, renal disease, and vitamin D_3 toxicity. It may also occur with excessive egg laying, but the pathogenesis is unclear. Mineral can be deposited in areas of myocarditis or myofiber necrosis of any etiology.

Grossly there are gray-white streaks and patches in the pericardium, epicardium, and/or myocardium. Gross differentiation from urates may not be possible, and both may be present in some cases. A spectrum of histologic changes can be seen, depending on the duration of the lesion. Evidence of primary inflammation or degeneration can coexist with myofibers containing a fine basophilic stippling along the cross striations. In some areas, there may be almost complete effacement of myofibers by mineral (Figs. 1.17 and 1.18).

Fat Infiltration. Epicardial fat with some infiltration can be seen in birds, but it can be excessive, usually associated with an obese bird. Grossly the fat appears normal, but histologically there can be deep infiltration of the myocardium.

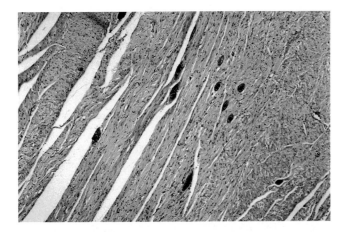

1.16.   Multiple cysts of **Sarcocystis sp.** *in the myocardium. Inflammation is usually not seen.*

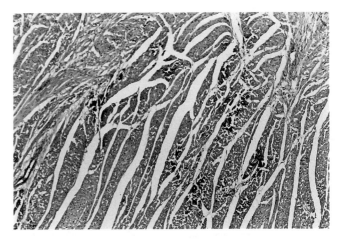

1.17.   Multiple foci of myofiber mineralization in a bird with vitamin E deficiency.

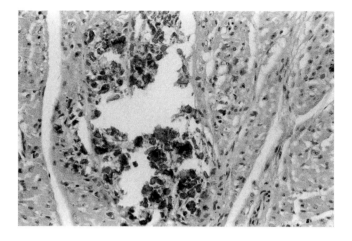

1.18. Severe myofiber necrosis and mineralization as a part of systemic changes in vitamin D toxicity.

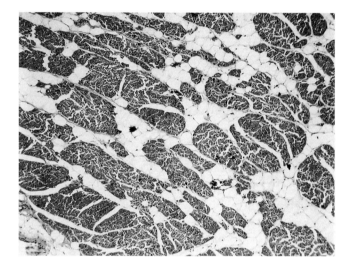

1.19. Severe myocardial fatty change probably associated with long-term feeding of a high-fat diet.

Excessive amounts of fat may be a factor in heart failure, and the condition is seen in birds that die suddenly, with no other morphologic change to explain death (Fig. 1.19).

Lipofuscin. This is an intralysosomal pigment associated with excessive oxidation and polymerization of unsaturated fatty acids. It may accumulate in cells, including cardiac myocytes, secondary to a variety of disease processes. Although usually indicating emaciation or chronic disease, it is sometimes seen in young birds with acute clinical disease, possibly indicating a more chronic process than was expected. It is usually considered an incidental necropsy finding. If severe, the myocardium may have a brown discoloration. Microscopically, fine yellow-brown pigment is seen, primarily near the nucleus, but more diffuse in severe cases. One form of lipofuscin, ceroid, may occur in vitamin E deficiency.

Cardiomyopathy. Three forms of cardiomyopathy are usually described in mammals: hypertrophic, dilated, and restrictive. We have seen examples of the first two in pet birds. In both cases, the diagnosis is usually made on gross examination. Hypertrophic cardiomyopathy is characterized by ventricular thickening that leads to a diminution in ventricular volume. Dilated cardiomyopathy presents usually as a left-sided problem, with the left ventricle thin and flabby. In both cases, there may be no histologic change noted without quantitative morphometry and comparison to an age- and sex-matched bird of the same species. In some cases of dilated cardiomyopathy, the myofibers may appear obviously thin, with loss of sarcoplasmic detail, and, in some chronic cases, there has been evidence of fibroplasia, possibly indicating a previous insult. Restrictive cardiomyopathy is characterized by endocardial disease and fibrosis and could theoretically follow a variety of endocardial diseases, but we have not seen well-documented cases in pet birds.

Myocardial Degeneration. This may be the result of a vitamin E and/or selenium deficiency, vascular problems, and some toxicities. In many pet bird cases, the exact underlying problem is not determined. The gross appearance of an affected heart varies from having white streaks and patches to large pale areas (Fig. 1.20). In some chronic cases, the foci may appear as depressed areas. If there has been mineralization, affected areas are gritty when cut. Hydropericardium may be present.

Early histologic changes include contraction band formation, cross-striation loss, swelling, and hyalinization (Fig. 1.21). With progression, there is granulation, necrosis, and segmental fragmentation of myofibers. Microscopic mineralization may be seen, and, in chronic lesions, myofiber shrinkage and fibrous connective tissue proliferation are noted. No appreciable inflammatory response is seen (Fig. 1.22).

Myocardial degeneration is a prominent feature of a fatal disease of great-billed parrots. Also affected are the

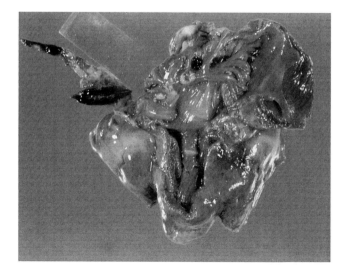

1.20. Myocardial degeneration due to vitamin E deficiency. Pale streaks and foci extend into the myocardium and on the epicardial and endocardial surfaces.

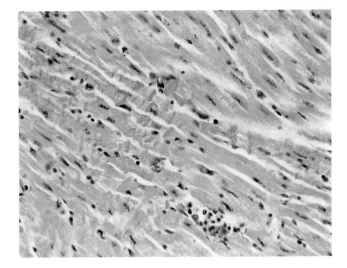

1.21.   Contraction band formation and early myofiber fragmentation.

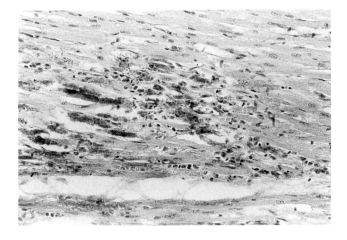

1.22.   Necrosis of myofibers and severe mineralization in chronic nutritional myodegeneration.

white matter and Purkinje cells of the cerebellum and skeletal muscles. The etiology is not known, but the lesions closely resemble those seen in poultry with vitamin E deficiency.

Endocardiosis. Noninflammatory swelling of true heart valves occurs occasionally. The cause is usually not determined. Affected valves are grossly swollen and usually smooth and firm. Histologically there may be hemorrhage, fibrous tissue proliferation, deposition of mucinous material, and cartilaginous metaplasia.

Heterotopic bone is seen sporadically in the myocardium. Its cause is usually not determined. Grossly the myocardium may feel gritty and histologically there is well-differentiated bone (Fig. 1.23).

MYOCARDIAL TOXICITY

Although a variety of drugs and chemicals are potentially cardiotoxic in birds, there are very few documented cases.

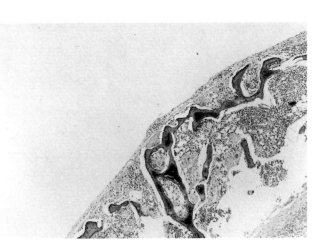

1.23.   Diffuse production of heterotopic bone in the atrium of the heart.

Natural and experimental poisoning by avocados is seen in ostriches, canaries, cockatiels, and budgerigars. Gross lesions include subcutaneous edema and hydropericardium. Histologic lesions include myofiber degeneration and variable inflammation. Heterophils are seen in affected ostriches, but the lesion in canaries is characterized by nonsuppurative inflammation (Fig. 1.24). The toxic principle has not been determined.

PROLIFERATIVE DISEASE OF THE MYOCARDIUM

Hypertrophy

Hypertrophic cardiomyopathy as a specific condition has already been discussed. Sporadic cases of myofiber hypertrophy are seen secondarily as compensatory responses to conditions that lead to an increased preload. These changes include pulmonary disease, vascular disease, congenital anomalies, and possibly chronic renal disease. Grossly the affected portion of myocardium is thickened and the lumen of the affected ventricle(s) is reduced. His-

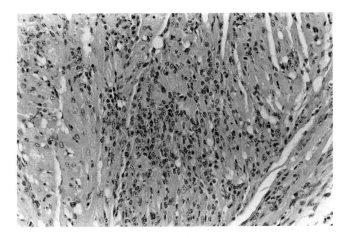

1.24.   Myodegeneration, sarcolemmal proliferation, and nonsuppurative inflammation in a bird with avocado toxicity.

tologically myofibers may appear to be normal, and without quantitative morphometry change can be difficult to discern. In more advanced cases, fibers may be thickened and lose their typical parallel appearance, and their nuclei may be enlarged.

Neoplastic Disease

Several types of tumor are seen in the heart of birds. Rhabdomyoma or rhabdomyosarcoma is usually pale and firm grossly and may be multiple. Microscopically, strap and fusiform cells and cross striations are seen in routine sections of benign tumors. Sarcomas contain cells that may be fusiform, stellate, or straplike, and cross striations are usually not present with hematoxylin-eosin-stained sections. Immunohistochemistry is often needed to prove the tumor is of striated muscle origin. Cell nuclei are enlarged and vesicular and may be multilobulated. Giant cells are often present. Rhabdomyosarcomas are infiltrative into surrounding myocardium.

Hemangiomas and hemangiosarcomas are found in the myocardium as red-black masses that may be friable and bleed easily. Histologically, benign tumors are comprised of well-differentiated vascular channels. Although histologically benign, these lesions interfere with normal cardiac function and do not have a benign behavior. Sarcomas are less well differentiated and may contain vascular channels lined by poorly defined endothelium, as well as solid foci.

We have seen primary fibrosarcomas of the myocardium. These tumors present as firm gray-white masses comprised of interlacing bundles and whorls of fibroblasts. Mitotic figures are typically abundant (Fig. 1.25).

Lymphosarcoma may involve the myocardium alone, or the heart may be involved as part of a generalized disease. Grossly the tumor is yellow-white or gray and may be diffuse or in multiple masses. Histologically lymphosarcoma is comprised of moderately undifferentiated pleomorphic lymphoid cells with variable mitotic activity (Fig. 1.26). They form infiltrative sheets in the myocardium. Occasionally, varieties appear to be primarily histiocytic (Fig. 1.27).

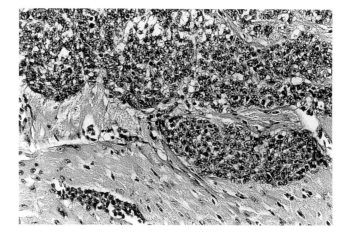

1.26.   Lymphosarcoma infiltrating and effacing the myocardium.

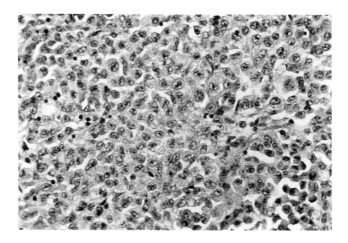

1.27.   Myocardial histiocytosis. Compare the cell morphology with Figure 1.26.

Malignant melanoma may be found in the avian heart and is usually metastatic. These tumors are brown-black and may be multiple. Microscopically, poorly differentiated melanocytic cells form nests and sheets within the myocardium.

Other metastatic tumors are rarely seen in the avian heart, but we have noted metastatic proventricular carcinoma in the epicardial lymphatics in a few birds.

THE MORPHOLOGY OF HEART FAILURE

A variety of conditions have been described that lead to heart lesions and subsequent death in birds. In addition, there have been many cases of pet birds whose presenting clinical sign was sudden death. In many of these cases, there is no gross or microscopic lesion. Sudden cardiac failure may be the underlying cause in many of these cases, and a careful and complete necropsy, as well as an investigation into the environment and husbandry of the bird, may be necessary to try and reach a conclusion as to possible cause.

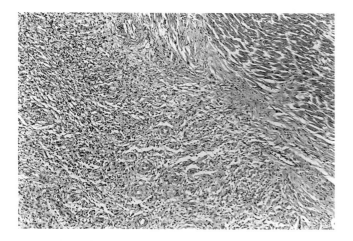

1.25.   Fibrosarcoma replacing myofibers of the ventricle.

The mechanism leading to acute cardiac death in any animal is often the creation of ventricular fibrillation or asystole. Factors influencing fibrillation include a long QT interval, hypokalemia, acidosis, imbalance in sympathetic/parasympathetic stimulation with a sympathetic dominance, and emotion. With sympathetic dominance, there is an exaggerated catecholamine reaction, reduced oxygen supply to the myocardium, and muscle spasm. The cardiac conduction system is described as anaerobic, with every cell functioning in an all-or-nothing capacity. Only a few cells are required for functioning, and problems can persist for some time until some insult leads cardiac failure. In chickens and turkeys, abnormal calcium regulation plays a part in the pathophysiology of heart failure. Although studies have not been done in pet birds, the mechanism may be similar.

Internal factors to consider in evaluating possible acute heart failure include disease in almost any other organ. In particular, there may be a relationship between the adrenal gland and the heart that leads to sudden death. With stress, there is an increase in interrenal cell (avian analog of cortical cells) hormone production that increases target organ sensitivity to the beta-adrenergic effects of epinephrine, leading to cardiotoxicity.

External factors may be obvious, such as a high-fat or other improper diet leading to obvious heart lesions. Less obvious is the possibility of the water supply being artificially softened, possibly causing electrolyte (potassium and magnesium) imbalances. In humans, soft water is apparently associated with cardiac problems. Although not documented in birds, evaluation of the water supply could be considered in ruling out unexplained sudden death.

The oculocardiac reflex results from pressure on or within the eyeball or stretching of ocular muscles. This results in a trigeminovagal reflex that leads to slowing of sinus rhythm and decreased conduction and contractility. This reflex has caused sudden cardiac failure in a pet bird.

Nonspecific stress is difficult to quantify and may be of different types and intensity. It is a factor in birds, particularly those in large aviary situations. Physical stress may be suspected if the owner is a good observer, but the possibility of mental or emotional stress as documented in humans is difficult to affirm. If environmental conditions include overcrowding, noise, and species/size mixture, some of the birds may certainly become stressed and die suddenly of no apparent cause.

VASCULAR DISEASE

Inflammatory Disease

Arteritis, phlebitis, and lymphangitis are infrequently encountered in pet birds. Bacterial infections can result in associated vasculitis in any organ. Histologically there is necrosis of the vessel wall and a response comprised primarily of heterophils. Microorganisms may or may not be present.

Mycobacterial arteritis is seen associated with lesions involving the pericardium and base of the heart. Lesions are similar to those that are seen in other parts of the heart (Fig. 1.28).

Fungi, such as *Aspergillus* sp., commonly invade the vasculature, resulting in the wide dissemination of fungal emboli that can cause vasculitis within any organ. In addition to necrosis and a pleocellular inflammatory infiltrate involving the vessel wall, organisms are usually present in the lumen and wall of the involved vessel or vessels.

Although not common in pet birds, paramyxovirus 1 (PMV-1), and togavirus (western equine encephalomyelitis or WEE) can cause vasculitis. Grossly, in both infections, there will be hemorrhages, particularly in the serosa of the gastrointestinal tract. Histologically, vascular lesions of both infections are similar. Hemorrhage and edema are associated with hyalinization and degeneration of blood vessel walls, endothelial necrosis, possible thrombosis, and a variable mononuclear inflammatory infiltrate (Fig. 1.29).

Noninflammatory Disease

Aneurysmal dilatation of blood vessels is not common in pet birds. Occasional uncomplicated aneurysms are noted as variably sized dilatations in arteries. Histologically they are characterized by attenuation of the media, and there is usually no indication as to underlying cause, but they may be associated with atherosclerotic plaques.

Dissecting aneurysm is found in many avian species but is most often seen in the turkey and occasionally seen in the ostrich. These lesions are usually considered to be associated with a copper deficiency. A copper-dependent enzyme, lysly oxidase, is needed for connective tissue cross-linking of collagen and elastin in artery walls. Aneurysms begin with necrosis of elastin and arterial smooth muscle in the media, with subsequent hemorrhage and longitudinal dissection within the artery. Grossly there is dilatation and hemorrhage, and, on section, the dissecting band of hemorrhage is noticeable.

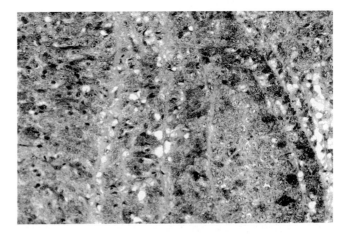

1.28.   Acid-fast stain of diffuse infiltration of the artery wall by large macrophages containing acid-fast bacteria in a bird with mycobacteriosis.

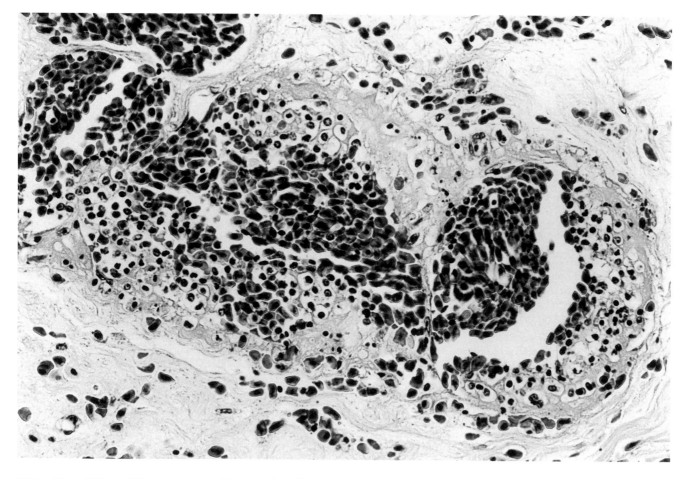

1.29. Vasculitis and degeneration of the vessel wall due to togavirus infection.

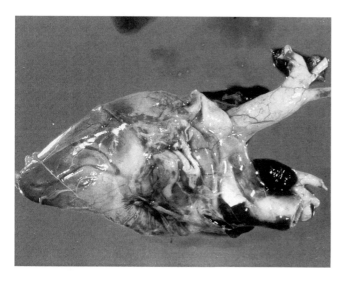

1.30. Ruptured aortic aneurysm with associated severe hemorrhage.

Affected arteries may rupture (Fig. 1.30), with hemorrhage and clots noted in adjacent tissue and spaces. Thrombosis may also be present. Microscopically there is elastic tissue necrosis, acid mucopolysaccharide material deposition, hemorrhage, and variable inflammation that separate the arterial media.

Atherosclerosis. This is seen most often in Amazon parrots, particularly the blue-front Amazon parrot, African grey parrots, and macaws, although it occurs sporadically in a variety of species. Birds can be of any age, but most are 8 or more years old and many are more than 15 years old. Birds may die suddenly and be in excellent condition or be obese. Somewhat less commonly, atherosclerosis may cause a chronic disease that results in a loss of condition. Often there is a history of birds going through periods of a loss of awareness of their surroundings in the days or weeks prior to their death. Many birds have a history of being fed a diet rich in fat.

The lesion can be found in the aorta, brachiocephalic trunks, and pectoral and carotid arteries. Carotid artery involvement is relatively rare. Grossly the arterial wall is variably thickened and yellow (Fig. 1.31) and contains roughened yellow intimal plaques. Microscopically the appearance of these plaques depends on the chronicity of the condition. The lesion begins in the media. In early stages, there is fragmentation of the elastica and cell proliferation resulting in thickening of the media. Advanced lesions are characterized by the foam cells, which have distended cytoplasm that contains lipid and cholesterol clefts. These cells undergo necrosis, and extracellular lipid and amorphous ground substance are found within the atheroma. There can be microhemorrhage, chondroid

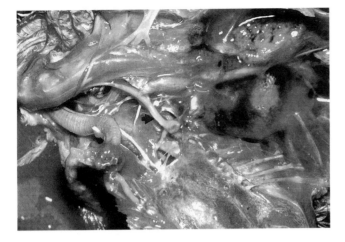

1.31.   Typical atherosclerosis. Artery walls are thickened and discolored (arrow).

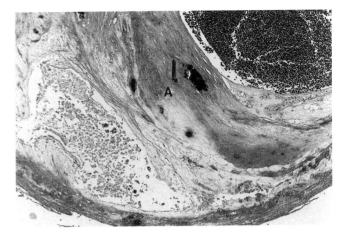

1.33.   Severe arterial thickening due to atherosclerosis. Note the early chondroid metaplasia (A) and canalization.

metaplasia, fibrosis, and mineralization (Figs. 1.32 and 1.33).

Many birds die because of a decreased blood supply to the brain as a result of severe narrowing of the carotid arteries. Infarction of the pectoral muscles occurs but is relatively rare. Likewise, it is rare to see ischemic disease of the heart. Atherosclerosis can lead to aneursymal dilatation of the arteries. More commonly, it causes increased arterial resistance that affects the heart. Early changes in the heart include hypertrophy of the left ventricle, followed by left ventricular dilation, dilation of the left atria, right-heart dilation, and right-heart failure. Right heart failure causes congestion, atrophy, and subsequently cirrhosis of the liver.

Mineralization. Mineralization of blood vessels with no other morphologic change is seen in cases of severe renal failure, chronic dietary imbalance of calcium and phos-

phorus, and vitamin D_3 toxicity. The change is typically in arteries or arterioles and can be found in any organ or tissue. The only gross indication may be a gritty feel to the tissue if the lesion is widespread or associated with other soft tissue mineralization. In larger arteries, raised, firm, irregular plaques may be seen that are usually gray-white and may be have a shiny appearance. Histologically, all or part of the vessel wall may be affected (Fig. 1.34).

Amyloidosis. Among pet birds, amyloidosis is more common in the small passerines species but can occasionally be seen in other birds. Amyloid is deposited in a number of soft tissues and, in some cases, is found in the walls of blood vessels. This condition is usually not detected grossly. Histologically, affected vessels have a thickened media that has an amorphous, smooth appearance that is eosinophilic or amphophilic on hematoxylin-eosin stain. As in mammals, it is birefringent when stained with Congo red and viewed with polarized light (Fig. 1.35).

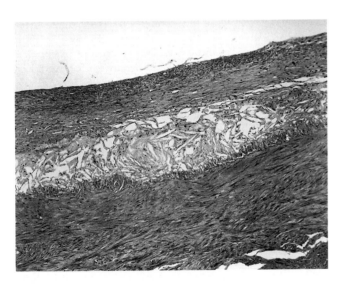

1.32.   Early atherosclerotic lesion with foam cell and cholesterol cleft formation.

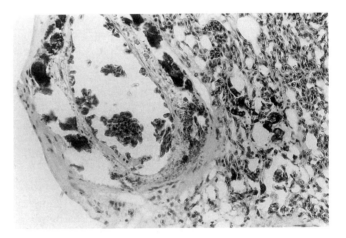

1.34.   Mineralization of the arteriolar wall associated with a generalized problem due to chronic renal disease.

Thrombosis. Septic and nonseptic thrombi may be found in any tissue, depending on their cause. Septic thrombi are often associated with valvular endocarditis, and bacteria may be present. Fungal infection that involves blood vessels may also lead to thrombi. Secondary changes include infarcts and infection/inflammation in the involved tissue.

Proliferative Lesions. Hemangioma and hemangiosarcoma can occur in any organ but are most common in the skin and subcutis. Hemangiomas are usually deep red or black and have a smooth surface (Fig. 1.36). They are comprised of numerous fairly regular vascular channels lined by well-differentiated endothelium (Fig. 1.37). Occasionally, they are associated with adipose tissue proliferation leading to a tumor that has been called hemangiolipoma.

Hemangiosarcomas may be red-brown and have a roughened appearance with indistinct borders. They contain moderately undifferentiated or poorly differentiated endothelium and irregular vascular channels, as well as solid foci (Fig. 1.38).

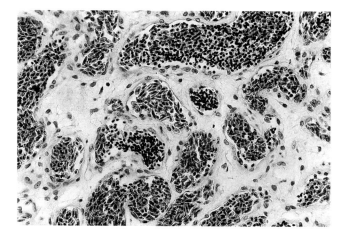

1.37. Typical appearance of hemangioma. Well-differentiated endothelial cells line the vascular channels.

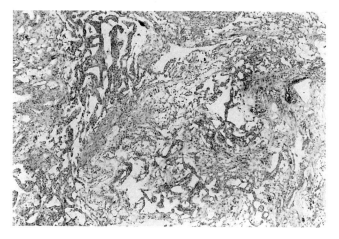

1.38. Poorly defined vascular channels and solid foci in hemangiosarcoma.

Lymphangiomas are similar to hemangiomas, being lined by fairly well differentiated endothelial cells. No erythrocytes are found in the channels, however (Fig. 1.39).

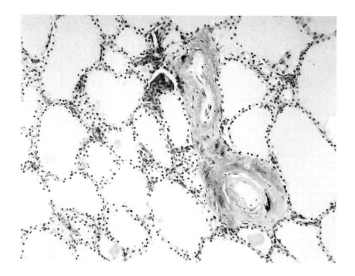

1.35. Amyloidosis of the arteriolar walls in the thyroid gland.

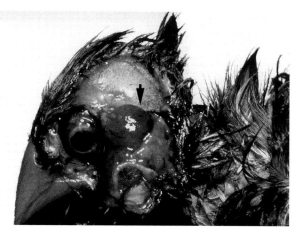

1.36. Red-brown mass typical of cutaneous and subcutaneous hemangioma (arrowhead).

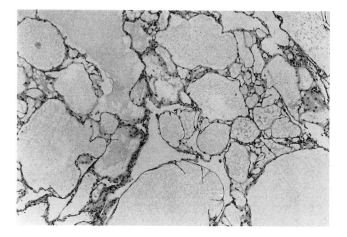

1.39. Lymphangioma comprised of dilated lymphatic channels containing proteinaceous material.

ADDITIONAL READING

Bachmaier K, Neu N, de la Maza LM, Pal S, et al. 1999. Chlamydia infections and heart disease linked through antigenic mimicry. Science 283:1335–1339.

Baptiste KE, Pyle RL, Robertson JL, Pierson W, et al. 1997. Dissecting aortic aneurysm associated with a right ventricular arteriovenous shunt in a mature ostrich. (*Struthio camelus*). J Avian Med Surg 11:194–200.

Beehler BA, Montali RJ, Bush M. 1980. Mitral valve insufficiency with congestive heart failure in a pukeko. J Am Vet Med Assoc 177:934–937.

Burger WP, Naude TW, Venrensburg IBJ, et al. 1994. J S Afr Vet Assoc 65:113–118.

Conrad AD, Consigli RA, Conrad GW. 1993. Infection with the avian polyomavirus, BFDV, selectively affects myofibril structure in embryonic chick ventricle cardiomyocytes. J Exp Zool 267:253–266.

Duncan A, Fitzgerald SD. 1997. Clinical challenge. J Zoo Wildl Med 28:501–503.

Freeman KP, Hahn KA, Adams WH, et al. 1999. Radiation therapy for hemangiosarcoma in a budgerigar. J Avian Med Surg 13:40–44.

Gaskin JM, Homer BL, Eskelund DK. 1991. Preliminary findings in avian viral serositis: A newly recognized syndrome of psittacine birds. J Assoc Avian Vet 5:27–34.

Greenacre CB, Mann KA, Latimer KS, Ritchie BW. 1993. Adult filarioid nematodes (*Chandlerella* sp.) from the right atrium and major veins of a Ducorps' cockatoo (*Cacatua ducorpsii*). J Assoc Avian Vet 7:135–137.

Harari J, Miller D. 1983. Ventricular septal defect and bacterial endocarditis in a whistling swan. J Am Vet Med Assoc 183:1296–1297.

Hargis AM, Stauber E, Casteel S, Eitner D. 1989. Avocado (*Persea americana*) intoxication in caged birds. J Am Vet Med Assoc 194:64–66.

Helfer DH, Schmitz JA, Grumbein SL, Lowenstine L. 1981. Myocarditis-encephalopathy in canaries. In: Proceedings of the 30th Western Poultry Disease Conference, Davis, CA, p 92.

Isaza R, Buergelt C, Kollias GV. 1992. Bacteremia and vegetative endocarditis associated with a heart murmur in a blue-and-gold macaw. Avian Dis 36:1112–1116.

Johnson JH, Phalen DN, Graham DL, et al. Atherosclerosis in parrots. In: 1992 Annual Conference of the Association of Avian Veterinarians, New Orleans, LA, pp 87–93.

Kim CS, Davidoff AJ, Maki TM, et al. 2000. Intracellular calcium and the relationship to contractility in an avian model of heart failure. J Comp Physiol [B] 170:295–306.

Oglesbee BL, Oglesbee MJ. 1998. Results of postmortem examination of psittacine birds with cardiac disease: 26 cases (1991–1995). J Am Vet Med Assoc 212:1737–1742.

Page CD, Schmidt RE, English JH, et al. 1992. Antemortem diagnosis and treatment of sarcocystosis in two species of psittacines. J Zoo Wildl Med 23:77–85.

Phalen DN, Hays HB, Filippich LJ, et al. 1996. Heart failure in a macaw with atherosclerosis of the aorta and brachiocephalic arteries. J Am Vet Med Assoc 209:1435–1440.

Pipo R, Broadstone RV, Murphy CJ. 1996. Lethal oculocardiac reflex in a cockatiel. Vet Comp Ophthalmol 6:27–29.

Puette M, Latimer KS, Norton TM. 1995. Epicardial keratinaceous cyst in a tawny frogmouth (*Podargus strigoides plumiferus*). Avian Dis 39:201–203.

Randolph JF, Moise NS, Graham DL, Murphy CJ. 1984. Bacterial endocarditis and thromboembolism of a pelvic limb in an emu. J Am Vet Med Assoc 185:1409–1410.

Riddle C. 1987. Avian histopathology. Lawrence, KS: Allen, pp 31–36.

Speer B. 1993. Selected avian pediatric viral diseases. In: Fudge A, ed. Seminars in avian and exotic pet medicine, pp 125–135.

Vanhooser SL, Stair E, Edwards MR, Carter C. 1994. Aortic rupture in ostrich associated with copper deficiency. Vet Hum Toxicol 36:226–227.

Vice CAC. 1992. Myocarditis as a component of psittacine proventricular dilatation syndrome in a patagonian conure. Avian Dis 36:1117–1119.

Vink Nootebooom M, Schoemaker NJ, Kik MJL, et al. 1998. Clinical diagnosis of aneurysm of the right coronary artery in a white cockatoo (*Cacatua alba*). J Small Anim Pract 39:533–537.

Wack RF, Kramer LW, Anderson NL. 1994. Cardiomegaly and endocardial fibrosis in a secretary bird (*Sagittarius serpentarius*). J Assoc Avian Vet 8:76–80.

Wallach JD, Glieg GM. 1969. Frostbite and its sequelae in captive exotic birds. J Am Vet Med Assoc 155:1035–1038.

2 Respiratory System

NORMAL STRUCTURE

The cere is the thickened portion of integument that straddles the base of the nasal region. It may be feathered or bare, and it may or may not contain the nares (nostrils). In psittacines, the nares are located dorsally within the cere. Cockatiels have a well-developed cere compared to Amazon parrots. The cere of an Amazon is covered with tiny feather bristles (setae). Pigeons have well-developed ceres above the horn (rhinotheca) of their bills and behind the nares.

The vestibule of the nare is lined by a uniquely structured, keratinized, stratified squamous epithelium. The epidermis arises from a one to two layer thickness of basal cells—the stratum basale—that supports columns of epithelial cells, producing a corrugated surface. The uppermost cells in each column have pyknotic nuclei. The vestibular epithelium blends with the epidermis on the inner side of each nostril.

Many species of parrots and galliformes have an operculum just inside the cere. It is a rounded, keratinized structure that may act as a baffle to deflect and prevent inhalation of foreign material. The external nares open into the nasal cavity, which is tubular and separated into right and left chambers by the nasal septum. The nasal cavity has a threefold function of olfaction, filtration of airborne debris, and thermoregulation. Along the lateral walls of the nasal cavity are scrolls of cartilaginous and bony nasal conchae. The nasal conchae increase the surface area of the nasal cavity and, in most psittacines, are divided into three regions. The rostral concha is highly vascular and lined with stratified squamous epithelium. The middle and largest section has a mucociliary lining, and its cavity is continuous with the nasal cavity. The caudal section is lined by olfactory epithelium and does not open into the main nasal cavity. The olfactory epithelium is a pseudostratified columnar epithelium comprised of basal, olfactory, and supporting cells. This caudal section connects dorsally with the infraorbital sinus. African grey parrots—Falconiformes—and swifts do not have a definitive caudal nasal concha.

The infraorbital sinus is a large cavity under the skin primarily in the lateral region of the upper jaw. The right and left sinuses communicate in psittacines but not passerines. The infraorbital sinuses have openings directly into the nasal cavity or dorsally into either the middle or caudal nasal conchae. Numerous diverticula from the sinus extend around the eye and ear, into the maxillary and mandibular beak and pneumatized sections of skull. These diverticula communicate with the cervicocephalic air sac at its caudal-most extent. In Amazon parrots, the diverticula can extend as far caudal as the seventh cervical vertebra. Stratified squamous epithelium lines the rostral infraorbital sinuses, and ciliated columnar epithelium with a few mucous glands are found caudally. Because of its position and poor drainage, this sinus is often involved in diseases of the upper respiratory tract.

The nasal cavity opens into the oropharynx via the choana, a median slitlike structure in the palate. The mucosa changes from the pseudostratified ciliated columnar cells with intraepithelial mucous glands of the nasal cavity to the stratified squamous epithelium of the palate. The palate surrounding the choanal slit is covered with keratinized papillae and supports the submucosal salivary glands.

The rima glottis is the laryngeal opening into the trachea. The larynx is comprised of four laryngeal cartilages. The cricoid cartilage is scoop shaped, with left and right lateral wings. The procricoid is small and articulates with cricoid wings on the dorsal midline. The two arytenoid cartilages form the margins of the glottis.

Closed cartilage rings that are shaped like overlapping signet rings form the avian trachea. The trachea is longer and wider than in a comparably sized mammal. There are some species variations of the trachea. Curassows and spoonbills have long tracheal coils between skin and pectoral muscle. In penguins and toucans, the trachea is divided at the cranial end of the neck into left and right tubes by a medium cartilaginous septum. Emus and ruddy ducks have an inflatable saclike diverticulum.

The syrinx is at the tracheal bifurcation within the thorax. The majority of birds have a tracheobronchial syrinx. Male ducks of subfamily Anatinae have a syringeal bulla that is an asymmetric dilation on the left side of the syrinx. Two primary bronchi form at the tracheal bifurcation, and they again branch into approximately 20 secondary bronchi.

The normal tracheal mucosa consists of ciliated pseudostratified columnar epithelium and mucus-producing goblet cells. The goblet cells are arranged as intraepithelial simple alveolar mucous glands in the proximal trachea and are more prominent as individual goblet cells in the distal trachea. The syrinx is lined by a stratified squamous epithelium. The primary and secondary bronchi are also lined with a pseudostratified ciliated epithelium and variable number of goblet cells.

The secondary bronchi give off a large number of small, tertiary bronchi that have a constant mean internal diameter. These tertiary bronchi, which are also known as parabronchi, anastomose with other tertiary bronchi. The walls of tertiary bronchi are thin, lined with squamous epithelium, and have thin underlying bands of smooth muscle (atrial muscles). These walls are perforated by numerous openings leading into small sacculations in the bronchial walls (atria). These atria are lined with flat or cuboidal epithelium. The atria are separated by atrial septa. Funnel-shaped infundibula from the floor of the atria open into the air capillaries.

The air capillaries branch and freely anastomose with each other and are surrounded by a network of blood capillaries. This is the site of gaseous exchange. The blood-gas barrier is formed by endothelial cells, a common basal lamina comprised of a thin, electron-dense air capillary membrane that is frequently fused with a thicker, more lucent, blood capillary membrane, and the squamous epithelial cells of the air capillaries. The epithelial cells of the air capillaries have very thin cytoplasmic extensions, reminiscent of the mammalian type I pneumocyte. Macrophages are not normally found in air capillaries.

There are two functional, but not distinctly anatomic, systems of the avian lung. The phylogenetically primitive paleopulmonic lung includes the cranial pulmonary air sacs. This functional unit is present in all birds, and the airflow is unidirectional. The neopulmonic lung includes the caudal pulmonary air sacs, and air changes direction with each phase of breathing.

Air sacs are thin-walled structures with limited vascularity. They are an adaptation for more efficient respiration, insulation, and buoyancy in some birds. There are nine air sacs in pet birds: the unpaired clavicular, and the paired cervical, anterior thoracic, posterior thoracic, and abdominal air sacs. The clavicular air sac extends into the humerus, coracoid, scapula, and clavicle. It runs adjacent to a main ventral nerve to the wing. Inflammation of this air sac can result in paresis of the wing.

The cervical air sacs are between the lungs, dorsal to the esophagus, and have extensions into the vertebrae. The cranial thoracic air sacs lie in the dorsolateral thoracic cavity. The caudal thoracic air sacs are caudal to the cranial thoracic. The abdominal air sacs penetrate into the intestinal peritoneal cavity. Except for the abdominal sacs, each air sac is connected directly to a secondary bronchus. The abdominal sac connects to a primary bronchus. The lining of the air sacs is a simple squamous epithelium with a basement membrane and underlying connective tissue. The air sacs have a similar histologic appearance to the peritoneum.

The cervicocephalic air sac is not part of the pulmonary air-sac system and is not used in gas exchange. It may function as insulation, as buoyancy control, or perhaps to support the head during sleep or flight. There are two divisions—the cephalic and cervical portions—and it connects to the caudal infraorbital sinus. The cephalic division is not found in macaws. The cervical portion extends around the tympanic area and extends in two columns bilaterally down neck. It is lined with single layer of low cuboidal or flat squamous cells.

RESPIRATORY DISEASE

Upper Respiratory System
Congenital Disease. Choanal atresia is described in African grey parrots and an umbrella cockatoo (*Cacatua alba*). A persistent membrane or bony plate at the palate of the nasal cavity results in a closed choanal slit. This blocks the normal drainage of nasal secretions into the oral cavity. Young birds will present with a chronic nasal or ocular discharge, and, in some cases, the infraorbital sinuses will be distended with clear secretions.

Infectious Disease

Bacterial Disease. A number of gram-negative bacteria and occasionally gram-positive organisms can cause a bacterial sinusitis. Acute sinusitis is characterized by a serous discharge, with swelling and redness in the orbital area and nares (Fig. 2.1). Histologically there is a thickening of the nasal mucosa or sinus membranes due to infiltrating heterophils, lymphocytes, and plasma cells, as well as hemorrhage, fibrin deposition, and tissue edema (Figs. 2.2 and 2.3).

Chronic infections are generally more common in cockatiels, Amazons, macaws, and African greys. They are

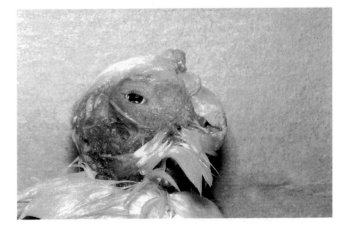

2.1.   *Marked swelling and feather loss secondary to sinusitis.*

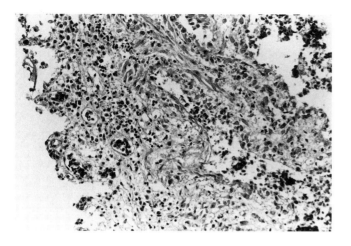

2.2. Diffuse necrosis and loss of mucosa in a bird with bacterial sinusitis.

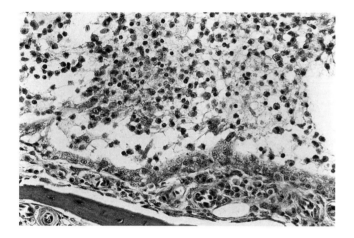

2.3. Bacterial sinusitis. Detail of a pleocellular inflammatory response.

associated with a mucopurulent discharge and variable tissue distortion of the nares and beak or swelling of the periorbital sinuses and choanal slit region. There is loss or blunting of the palatine papilla and the formation of small pyogranulomas or granulomas in the mucosa. The majority of chronic cases will have a focal lesion within the nasal cavity or diverticula of the infraorbital sinuses. Chronic bacterial or fungal granulomas, inflammatory polyps, unorganized caseous material, and mucoceles have been described.

The sunken-eye syndrome of macaws is associated with chronic bacterial sinusitis. The enophthalmia that occurs appears to be a sequela of an infection in the infraorbital sinus diverticula around the eye. *Escherichia coli*, *Klebsiella* species, and *Haemophilus* species have been isolated from these cases. Examination of the globes and periorbital soft and bony tissue is recommended.

Another specific syndrome attributed to a bacterial sinusitis is the lockjaw syndrome of cockatiels. A number of microorganisms have been isolated from the sinuses of affected birds, including *Bordetella avium*, *Klebsiella* species, *Aeromonas* species, *Pseudomonas* species, *Enterococcus* species, *Staphylococcus* species, *Streptococcus* species, and *Bacillus* species.

The disease generally affects young cockatiels 3 to 10 weeks of age. They initially develop a nasal and ocular discharge and swollen periorbital tissues that progress to an inability to open the beak. This results in death. Nasal passages, sinuses, and air spaces within cranial bones will contain inflammatory exudates consisting of fibrin, heterophils, and histiocytes. Histologic sections through the skull will have a necrotizing rhinitis and sinusitis, as well as pleocellular and fibrosing myositis of the jaw muscles. Osteomyelitis of the cranial bones and perineuritis are often present. The lesions in the sinuses and adjacent muscles of the temporomandibular joint are the most significant. Rarely, peracute hepatic necrosis, chronic hepatic fibrosis, splenic lymphocytic depletion, and subacute pneumonia with air sacculitis are present.

An unidentified spirochete has been associated with upper respiratory infections in cockatiels. The birds develop excess mucus of the choanae and trachea. There is an acute mild nasal sinusitis, and a thin gram-negative spirochete can be identified by exfoliative cytology. The significance of the bacteria is unknown. It is speculated that the spirochete may interfere with normal ciliary function of the upper respiratory tract.

Mycotic Disease. Members of the genus *Aspergillus* and the class Zygomycetes are capable of causing localized and/or disseminated disease. This group is characterized by the formation of hyphae in tissue.

Aspergillus is a ubiquitous, opportunistic fungus that grows readily in moist environments and on substrates such as wood shaving, corncob bedding, and seed hulls. It can be isolated from bird feces. *Aspergillus fumigatus*, *A. flavus*, *A. glaucus*, *A. oryzae*, *A. niger*, and *A. nidulans* have all been isolated from lesions in avians. *Aspergillus fumigatus* is the most common.

At least 11 species of the class Zygomycetes are regarded as medically important. The class includes the order Mucorales, containing the genera of the bread molds, such as *Mucor*, *Rhizopus*, and *Absidia*. This order is unique in that the hyphae are nonseptate or rarely septate. They are widespread in nature, thriving in organic material. They are also common laboratory contaminants. Infections involving *Rhizopus*, *Mucor*, and *Absidia* are reported in birds, although they are uncommon and usually associated with an underlying disease condition. The most common route of infection is by inhalation of the spores. There is a reported affinity of Zygomycetes to localize within blood vessels and the heart.

Localized lesions have been described in the trachea, bronchi, sinus, nasal cavity, and body cavity. In nasal cavity infections, the respiratory region of the nose is more susceptible than the vestibular region. Most mycotic rhinitis infections in psittacines start unilaterally and have a mucopurulent discharge. The fungal organisms tend to invade the sinuses, blood vessels, turbinate cartilages, and nasal bones. Mats of the fungal hyphae are supported within necrotic debris, hemorrhage, fibrin deposition, edema, and mixed inflammation. Cases of acute rhinitis or sinusitis have a large number of viable and degenerate heterophils.

More chronic lesions will have perivascular clusters of lymphocytes and plasma cells and hyphae associated with multinucleated giant cells and epithelioid macrophages. The underlying lesions may suggest mucosal epithelial metaplasia of vitamin A deficiency or foreign material lodged within the nasal or infraorbital sinus.

Cryptococcal sinusitis, also known as turulosis or European blastomycosis, is caused by the saprophytic yeast *Cryptococcus neoformans*. There are two varieties of *Cryptococcus neoformans*. *Cryptococcus neoformans* var. *neoformans* has been recovered from a variety of environmental substrates, including fruit, vegetables, nonpasteurized milk, and hay. It is commonly isolated from the feces of birds, especially poultry and pigeons. Avian feces contain creatinine that the fungus uses as a source of nitrogen. This variety grows poorly at temperatures higher than 40°C. *Cryptococcus neoformans* var. *gattii* is associated with the flowers of the *Eucalyptus camaldulensis* (red river gum) and *E. tereticornis*. The *gattii* variety grows poorly at temperatures higher than 37°C.

Cryptococcus neoformans infrequently causes disease in birds, possibly due to the protection by their normal bacterial microflora and high body temperature. The respiratory tract appears to be the portal of entry, possibly because the upper respiratory tract has a lower mean temperature that may be predisposed to colonization. Dissemination to the central nervous system is not unusual with this fungus. The lesions are of a myxomatous gelatinous tan to white material within the nasal and infraorbital sinuses, lungs, air sacs, and brain.

On exfoliative cytology, the organisms are narrow-based budding round yeast with a thick capsule. India-ink stains demonstrate the large heteropolysaccharide capsule. Histologically the numerous yeast appear as "soap bubbles" separating the tissue's elements. They have infrequent narrow based budding and are 5 to 15 μm in diameter. A variable and generally mild infiltration of heterophils, lymphocytes, plasma cells, and macrophages will be present (Fig. 2.4). Mucicarmine stain will help visualize the typical thick outer capsule.

Noninfectious Disease. Pet birds that are on a primary seed or cereal grain diet or have intestinal mucosal lesions that interfere with conversion of carotenoids to vitamin A may develop vitamin A deficiency. Vitamin A deficiency results in epithelial squamous metaplasia, which is manifested as hyperkeratosis of oral cavity, conjunctiva, nasal lacrimal duct, upper alimentary tract, and respiratory tract (Fig. 2.5). In large parrots, the epithelial changes will appear when vitamin A concentrations in the liver decrease below 50 IU/g.

Keratinizing epithelium that blocks the ducts of submucosal mucous glands is the typical lesion. These

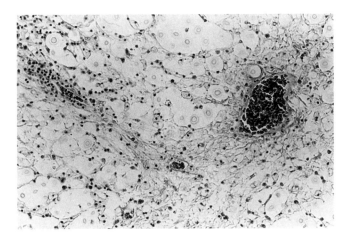

2.4. Sinusitis due to Cryptococcus sp. Note the numerous organisms and minimal inflammatory response.

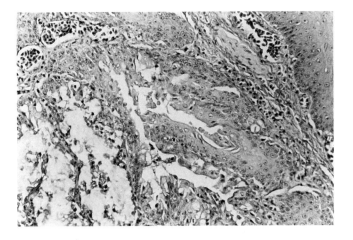

2.5. Metaplasia of pharyngeal and glandular mucosa in a bird fed a vitamin A–deficient diet.

glands enlarge and become secondarily infected, resulting in large keratin granulomas within the nasal or oral cavity. Some birds, especially African grey parrots, develop massive keratin rhinoliths that distort the nares and nasal sinus. The squamous metaplasia also alters the mucosal defenses, predisposing the bird to fungal and bacterial infections primarily of the respiratory tract.

Neoplastic Disease

Nasal/Sinus Carcinoma or Adenocarcinomas. Carcinoma and adenocarcinoma of the upper respiratory system may arise from the nasal or sinus mucosa or from glandular epithelium. These tumors can become quite large, leading to distortion of the skull. They may impinge upon the brain in severe cases. Grossly the tumor is gray-white, firm, and nodular (Fig. 2.6). Histologically infiltrative cords and nests of neoplastic cells are usually seen within a moderate amount of stroma (Fig. 2.7).

Squamous Cell Carcinoma. Squamous cell carcinoma (SCC) is a malignant tumor comprised of nests and infil-

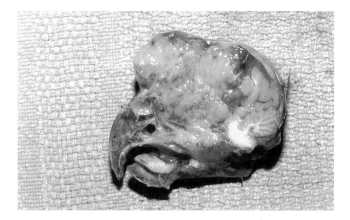

2.6.   Nasal/sinus carcinoma with extension into the skull and brain.

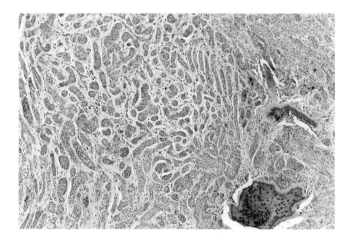

2.7.   Nasal/sinus carcinoma. Numerous trabecular structures and nests are separated by moderate stroma.

trative cords of moderately undifferentiated to poorly differentiated squamous cells that frequently form central cores of compressed, laminated keratin ("keratin pearls"). In pet birds, the primary sites for SCC are the skin and upper gastrointestinal tract, including the beak, oral cavity, esophagus, crop, and proventriculus. SCC is a common tumor in budgerigars.

SCC in the nasal sinuses and oral cavity has poorly defined borders and is associated with hemorrhage and necrosis of the surrounding tissues. It is commonly associated with chronic stomatitis, and caseous material may be found within the mass. It is a locally aggressive tumor that tends to recur. There are few reports of metastases.

Fibrosarcoma. Fibromas and fibrosarcomas are tumors that originate from fibrous connective tissue and are common neoplasms in pet birds. Fibromas are not reported in the upper respiratory tract, and fibrosarcomas are rarely described within the nasal infraorbital sinuses. The common sites of occurrence include the limbs, face, beak, syrinx, liver, small intestine, cloaca, spleen, air sacs, and lungs. Fibrosarcomas are gray-to-white firm masses with irregular and indistinct borders. Fibrosarcomas are locally

invasive, rarely metastasize, and have a moderate to high potential for recurrence, giving them a guarded prognosis.

Lymphosarcoma. Multicentric lymphosarcoma is the most common lymphoid neoplasia in psittacine and passerine birds. Lymphosarcoma may be more common in canaries, with an increased prevalence in males. However, male canaries, due to their popularity as songsters, may be the most common sex presented to veterinarians. Lymphoid neoplasms have been reported in many psittacine species. The reported ages of birds at the time of diagnosis ranged from 5 months to 30 years, with an average of 8 years.

A leukemic blood profile is uncommon in psittacine birds with lymphoid neoplasia. Canaries tend to have leukocytosis and lymphocytosis. Anemia (packed cell volume < 35%) is common.

Diffuse or nodular involvement is characteristic of pet bird lymphosarcoma. Organs typically infiltrated include liver, spleen, kidneys, skin, bone, gastrointestinal tract, thyroid gland, oviduct, lungs, sinus, thymus, testes, brain, mesentery, trachea, fat, periorbital muscles, and pancreas. In the upper respiratory tract, Amazon parrots more commonly present with a mass in the choana, and African grey parrots develop a periorbital mass. Grossly the lesions are firm and gray-white. Histologically normal tissue is effaced by a diffuse sheet of immature lymphoid cells. Mitotic activity is variable.

Although lymphosarcoma in chickens commonly is associated with retrovirus (avian leukosis virus) or herpesvirus (Marek's) infection, there is no evidence to date of a viral link to the tumor formation in pet birds. Recent molecular investigations suggested a retroviral cause for multicentric lymphosarcoma in a starling. Retrovirus-induced lymphosarcoma has been suspected in other passerines but remains to be proven.

Malignant Melanoma. This has been recognized in the nasal sinuses as part of an infiltrative tumor involving the oral cavity and beak of African grey parrots (chapter 3). The tumor masses are black and firm. The infiltrative, deeply pigmented, melanocytic neoplasm is arranged in clusters and packets. The cells are round to ovoid, with an eosinophilic cytoplasm containing small to moderate amounts of brown granular pigment. The cell nuclei are pleomorphic, with a vesicular and marginated chromatin and variably prominent nucleoli. The cells have negative S-100 protein immunoreactivity.

Trachea
Viral Disease

Herpesvirus. Herpesviruses are enveloped DNA virions that measure approximately 120 to 200 nm in diameter. The three viral subfamilies are alpha herpesvirus, beta herpesvirus, and gamma herpesvirus. Members of the alpha herpesvirus are associated with rapid viral replication, cytolysis, and ability to establish latent infection. Infectious laryngotracheitis in chickens, Pacheco's disease, Amazon tracheitis virus, and parakeet herpesvirus are caused by alpha herpesvirus. Amazon tracheitis virus and parakeet herpesvirus have a tissue tropism for the respiratory tract. The Amazon tracheitis virus is believed to be a variant of the infectious laryngotracheitis virus. A herpesvirus causing similar lesions to those seen with the Amazon tracheitis virus are reported in brown-throated conures (*Aratinga pertinax*). This virus was positive with an in situ probe derived from a Pacheco's disease virus, suggesting that the Pacheco's disease virus and the virus in the conures are genetically similar.

The defining lesions of Pacheco's virus are massive hepatic and splenic necrosis with syncytial cells, and eosinophilic intranuclear inclusion bodies. Occasionally, intranuclear inclusions and necrotic lesions have been described in a variety of other tissues. Outside of the liver and the spleen, the pancreas, crop, and intestine are most likely to contain lesions. Less commonly, kidney, endocrine organs, or cloaca are involved. It is unusual for Pacheco's disease to affect the respiratory system, but, when it does, the intranuclear inclusions have been observed in epithelial and syncytial cells of the larynx, trachea, and bronchi.

The herpesvirus outbreaks that primarily target the respiratory tract (Amazon tracheitis like virus) have been recognized in Amazon parrots, brown-throated conures, Bourke's parakeets (*Neopsephotus bourkii*), whiskered lorikeets (*Oreopsittacus arfaki*), and rosellas (*Platycercus* species). The tracheal mucosa and lungs appear edematous and congested. The histologic lesions range from the severe hemorrhagic or fibrinonecrotic inflammation that primarily affects the upper respiratory tract to a proliferative bronchitis with mild necrosis and syncytial cell formation. Type A nuclear inclusion bodies can be found in bronchial epithelial and syncytial cells (Fig. 2.8).

Cytomegalic Virus. Finch cytomegalovirus is a host-specific beta herpesvirus that appears to be a disease primar-

ily of finches, especially Gouldian finches, and is characterized by high mortality, conjunctivitis, tracheitis, and bronchitis. The prominent gross lesion is a hyperemic and edematous conjunctiva. The air sacs may be thickened with fibrin. The conjunctivae, syrinx, and bronchi will all have a hyperplastic epithelium with cytomegaly and karyomegaly (Fig. 2.9). The esophagus and nasal conchae have focal diphtheritic lesions with the characteristic inclusion bodies. The viral inclusions are large intranuclear basophilic inclusion bodies within cytomegalic cells.

Polyomavirus. Polyomavirus, a nonenveloped DNA virus in the Papovaviridae family, commonly results in a pansystemic disease of nestling budgerigars and other psittacines. The most consistent lesions of polyomavirus include hepatic necrosis, membranous glomerulopathy, variable karyomegaly of hepatocytes and renal tubular epithelial cells, and large clear to basophilic

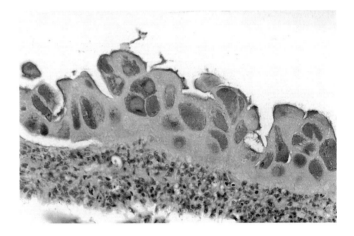

2.9.   A finch with cytomegalic herpesvirus infection. There is marked mucosal proliferation with karyomegaly and intranuclear inclusion body formation.

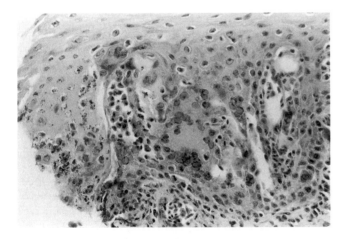

2.8.   Pharyngeal necrosis and intranuclear inclusion body formation in herpesvirus (possible Amazon tracheitis) infection.

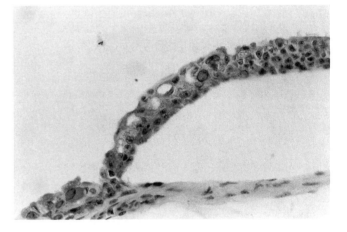

2.10.   Polyomavirus infection leading to tracheal mucosal proliferation and intranuclear inclusion body formation. The changes are not as severe as those seen in cytomegalic herpesvirus infection and are unusual in polyomavirus infection.

intranuclear inclusion bodies of the splenic periarteriolar sheaths. The intranuclear inclusions have rarely been recognized within the bursa of Fabricius and the mucosa of the trachea, crop, and proventriculus (Fig. 2.10).

Mycotic Disease. The fungal organisms associated with cases of mycotic tracheitis are the same as those producing mycotic sinusitis. Localized fungal lesions have been described in the trachea bronchi, sinus, nasal cavity, and body cavity. The lumen of the trachea, syrinx, or bronchi will be partially to completely occluded with a white to cream-colored fibrinocaseous plug (Fig. 2.11). In the trachea and bronchi, the fungal mycelia penetrate the walls and combine with inflammatory cells to form caseous, granulomatous nodules (Fig. 2.12).

The syrinx is a common site of primary infection. Many pet birds will have a history of unsupplemented all-seed diet, suggesting that hypovitaminosis A was a predisposing factor to the development of the tracheal lesions.

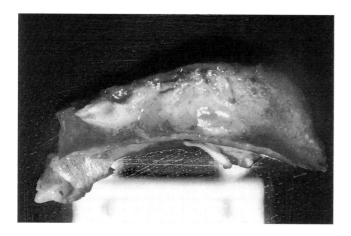

2.11. Severe tracheal aspergillosis with blockage of the lumen by exudate.

Parasitic Disease

Protozoal Disease. Trichomonads are flagellated protozoa that are primarily enteric pathogens. Several closely related organisms have been isolated from lesions in the upper respiratory tract of birds. *Tetratrichomonas anatis* was isolated from the swollen infraorbital sinus, the nasal sinus, trachea, and the lower small intestine in ducklings. It is associated with a mucoid fibrinopurulent sinusitis and catarrhal rhinitis and tracheitis. There is marked hyperplasia of mucous cells in the epithelium, with excessive mucofibrinous exudate and many desquamated epithelial cells. Heterophils, some mononuclear cells, and erythrocytes are also present. Large numbers of pyriform-shaped protozoa stained purplish red with hematoxylin-eosin are seen in the exudate.

Trichomonas gallinae, normally a pathogen of the digestive tract of Columbidae and raptors, is found within lesions of the respiratory sinuses and trachea of these species. The mucosa is covered with superficial dry caseous diphtheritic membranes, and caseous material fills the tracheal lumen. Another common location for these lesions is the pharynx. These lesions are often large and caseous and may obstruct the choanal slit or the glottis. Trichomoniasis species are also associated with necrotic, caseated masses in the trachea of psittacines (Fig. 2.13). These protozoa are best visualized on wet mount preparations. The exudates from infraorbital sinuses and intestinal contents will have many motile protozoa with an undulating membrane and flagella. They are pear shaped, 12.20 μm long, and 8 to 12 μm wide, with a distinct nucleus.

Nematodes. *Syngamus trachea*, also commonly known as the "gapeworm," has been reported in psittacine birds only once. This nematode parasite inhabits the trachea, bronchi, and bronchioles of waterfowl, game birds, Galliformes, and occasionally kestrels and Columbiformes. It also commonly affects American robins. It is a large, robust, bright-red helminth that appears Y shaped because the

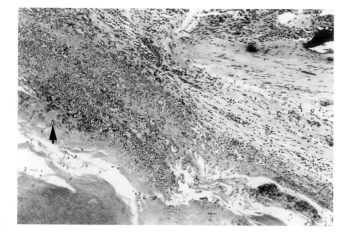

2.12. Tracheal/syringeal aspergillosis. Severe inflammation, fibroplasia, and exudate formation. A few organisms can be seen (arrowhead).

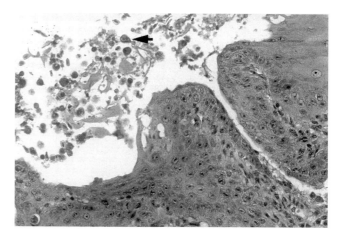

2.13. Trichomoniasis of the trachea. The mucosa is thickened, and organisms are seen within the lumenal exudate (arrowhead).

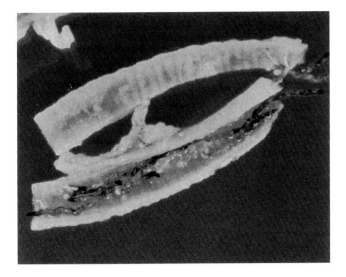

2.14. Syngamus sp. *and exudate within the tracheal lumen.*

male is attached to the female. (Fig. 2.15). The life cycle is direct, although earthworms and cockroaches may serve as transport hosts. They produce large, ellipsoidal, operculated eggs that can be identified on fecal parasitic examinations and direct smears of the oral cavity.

Grossly the trachea will be hemorrhagic with many nematodes and eggs (Fig. 2.14). The lungs are firm, with irregular focal yellow areas of the parenchyma. The air sacs can be thickened and covered with yellow material (fibrin). The nematodes are associated with intense mixed inflammatory cell inflammations and associated hemorrhage, fibrin deposition, and edema (Fig. 2.15). Multinucleated giant cells and a large number of macrophages commonly aggregate around the eggs.

Sternostoma tracheacolum, a parasitic rhinonyssid mite, is the tracheal mite of canaries and Gouldian finches (*Erythrura gouldiae*). It is presumed to have a direct life

cycle passing from parents to chicks. Aviculturists will use society finches to raise Gouldians in order to raise mite-free chicks. Air-sac mites are generally distributed throughout the respiratory system, especially in juvenile birds. Mites attach to the mucosa by embedding their legs into the connective tissue. Mucus from the host will coat the mites. They are recognized as small black masses within the lumen of the trachea. The tracheal lesion associated with the mite is mucosal epithelial necrosis as well as mucosal hyperplasia with mixed inflammation. Heterophils, lymphocytes, and plasma cells will accumulate in the submucosa and extend between the tracheal rings. Mites have a brown, slightly refractile cuticle, segmented legs, and bands of striated skeletal muscle within the body cavity.

Inhaled Toxins/Irritants. Exposure to gases produced by undiluted sodium hypochlorite (5% chlorine bleach) appears to induce tracheal lesions that can result in death. Days after the initial lesion of tracheal hyperemia, multifocal diphtheritic membranes and caseous material covering the tracheal mucosa develop. These birds may also have yellowish, cloudy air sacs.

The histopathologic lesions of the trachea include epithelial deciliation, ulceration, squamous metaplasia, and epithelial hyperplasia. Death is considered to be the result of hypoxia secondary to blockage of the trachea or pulmonary congestion and, in some cases, sepsis secondary to invasion of bacteria through the altered tracheal mucosa.

Inadvertent inhalation of ivermectin diluted 1:10 with propylene glycol can result in respiratory distress and a necrotizing tracheitis. It was unknown whether the inhaled ivermectin or a carrier is responsible.

Foreign bodies lodging in the trachea are not an uncommon problem, although there are rare reports in the literature. In cockatiels, millet seeds are the most common foreign bodies to become lodged at the tracheal bifurcation. Acutely the mucosa of the trachea becomes

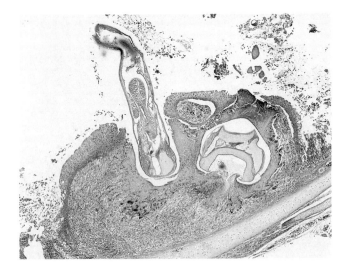

2.15. Tracheal infection by Syngamus sp. *Note the swelling and inflammation associated with attachment of the parasites.*

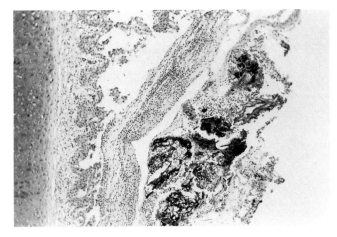

2.16. Foreign-material inhalation leading to an inflammatory response and fibrin production. Partial or complete tracheal blockage can occur.

edematous, and heterophils infiltrate within the first few hours. As time passes, mixed cellular infiltrates, vascular compromise, and necrosis occur (Fig. 2.16).

Neoplastic Disease. Internal papillomatosis results in proliferative, gray-white growths on mucous membranes. Histologically they are frondlike projections of hyperplastic epithelium supported by thin, inflamed, fibrovascular stromal stalks. Mitotic activity is primarily in the polygonal basal cells, and mucin-producing cells may be present in the lining epithelium. The fibrovascular stroma will have varying infiltrates of plasma cells, lymphocytes, and heterophils. The lesions closely resemble those caused by papillomaviruses in mammals. To date, evidence for a papillomavirus in these lesions has not been found. However, many, possibly all, birds with internal papillomatosis are concurrently infected with one of the Pacheco's disease viruses. The role that these viruses play in the pathogenesis of this disease remains to be determined. Reported sites include the oropharynx, choanal cleft, conjunctiva, larynx, esophagus, crop, proventriculus, ventriculus, nasal mucosa, nasolacrimal duct, bile ducts, pancreatic ducts, and cloaca. Two of the most common sites for these lesions is the mucosa on the margins of the choanal slit and the mucosa of the glottis. Large papillomas in this location can interfere with breathing.

This disease affects New World psittacines, especially the macaws, Amazons, and hawk-headed parrots. The age range in a series of Amazons was from 18 months to greater than 15 years. There is a cyclic regression and recurrence. There is a suggested association in psittacines between papillomatosis and bile duct and pancreatic duct tumors.

Tracheal Osteochondroma. Tumors of the trachea are rare in birds. Tracheal osteochondroma, which is the most common tracheal tumor of dogs, was recognized in a psittacine bird. The tumor resulted in tracheal stenosis. The irregularly formed cartilage was ossified and protruded into the submucosal layer, and the cells were well differentiated.

LOWER RESPIRATORY SYSTEM

Lung
Infectious Disease

Polyomavirus. The common gross lesions of polyomavirus are hepatomegaly with necrotic foci, splenomegaly, an enlarged bursa of Fabricius with serosal hemorrhages, and widespread petechial and ecchymotic hemorrhages. In the classic cases of avian polyomavirus, there are either no histologic changes in the lungs, or the interstitium of the lung is expanded with mononuclear inflammatory infiltrates. Rarely large pale basophilic intranuclear viral inclusions can be identified within this mononuclear population (Fig. 2.17). Recently another form of avian polyomavirus was recognized in cockatoos.

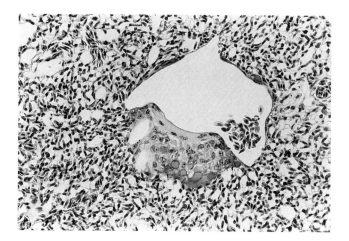

2.17. *Bronchiolitis due to polyomavirus infection. Note the karyomegalic nuclei and minimal early inflammation.*

These birds have a chronic illness and are often poorly grown and emaciated. Grossly their lungs are moist and may have a decreased buoyancy. Histologically there is a diffuse interstitial pneumonia. There appears to be a proliferation of type II pneumocytes, and there is severe pulmonary edema and numerous viral inclusions.

Herpesviruses. The Amazon tracheitis virus, parakeet herpesvirus, and possibly other herpesviruses may cause pneumonia. (See section on diseases of the trachea.) The gross pulmonary lesions are edema and congestion. Within the lung, intranuclear inclusions are observed in epithelial and syncytial cells of the bronchi. Amazon tracheitis virus is generally associated with severe hemorrhagic or fibrinonecrotic inflammation that primarily affects the upper respiratory tract as well as the lung (Fig. 2.18). Parakeet herpesvirus results in a proliferative bronchitis with mild necrosis and syncytial cell formation.

Poxvirus. Avipoxviruses are epitheliotropic viruses that have cutaneous, mucosal, and systemic presentations.

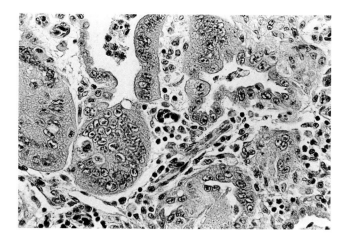

2.18. *Pneumonia associated with Amazon tracheitis virus. There is inflammation and epithelial proliferation with syncytial cell formation.*

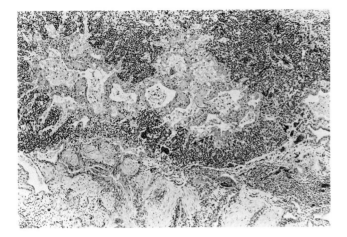

2.19.   Bronchopneumonia due to systemic poxvirus infection. Variable epithelial proliferation is associated with congestion, as well as inflammatory response and fibrin deposition within airways.

Canary poxvirus, a virulent avipoxvirus, generally presents as a systemic infection and can cause up to 100% mortality in susceptible canary flocks. Upper respiratory tract disease, pneumonia, air sacculitis, and splenomegaly may be evident.

Histologically pox is characterized by marked epithelial hyperplasia and vacuolar degeneration of airway epithelial cells associated with small numbers of mixed inflammatory cells (Fig. 2.19). Scattered areas of coagulative necrosis may be present within the mucosa. Rarely the virus forms eosinophilic intracytoplasmic inclusion bodies (called Bollinger bodies in histologic sections and Borrel bodies in impression smears) (Fig. 2.20).

Bacterial Pneumonia. This can occur from either inhalation of the bacteria or as part of a septicemic process. With the exception of some virulent bacterial organisms, most cases of bacterial pneumonia due to a systemic

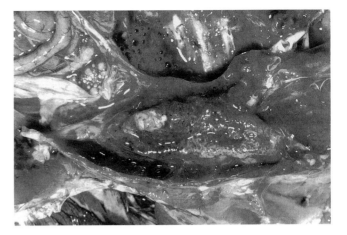

2.21.   Bacterial pneumonia. Generalized discoloration and a focus of abscess formation are seen.

process are secondary to underlying viral infections or other diseases such as malnutrition. Grossly both processes will produce dark red lungs, occasionally with foci of abscessation (Fig. 2.21).

With inhalation, the bacteria can be seen within the lumen of bronchioles admixed with fibrin, small numbers of inflammatory cells, usually heterophils, and some hemorrhage. The inflammation, hemorrhage, and fibrin may extend into the surrounding air capillaries.

The bacterial pneumonia of a systemic process generally results in diffuse lesions that efface significant portions of the lung. Abundant hemorrhage, congestion, fibrinopurulent exudates, and scattered bacteria are noted (Figs. 2.22 and 2.23). Bacteria may be identified within the cytoplasm of macrophages or within the lumen of vascular spaces, indicating a bacteremia (Fig. 2.24).

Nocardia. *Nocardia* is a gram-positive bacterium with branching filaments and an irregularly granular and beaded appearance. It is variably acid fast. Pathogenic nocardia grow as saprophytes in the soil. The most com-

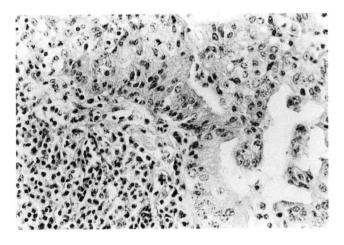

2.20.   Detail of poxvirus-induced pneumonia. Note the epithelial proliferation and inflammatory response. Inclusion body formation is inconsistent.

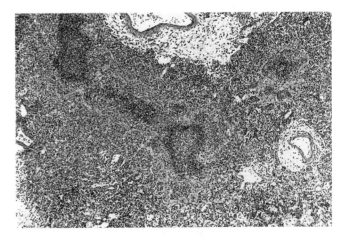

2.22.   Severe bacterial pneumonia. Diffuse effacement of pulmonary parenchyma by inflammatory cells is seen.

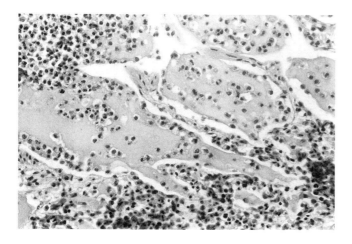

2.23. *Detail of fibrin deposition and inflammatory infiltrate in bacterial pneumonia.*

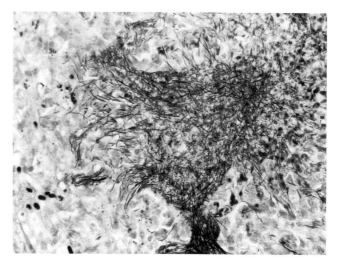

2.25. *Pneumonia due to* Nocardia *sp. A gram-stained section with numerous filamentous organism is seen.*

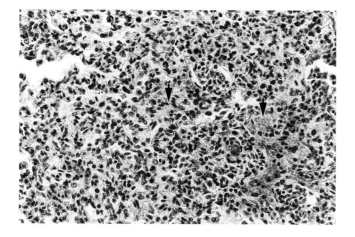

2.24. *Pneumonia due to* Pseudomonas *sp. in an immunocompromised bird. Note the numerous free and phagocytosed bacteria (arrowheads).*

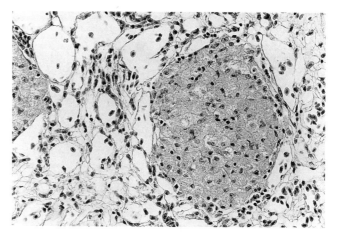

2.26. *Early pulmonary mycobacteriosis with formation of discrete granulomas. Large macrophages contain organisms that are better visualized with acid-fast stains.*

mon isolate from birds is *Norcardia asteroides*. There are rare case reports of infections in birds. In most avian cases, the primary site of infection appears to be the respiratory tract, with secondary involvement of other organs. The lung may have red-to-pink mottling, and the air sacs can appear thickened. The lungs and other tissues will also have multiple grayish white nodular lesions.

Histologically the lungs and other organs with the nodular lesions contain multiple, often confluent granulomas with central necrosis. The delicate filamentous bacteria are visible in the necrotic centers (Fig. 2.25). These organisms are acid fast when stained with Fite-Furaco. A mild fibrinous air sacculitis may also be recognized.

Mycobacteria. Mycobacteria are gram-positive, rod-shaped bacteria that stain with all acid-fast stains (Fig. 2.26). In pet birds, *M. avium* is most common although *M. genevense* is frequently recognized. It is a slow-spreading,

usually chronic infection of semimature to mature birds. The main portal of entry is the gastrointestinal tract, where the organisms penetrate the mucosa, colonize under the serosa and, once in the vascular system lodge in the liver, spleen, and bone marrow.

The typical gross lesions are of organ enlargement, especially the liver and spleen, and a regional to diffuse thickening of the intestines. Multifocal to large, coalescing, firm, white masses may develop through the coelomic body cavity. In pet birds, the nodular masses (tubercles) do not calcify. The granulomas and granulomatous inflammation are commonly found in the liver, intestine, spleen, lung, air sacs, bone marrow and, uncommonly, kidney. The multifocal to coalescing granulomas will efface the normal architecture of the pulmonic parenchyma (Fig. 2.27).

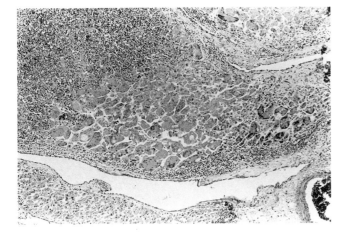

**2.27.   Severe pulmonary mycobacteriosis with efface-
ment of parenchyma and a pleocellular infiltrate that
includes giant cells.**

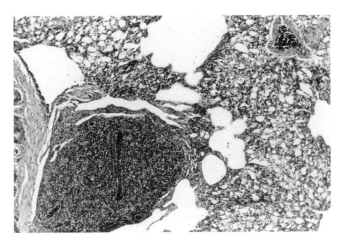

**2.29.   Pulmonary lymphoid nodule formation consis-
tent with Mycoplasma infection.**

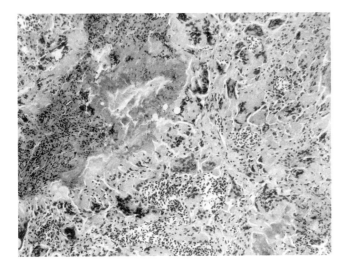

**2.28.   Chronic mycobacterial infection with formation
of a large granuloma with a necrotic center.**

A central core of granular eosinophilic matrix that is
surrounded by multinucleate giant cells, epithelioid
macrophages, and smaller numbers of infiltrating heterophils characterizes the granulomas (Fig. 2.28). Blood
vessels will have accumulations of perivascular plasma
cells and smaller numbers of lymphocytes with rare heterophils. Outlines of rod-shaped bacteria may be recognized within the cytoplasm of macrophages as well as
identified within the core of the granulomas on hematoxylin-eosin preparations.

***Mycoplasma* Pneumonia.** *Mycoplasma* infections of
pet birds are poorly documented, and the significance of
isolates from lesions is unknown. The lung can have lymphocytic infiltrates in the tertiary bronchial walls and in
the mucosa of secondary bronchi. The lymphocytic infiltrates may form prominent lymphoid nodules (Fig. 2.29).
Focal perivascular infiltrates of lymphoid cells in lung
parenchyma are also described.

Mycotic Pneumonia. *Aspergillus* species are the most common fungi causing pneumonia in birds. Aspergillosis presents in several forms in pet birds. The lesions depend on
the chronicity of the infection and the number of spores
inhaled. Colonization may be limited to the site of primary infection. The spores grow on the mucous membranes of the lungs and in the air sacs. It can occur as a
very acute systemic disease, due to an overwhelming dose
of fungal spores. It can present as a chronic infection of
the air sacs. In other forms, depending on the host's resistance, *Aspergillus* can be found in localized granulomatous
lesions of the sinuses, trachea, internal organs, or body
cavities.

The acute form results in multiple miliary granulomas
of the lungs and air sacs. It is usually seen in young birds,
raptors, waterfowl, poultry, and recent imports. Penguins,
pelagic waterfowl, gyrfalcons, and birds, such as the
ostrich, which originate from arid environments, are
extremely prone to aspergillosis if moved to a warm and
humid environment. Grossly the lungs appear dark red
and wet and contain numerous small, white miliary nodules. Histologically these are multifocal to coalescing foci

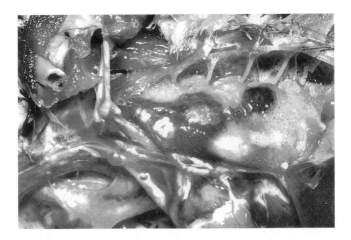

**2.30.   Severe pneumonia due to a fungus consistent with
Aspergillus sp.**

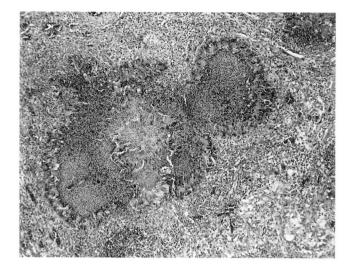

2.31.   Multifocal coalescing granulomas seen in mycotic pneumonia.

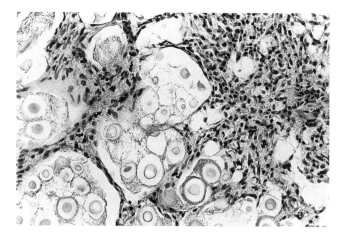

2.32.   Severe mycotic pneumonia due to Crypto-coccus sp.

of cell necrosis, hemorrhage, fibrin deposition, and edema. Large numbers of degenerate heterophils are present, as well as occasional fungal hyphae. These hyphae are usually branching and have internal septations (Figs. 2.30 and 2.31).

The chronic pulmonary and air-sac form is a slowly progressive disease. It occurs in immunocompromised birds exposed to persistent low levels of spores. Contributing factors can include recent importation, injuries, migration, inadequate nutrition, or long-term antibiotic therapy. Grossly the lesions include white-to-yellow plaques in the trachea, syrinx, bronchi, or on air sacs and other serosal surfaces, thickening of air sacs with or without caseous exudate, nodules in the lung parenchyma with caseous, consolidated, or necrotic centers, mycelial formation on air sacs or other serosal surfaces, and caseous nodules within organ parenchyma. From the air sacs, dissemination may occur following sporulation. Sites of secondary involvement include coelomic cavity, central nervous system, liver, intestines, kidney, pneumonic bone, adrenal glands, and spinal column.

Central necrotic cores surrounded by degenerate inflammatory cells and a variably thick capsule of multinucleated giant cells and epithelioid macrophages characterize the granulomas. Large number of fungal hyphae that have internal septations and branching can be identified.

Other fungi that produce tissue hyphae are associated with pulmonary granulomas and pneumonia. These include *Penicillium* species and the class Zygomycetes, such as *Mucor*, *Rhizopus*, and *Absidia* species. The hyphae of the Zygomycetes are recognized by the fact that they are nonseptate or rarely septate and do not dichotomously branch. The typical gross lesions consist of large granulomas in the lungs, free-growing sporulating mold in the air sacs, and emaciation. The granulomas efface the normal pulmonic architecture and are similar to those induced by *Aspergillus* species.

Cryptococcus neoformans.   Pulmonary cryptococcosis is generally an extension from the sinus infection (see the section on sinuses). The narrow-based budding yeast fills the pulmonary airways and is usually associated with mild and mixed inflammation (Fig. 2.32).

Protozoal Pneumonia. *Sarcocystis* species are protozoa with an obligate two-host life cycle. At least six species of *Sarcocystis* infect birds. *Sarcocystis falcatula* appears to be the most significant in susceptible pet birds that are inadvertent hosts. The North American opossum is the definitive host, and cowbirds and grackles are the intermediate hosts. Asexual reproduction of the protozoa occurs within the intermediate host's endothelium. This stage can result in serious or fatal disease in aberrant hosts. In the normal host, schizogony is followed by formation of sarcocysts in muscles. The cysts are 20 to 25 μm long and may be macroscopically visible. They are packed with banana-shaped bradyzoites. The definitive host is infected when it eats the cysts within the muscle tissues. American or neotropical (Mexico, South, and Central America)

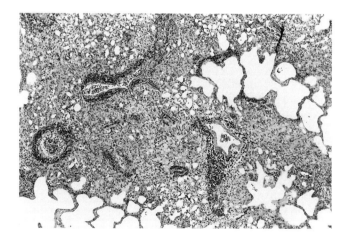

2.33.   Pneumonia due to Sarcocystis sp. Edema and air capillary collapse are seen, and a dense lymphoplasmacytic infiltrate is seen around the blood vessels.

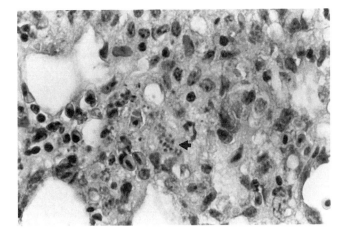

2.34. *Meronts of* **Sarcocystis** *sp. These can be found in the endothelial cells of the lung (arrow).*

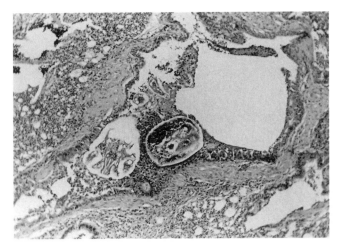

2.35. *Inflammation and exudate in a secondary bronchus of a bird with respiratory mite infection.*

psittacines are usually resistant to disease as adults, but clinical disease sometimes occurs. Old World psittacine birds of Australia, Asia, and Africa are highly susceptible to disease.

The primary gross lesion in susceptible species is severe pulmonary congestion, edema, or hemorrhage. Histologically the lungs will be congested with some fibrin deposition, edema, and hemorrhage within tertiary bronchi. Lymphocytes and plasma cells accumulate around blood vessels and bronchi (Fig. 2.33). Multiple aggregates or clusters of small elliptical or crescent-shaped structures compatible with protozoal merozoites can be seen throughout the pulmonary vessels (Fig. 2.34). The clusters formed are long and sinuous and may resemble microfilaria. The merozoites do not stain well with Brown and Brenn, periodic acid-Schiff, or Giemsa.

Mites. *Sternostoma tracheacolum* is the tracheal mite of canaries and Gouldian finches. (See the previous discussion in the trachea section.) Mites can be distributed throughout the respiratory system, especially in juvenile birds. Mites attach to the mucosa by embedding their legs into the connective tissue. Mucus from the host will coat the mites. The mites, when present in the lungs, remain within the lumen of the primary, secondary and, rarely, the tertiary bronchi.

The mites have a brown, slightly refractile cuticle, segmented legs, and bands of striated skeletal muscle within the body cavity. In these sections, there are peribronchial infiltrations of lymphocytes, plasma cells, and macrophages that efface the normal architecture of the adjacent pulmonary parenchyma and transmigrate across the mucosal surface. The lumen of bronchioles will fill with proteinaceous granular eosinophilic material, cell debris, viable and degenerate heterophils, and bacteria (Fig. 2.35). This inflammatory exudate extends out into the adjacent air capillaries. The mites may also stimulate epithelial hyperplasia.

Noninfectious Disease

Airborne Toxins. The best-documented reports of airborne pulmonary toxins are of those caused by inhalation of pyrolysis products produced from overheated polytetrafluoroethylene-coated cooking pans, stove tops, and coated heat lamps. The toxic products are made up of both gaseous and particulate materials. The acidic fumes cause direct damage to the delicate cell membranes of the lung tissue. The particulates are responsible for the necrotizing and hemorrhagic lesions. Other airborne toxins are aerosol sprays, cooking gas, carbon monoxide, tobacco smoke, and fumes from burned foods and cooking oils. Although the specific toxin is unknown, the operation of self-cleaning ovens has resulted in acute deaths. Compounds emitted from burned foods and other materials can be toxic.

Death after exposure to these airborne toxins is from acute pulmonary edema, hemorrhage, and shock. The birds consistently have severely congested lungs. Watery red fluid

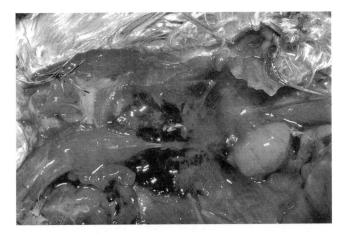

2.36. *Severe hemorrhage associated with inhalation toxicity. This is typical of teflon and other toxicities.*

may exude from the trachea and nares. Within the severely congested lungs, the lumen of the tertiary bronchi, atria, and air capillaries are filled with abundant pale eosinophilic proteinaceous edema fluid. Multifocal to coalescing hemorrhage in the pulmonary interstitium often extends into air spaces (Fig. 2.36). Pale-staining edema fluid accumulates around most arteries and veins. Cardiac lesions are described and are of multifocal degenerate myocytes with deeply eosinophilic cytoplasm and deeply basophilic nuclei. Transmission electron microscopy shows tracheal mucosal and tertiary bronchiolar epithelium degeneration and ulceration with necrosis of air capillary membranes.

Foreign-Material Inhalation. The inhalation of foreign material occurs most commonly in hand-fed nestling psittacine birds and sick birds that are being tube fed. The presence of the material will elicit an inflammatory response, with hemorrhage, congestion, fibrin accumula-

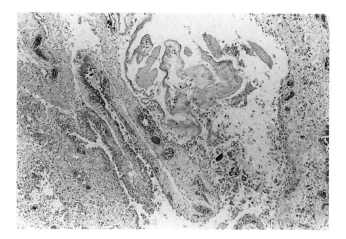

2.39.   Foreign-body pneumonia. The foreign material is surrounded by fibrin, necrotic debris, and inflammatory cells.

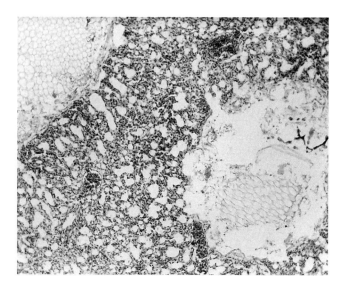

2.37.   Pneumonia associated with foreign-body inhalation.

tion, and edema. This will generally extend into the surrounding pulmonary parenchyma (Fig. 2.37). In peracute inhalation, little inflammatory reaction will be present, with a variable amount of congestion and edema (Fig. 2.38). More chronic lesions will result in accumulations of lymphocytes, macrophages, and multinucleated giant cells (Fig. 2.39).

Chronic Obstructive Pulmonary Disease (Macaw Pulmonary Hypersensitivity). Chronic obstructive pulmonary disease (macaw pulmonary hypersensitivity) with polycythemia appears most common in the blue and gold macaw. Early diagnosis is difficult due to the reserve capacity of avian lungs and relative inactivity of macaws in aviaries. The lung lesions are generally advanced when polycythemia occurs. Grossly the lungs have a firm, rubbery texture and are moderately congested. Histologically there is extensive consolidation and a thickened interstitium with eosinophilic material and fibrous tissue with a mixed

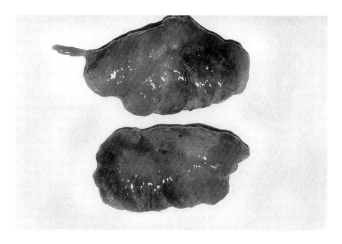

2.38.   Acute foreign-body inhalation. Note the congestion and lack of inflammatory response.

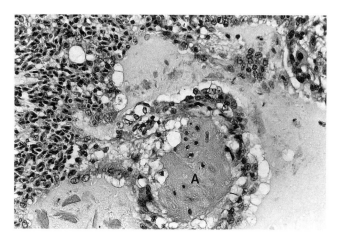

2.40.   Hypersensitivity-induced pneumonitis in a blue and gold macaw. Note the edema. There is mild inflammation and hypertrophy of atrial muscle (A).

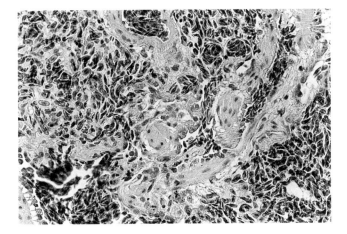

2.41. *Severe congestion and air capillary collapse in a blue and gold macaw with hypersensitivity-induced pneumonitis.*

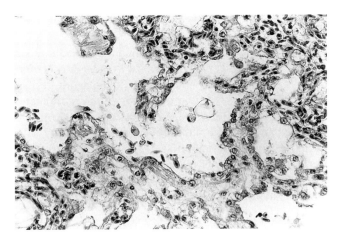

2.43. *Macrophages and minimal erythrophagocytosis in the lung of a bird with congestive heart failure.*

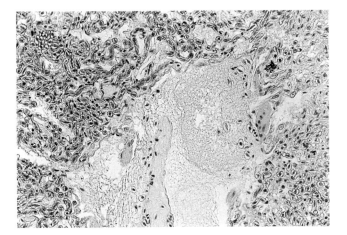

2.42. *Acute vaccine-induced pulmonary collapse and congestion. Proteinaceous fluid is seen in bronchioles.*

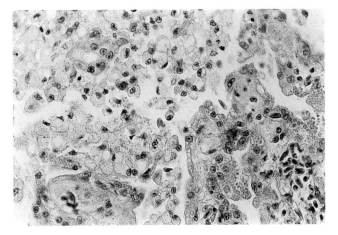

2.44. *Endogenous lipid pneumonia. The exact cause is often not determined, but many birds with this condition have chronic hepatic disease.*

cellular infiltrate. There is partial or complete obliteration of the tertiary lumen. The prominent lesion is the atrial smooth muscle hypertrophy and some atrial loss due to fusion and epithelial bridging (Fig. 2.40). Uncommonly, there is a proliferation of parabronchial lymphoid tissue and lymphoid nodule formation (Fig. 2.41).

Vaccine-Induced Reaction. A pulmonary lesion that has been associated with vaccine reactions in pet birds is suspected to be an anaphylactic reaction or type I hypersensitivity. Death occurs within minutes after the vaccination. The lungs are congested, and there is loss of the air capillary lumen due to collapse. Lacy, pale eosinophilic proteinaceous fluid can be identified within the bronchiole lumens (Fig. 2.42).

Heart Failure Lung. Chronic pulmonary congestion can lead to capillary bleeding, which results in heart failure cells and hemosiderin-laden macrophages. With pulmonary congestion, the capillaries become engorged and may rupture, resulting in intra-air capillary hemorrhages.

The erythrocytes break down and are phagocytosed by pulmonary histiocytes. Cytoplasmic granular golden brown pigments or occasionally intracytoplasmic erythrocytes can identify these cells (Fig. 2.43).

Endogenous Lipid Pneumonia. Lipid pneumonia is an incidental and uncommon lesion of pet birds. The etiology of the lesion is unknown, although in mammals it may represent a storage disease or acquired disorder due to reduced airway clearance. Many birds have concurrent atherosclerosis, liver disease, or other lesions in the respiratory tract. The gross appearance is of white foci typically subtending the pleura of the lungs. Histologically the tertiary bronchi are filled with proteinaceous fluids and histiocytic cells with foamy cytoplasm (Fig. 2.44).

Embolic Pneumonia: Yolk and Bone Marrow. Egg yolk pneumonia is similar to foreign-material inhalation pneumonia. The anatomy of the mesenteries provides access of the ovary and oviduct to the caudal abdominal air sacs. Any disease, trauma, or neoplasm of the reproductive

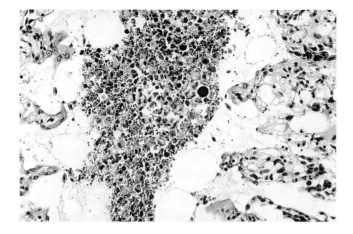

2.45. Retrograde yolk inhalation and pneumonia. In addition to yolk protein, there is edema and some fibrin deposition.

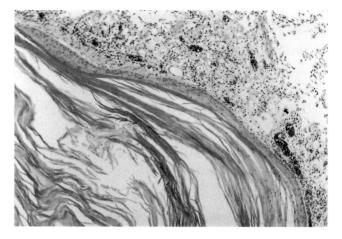

2.47. Severe squamous metaplasia of bronchial mucosa and hyperkeratosis in a bird with vitamin A deficiency.

tract during follicular development can result in the egg yolk material rupturing free into the intestinal mesenteric space. Any disease of the caudal air sacs allows the yolk into the respiratory system and inhalation into the lung.

The lungs, especially in the caudal fields, will be severely hemorrhagic and coated with the yolk. The yolk will be associated with hemorrhage, fibrin deposition, and edema (Fig. 2.45).

Pulmonary emboli from fat, bone marrow, and egg yolk have been recognized. These birds generally present in severe respiratory distress. On gross examination, the lungs will be diffusely and severely congested. The emboli are recognized as occlusions in pulmonary capillaries and arteries. The emboli may be associated with widespread, multifocal hemorrhages in tertiary bronchi and air capillaries. Bone marrow emboli are comprised of adipose connective tissue containing hematopoietic islands (Fig. 2.46). The egg yolk emboli, which are variably sized globular and amphophilic, may be the result of trauma and access of the egg yolk to the vascular system. Often an underlying cause of the yolk embolus is not determined.

Vitamin A. Pet birds that are on a primary seed or cereal grain diet or have intestinal mucosal lesions that interfere with conversion of carotenoids to vitamin A may develop vitamin A deficiency. Vitamin A deficiency results in epithelial squamous metaplasia, which will be manifested as hyperkeratosis of oral cavity, conjunctiva, nasal lacrimal duct, upper alimentary tract, and respiratory tract (nasal passages, sinuses, trachea, syrinx, and bronchi). This is characterized by the pseudostratified ciliated mucosal epithelium of the bronchi transforming into a stratified squamous epithelium (Fig. 2.47). In large parrots, the epithelial changes will appear after liver vitamin A decrease below 50 IU/g. The squamous metaplasia also alters the mucosal defenses, predisposing the bird to fungal and bacterial respiratory infections.

Pulmonary Proteinosis. Eosinophilic, amorphous, or crystalline material is occasionally noted within the lumen of tertiary bronchi and air capillaries. It is inter-

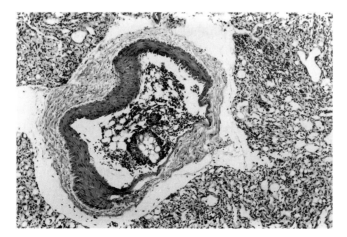

2.46. Bone marrow embolus in the lung. The cause may not always be determined.

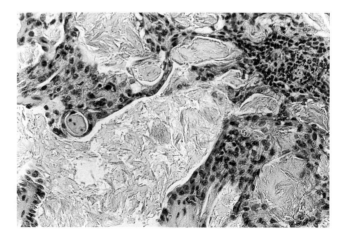

2.48. Pulmonary proteinosis/crystal formation. This is usually an incidental finding of undetermined cause, but it can involve large amounts of lung parenchyma in some cases.

preted as being proteinaceous, but its exact cause is not known. There is generally little to no inflammation. The significance of this uncommon lesion is also unknown (Fig. 2.48).

Pneumoconiosis. Pneumoconiosis (anthrasilicosis) is the focal accumulation of dust-laden macrophages in the interatrial septa of the tertiary bronchi. These lesions generally suggest exposure to airborne pollutants and appear incidental in sedentary pet birds. The lungs may have macroscopic miliary black foci, although usually the accumulations are not observed grossly. The histiocytic aggregates are located subtending the mucosa of the infundibula and atria of tertiary bronchi and around vessels. Rarely they occur in the lamina propria mucosae of primary and secondary bronchi. The histiocytes will have intracytoplasmic granular black pigments and refractile pale yellow crystalline material, which is birefringent with polarized light (Fig. 2.49). There may be infiltrates of lymphocytes and plasma cells associated with the nodules. These nodular lesions can also develop under the mucosal epithelium of the air sacs. When the crystalline material has been examined by transmission electron microscopy and x-ray spectra, most of the crystals are silicates. The silicates do not appear to elicit fibrosis in birds.

The death of a double yellow-headed parrot exposed to smoke from an oil furnace has been reported. It developed dyspnea and died 2 years later. Histologically its lungs were largely replaced by multifocal, coalescing granulomas comprised entirely of histiocytes, which contained fine back particles that were suspected to have originated from the smoke.

Pulmonary Mineralization. Mineralization of the basement membranes of the pulmonary capillaries is seen sporadically in pet birds. Excess dietary calcium or severe renal disease may predispose birds to the development of

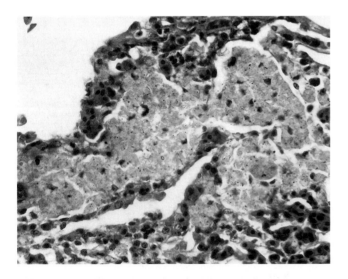

2.49. Pneumoconiosis. The partially birefringent pigment can be free or phagocytosed.

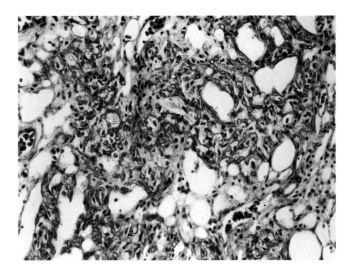

2.50. Diffuse mineralization of pulmonary basement membranes. This lesion is seen secondarily to several metabolic conditions and in vitamin D toxicity.

this lesion. Excess dietary vitamin D_3 has also been proposed to cause this lesion but was not found to do so in budgerigars fed diets containing excess D_3. Soft tissue mineralization may also be seen in the proventricular glands, myocardium, and kidney. The foci in the lungs are generally at the periphery and are characterized as linear, deeply basophilic granular material along the capillaries (Fig. 2.50). Hemorrhage into the pulmonary airways may occur.

Osseous Metaplasia. Small spicules of bone are occasionally found in the pulmonary parenchyma of older birds. These are small trabeculae or nodular foci of dense lamellar bone that expand and compress the adjacent parenchyma. The significance is unknown although the lesions appear to be incidental findings.

Neoplastic Disease

Fibrosarcoma. Fibromas and fibrosarcomas are tumors that originate from fibrous connective tissue and are common neoplasms in pet birds. Fibromas are not reported in the upper respiratory tract, and fibrosarcomas are rarely described arising from the air sacs and lungs. Fibrosarcomas are gray-to-white firm masses with irregular and indistinct borders. Fibrosarcomas are locally invasive, rarely metastasize, and have a moderate to high potential for recurrence, giving them a guarded prognosis.

Carcinoma. Primary pulmonary carcinomas are rare tumors of pet birds. The few cases reported may have arisen from the lung or the air sac. Grossly, multiple, slightly firm, tan-gray foci may be identified in the lungs. In cases suspected as arising from either the lung or air sac, there was extension of the lesion through the air sacs to bone, primarily of the right humerus. The patterns are variable from a trabecular and tubular neoplasm to a densely cellular sheet of pleomorphic cells (Fig. 2.51). The

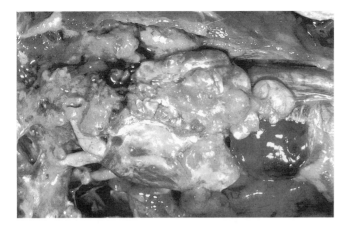

2.51.   Carcinoma arising in the lung/air sac and expanding to replace lung and surrounding tissue completely.

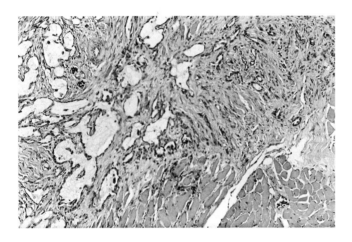

2.52.   Pulmonary carcinoma infiltrating into skeletal muscle of the body wall.

tumors are infiltrative and nonencapsulated (Fig. 2.52). The neoplastic cells are cuboidal to polygonal, with abundant eosinophilic cytoplasm and large round to oval nuclei. Cilia may be recognized on the apical pole.

Undifferentiated Pulmonary Tumors of Cockatiels. Massive discrete infiltrative pulmonary and air-sac tumors have been recognized in cockatiels. These tumors are large, firm, white-to-gray masses that replace areas of the lung. Often the bird dies when a tumor extends into the thoracic inlet, collapsing the interclavicular air sac and compressing the trachea. In some early cases, the tumor mass appears to arise from the mediastinal tissues. These tumors are so aggressive that they may invade vertebra, resulting in paralysis. The neoplasm is comprised of sheets of closely placed cells. The supporting stroma is of fibrous connective tissue and occasional islands of epithelial components. There are regions in these tumors with differentiation toward fibroblastic, adipocytic, or chondroblastic cell types. Rarely the tumor will appear to be a liposarcoma but will contain islands of the more characteris-

tic cells. Many cells have prominent karyomegaly and a pale intranuclear inclusion (Fig. 2.53). Electron microscopy suggests a virus that is morphologically consistent with polyomavirus within the nucleus (Fig. 2.54). Round foci of neoplastic cells compressing the surrounding parenchyma may also be seen in the spleen and less commonly in the liver and kidney.

Metastatic Tumors. Tumor metastases to the lungs of pet birds include adenocarcinoma and carcinoma from various primary sites, fibrosarcoma, hemangiosarcoma, liposarcoma, lymphosarcoma, melanoma, mesothelioma, and osteosarcoma (Fig. 2.55). Identification of the primary site may be necessary for diagnosis in the case of poorly differentiated neoplasms.

Air Sacs

Physical Agents/Trauma: Ruptured Air Sacs. Focal to diffuse subcutaneous pockets of air are most likely the result of a ruptured air sac. This condition has been described as secondary to trauma or from an underlying air-sac infection. A specific infectious etiology is seldom identified. Air-sac rupture is more commonly described in Amazons, macaws, and cockatiels. The sites are usually around the head, ear, dorsal cervical region, and the flanks.

Infectious Disease

Bacterial Infection. The same bacterial organisms that cause pneumonia can cause air sacculitis. Grossly there may be variable necrosis and yellow-white or gray exudate. Histologically the acute reaction is primarily heterophilic, with macrophages, lymphocytes, and giant cells increasing with chronicity.

Mycobacterial Infection. Air sacs can be involved in systemic mycobacteriosis. Air-sac disease is characterized grossly by yellow-white nodules and histologically by aggregates of macrophages with a foamy cytoplasm and small numbers of multinucleated giant cells that elevate as well as infiltrate and replace the respiratory epithelium (Fig. 2.56). Scattered plasma cells, lymphocytes, and rare heterophils will be seen in the connective tissue of the air sac.

***Chlamydophila* Infection.** Chlamydophilosis, also known as psittacosis, or parrot fever, and ornithosis in other bird species, is responsible for considerable morbidity, mortality, and production losses among pet birds. It is zoonotic and uncommonly causes a flulike condition and pneumonia in people. Chlamydiae are energy-dependent obligate intracellular parasitic agents. They are gram-negative, obligate intracellular bacteria that are susceptible to long-term tetracycline treatment.

Chlamydophila psittaci infections of the air sacs produce a diffuse cloudy opacification of air-sac membranes. Occasionally tan-yellow plaques may be seen. The histologic lesion is a fibrinous air sacculitis. An accumulation

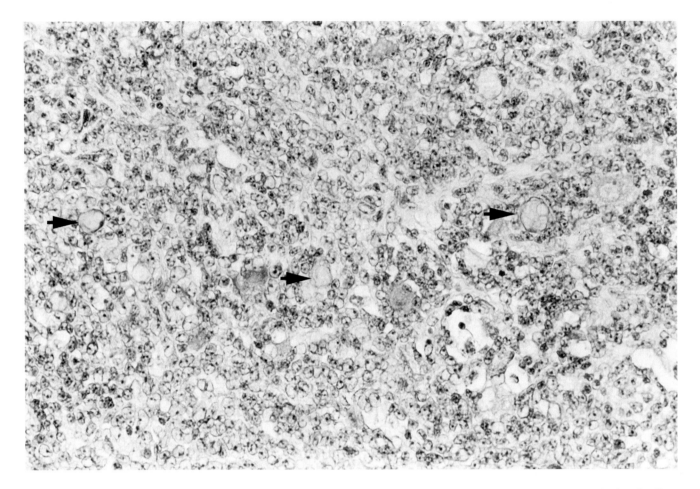

2.53.   Undifferentiated lung tumor with numerous karyomegalic nuclei containing pale intranuclear inclusion bodies (arrowheads). Polyomavirus particles are found in some of these nuclei.

of fibrin with an admixture of inflammatory cell debris thickens the air sacs (Fig. 2.57). The cells are primarily macrophages, lymphocytes, and plasma cells. Occasionally *Chlamydophila* organisms can be recognized as punctate basophilic structures within the cytoplasm of macrophages. There are several stains available to identify the intracellular organisms. The differential diagnosis for the air-sac lesions can include chronic bacterial infections, mycoplasma, and mycotic air sacculitis.

Mycotic Air Sacculitis. The etiologic agents of mycotic air sacculitis are the same as those of mycotic sinusitis. *Aspergillus* species and Zygomycetes are the common organisms seen. These fungi can be identified because they grow as hyphae in tissue.

The inflammation and growth of the fungi generally efface the air sacs (Fig. 2.58). Mats of the fungal hyphae are supported within necrotic debris, hemorrhage, fibrin deposition, edema, and mixed inflammation (Fig. 2.59). There are mixtures of heterophils, lymphocytes, and plasma cells. More chronic lesions will have perivascular clusters of lymphocytes and plasma cells. Fungal hyphae are associated with multinucleated giant cells and epithelioid macrophages. Conidiophores, the fruiting bodies of

the fungal organisms, may occur on the air sacs and can be used to identify the organism (Fig. 2.60).

Parasitic Infection. Nematodes can occasionally be found on the air sacs of birds. *Serratospiculum auraculata* is the best described and is a primitive filarioid, common in falcons. The infections appear incidental. The adults and eggs of *Cyathostoma* species, nematodes of the family Syngamidae, are found in air sacs, lungs, bronchi, and trachea of raptors in the Falconiformes and Strigiformes families. The major pathologic changes include a diffuse pyogranulomatous air sacculitis, pneumonia, and bronchitis. Necrotic inflammatory cells may surround dead nematodes or eggs (Fig. 2.61).

Trematodes are also occasionally found in the air sacs but are usually considered to be an incidental finding.

Neoplastic Disease

Air-Sac Carcinomas. These are rare tumors that are difficult to diagnose definitively as arising from the air sacs. The few cases described are in the large, mature psittacines. The initial presentation is of cystic masses or bony lesions primarily involving the right humerus. The cystic masses are fluid filled and have intraluminal, large, friable, gray-brown, mottled polypoid masses. Radiographs of the

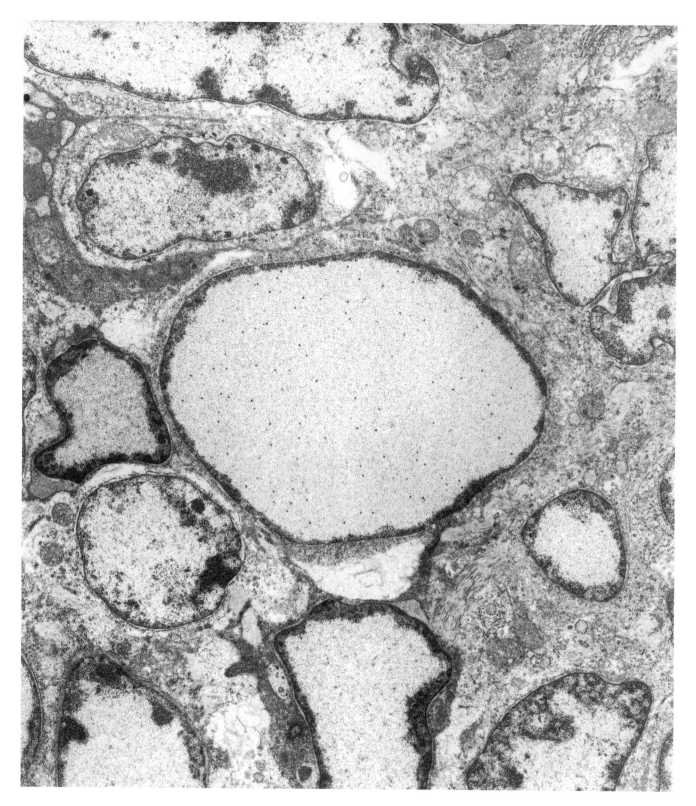

2.54. *Detail of karyomegalic nuclei (Fig. 2.53). The small dark foci are viral particles.*

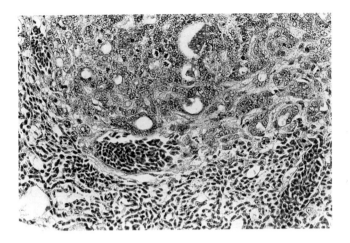

2.55.   *Metastatic renal carcinoma in the lung.*

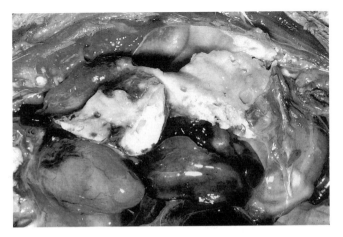

2.58.   *Severe caseous air sacculitis in a bird with aspergillosis.*

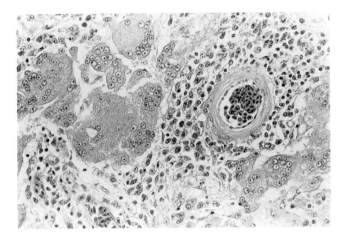

2.56.   *Chronic mycobacteriosis in an air sac. Plasma cells, macrophages, and giant cells are seen.*

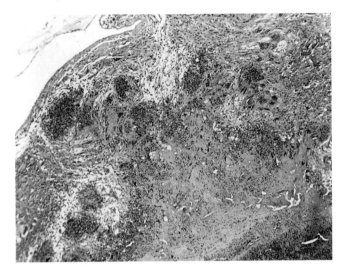

2.59.   *A thickened, necrotic air sac in aspergillosis.*

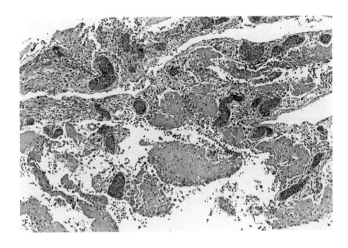

2.57.   *Congestion, fibrin deposition, and a diffuse inflammatory infiltrate in an air sac from a bird with Chlamydiophila infection.*

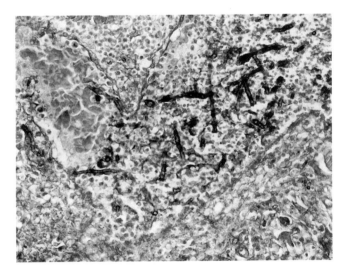

2.60.   *Air sacculitis due to fungus morphologically consistent with Aspergillus sp.*

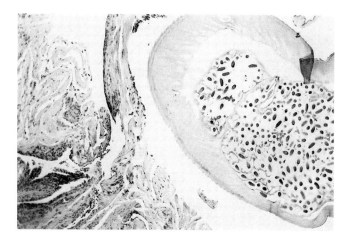

2.61.   A portion of a nematode within an air sac.

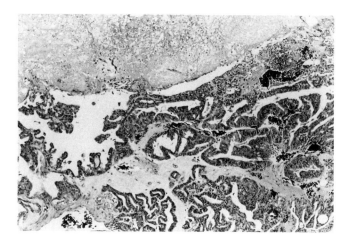

2.62.   Infiltrative air-sac adenocarcinoma.

humerus demonstrate deformed and proliferative new bone with areas of osteolysis. The tumors are poorly demarcated and nonencapsulated. They are comprised of variably sized acini, tubules, and papillary structures supported and separated by fine fibrous connective tissue. The neoplastic structures are lined by clumped cuboidal to short columnar epithelial cells. Rudimentary cilia may be identified on the apical pole of some cells (Fig. 2.62). Finding areas where the tumor is continuous with the air-sac reflection into the humerus and identifying it within the pulmonary parenchyma helps determine the origin.

ADDITIONAL READING

Andre JP, Delverdier M, Cabanie P, Bartel G. 1993. Malignant melanoma in an African grey parrot (*Psittacus erithacus erithacus*). J Assoc Avian Vet 7:83–85.

Andre J-P, Delverdier M. 1999. Primary bronchial carcinoma with osseous metastasis in an African grey parrot (*Psittacus erithacus*). J Avian Med Surg 13:180–186.

Bacciarini LN, Posthaus H, Pagan O, Miserez R. 1999. *Nocardia nova* causing pulmonary nocardiosis of black crakes (*Limnocorax flavirostra*). Vet Pathol 36:345–347.

Blandford TB, Seamon PJ, Hughes R, et al. 1975. A case of polytetrafluoroethylene poisoning in cockatiels accompanied by polymer fume fever in the owner. Vet Rec 96:175–178.

Boucher M, Ehmler TJ, Bermudez AJ. 2000. Polytetrafluoroethylene gas intoxication in broiler chickens. Avian Dis 44:449–453.

Brambilla C, Abraham J, Brambilla E, et al. 1979. Comparative pathology of silicate pneumoconiosis. Am J Pathol 96:149–170.

Brunner P, Meinl M. 1976 Fat-embolic vascular occlusions in avian lungs: Research of histologically determinable neutral fats in parrotlike birds (Psittaciformes). Vet Pathol 13:16–26.

Campbell TW. 1990. What is your diagnosis? J Assoc Avian Vet 4:168.

Clipsham RC, Britt JO. 1983. Disseminated cryptococcosis in a macaw. J Am Vet Med Assoc 183:1303–1305.

Colby SFM. 1998. What is your diagnosis? J Avian Med Surg 12:43–44.

Dennis PM, Heard DJ, Castleman WL. 2000. Respiratory distress associated with pulmonary fat emboli in an osprey (*Pandion haliaetus*). J Avian Med Surg 14:264–267.

Desmidt M, Ducatelle R, Uyttebroeck E, et al. 1991. Cytomegalovirus-like conjunctivitis in Australian finches. J Assoc Avian Vet 5:132–136.

Dorrestein GM, Buitelaar MN, Van der Hage MH, Zwart P. 1985. Evaluation of a bacteriological & mycological examination of psittacine birds. Avian Dis 29:951–962.

Dorrestein GM, Van der Hage M, Kik M, Beijer HA. 2001. Syngamus trachea: An unusual infection in vinaceous Amazons (*Amazona vinacea*). In: Proceedings of the Association of Avian Veterinarians, Orlando, FL, pp 59–65.

Ehrsam H, Hause RB. 1979. Nocardiose bei Blauflugel-konigssittichen (*Alisterus amboinensis hypophonus*). Schweiz Arch Tierheilkd 121:195–200.

Evans MG, Slocombe RF, Schwartz LD. 1988. Pulmonary silicosis in captive ring-necked pheasants: Definitive diagnosis by electron probe X-ray microanalysis. Vet Pathol 25:239–241.

Fenwick B, Takeshita K, Wong A. 1985. A Moluccan cockatoo with disseminated cryptococcosis. J Am Vet Med Assoc 187:1218–1219

Fitzgerald SD, Reed WM, Fulton RM. 1995. Development and application of an immunohistochemical staining technique to detect avian polyomaviral antigen in tissue sections. J Vet Diagn Invest 7:444–450.

Fitzgerald SD, Hanika C, Reed WM. 2001. Lockjaw syndrome in cockatiels associated with sinusitis. Avian Pathol 30:49–53.

Gibbons PM, Horton S. 2000. What is your diagnosis? J Avian Med Surg 14:60–64.

Hall RK, Bemis DA. 1995. A spiral bacterium found in psittacines. In: Proceedings of the Association of Avian Veterinarians, Philadelphia, PA, pp 345–347.

Harcourt-Brown N. 1999. Comparative avian surgical anatomy. Exotic DVM 1:35–40.

Harris D. 1999. Resolution of choanal atresia in African grey parrots. Exotic DVM 1:13–17.

Hillyer EV, Oroz S, Dorrestein GM. 1997. Respiratory System. In: Altman RB, Clubb SL, Dorrestein GM, Quesenberry K, eds. Avian medicine and surgery. Philadelphia: WB Saunders, pp 387–411.

Huff DG. 1993. Avian fluid therapy and nutritional therapeutics. Semin Avian Exotic Pet Med 2:13–16.

Irokanulo EOA, Makinde AA, Akuesgi CO, Ekwonu M. 1997. *Cryptococcus neoformans* var *neoformans* isolated from droppings of captive birds. J Wildl Dis 33:343–345.

Jones MP, Orosz SE, Richman LK, et al. 2001. Pulmonary carcinoma with metastases in a Moluccan cockatoo (*Cacatua moluccensis*). J Avian Med Surg 15:107–113.

Kennedy FA, Sattler-Augustin S, Mahler JR, Jansson PC. 1996. Oropharyngeal and cloacal papillomas in two macaws (*Ara* spp.) with neoplasia with hepatic metastasis. J Avian Med Surg 10:89–95.

King AS, McLelland J. 1984. Respiratory system. In: Birds: Their structure and function. Philadelphia: Bailliere Tindall.

Latimer KS, Niagro FD, Rakich PM, et al. 1997. Investigation of parrot papillomavirus in cloacal and oral papillomas of psittacine birds. Vet Clin Pathol 26:158–163.

Lavoie M, Mikaelian I, Sterner M, et al. 1999. Respiratory nematodiases in raptors in Quebec. J Wildl Dis 35:375–380.

Long P, Choi G, Silberman M. 1983. Nocardiosis in two Pesquet's parrots (*Psittrichas fulgidus*). Avian Dis 27:855–859.

McLelland JA. 1991. Respiratory system. In: A color atlas of avian anatomy. Philadelphia: WB Saunders, pp 95–123.

Nevarez J, Mitchell MA. 2001. What is your diagnosis? J Avian Med Surg 15:326–329.

Okoye JOA, Gugnani HC, Okeke CN. 1991. Experimental infection of chickens with *Nocardia asteroides* and *Nocardia transvalensis*. Avian Pathol 20:17–24, 1991.

Panigrahy B, Senne DA. 1991. Diseases of mynahs. J Am Vet Med Assoc 199:378–381.

Parnell MJ, Hubbard GB, Fletcher KC, Schmidt RE. 1983. *Nocardia asteroides* infection in a purple throated sunbird (*Nectarinia sperapa*). Vet Pathol 20:497–500.

Powers LV, Merrill CL, Degernes LA, et al. 1998. Axillary cystadenocarcinoma in a Moluccan cockatoo (*Cacatua moluccensis*). Avian Dis 42:408–412.

Pye GW, Bennett RA, Newell SM, et al. 2000. Magnetic resonance imaging in psittacine birds with chronic sinusitis. J Avian Med Surg 14:243–256.

Rombout PJ, Dormans JA, Van Bree L, Marra M. 1991. Structural and biochemical effects in lungs of Japanese quail following a 1-week exposure to ozone. Environ Res 54:39–51.

Roperto F, Borzacchiello G, Ungaro R, Galati P. 2000. Silicate pneumoconiosis in hens. J Comp Pathol 122:249–254.

Samour JH, Bailey TA, Cooper JE. 1995. Trichomoniasis in birds of prey (order Falconiformes) in Bahrain. Vet Rec 136:358–362.

Sileo L, Sievert RR, Samuel MD. 1990. Causes of mortality of albatross chicks at Midway atoll. J Wildl Dis 26:329–338.

Smith BL, Poole WSH, Martinovich D. 1973. Pneumoconiosis in the captive New Zealand kiwi. Vet Pathol 10:94–101.

Stoltz JH, Galey F, Johnson B. 1992. Sudden death in ten psittacine birds associated with the operation of a self-cleaning oven. Vet Hum Toxicol 34:420–421.

Takeshita K, Fenwick B, Wong A. 1986. Cryptococcosis in captive cockatoos. In: Proceedings Association of Avian Veterinarians, Miami, FL, pp 133–138.

Tidemann SC, McOris TS, Woinarski JC, Freeland WJ. 1992. Parasitism of wild Gouldian finches (*Erythrura gouldiae*) by the air-sac mite *Sternostoma tracheacolum*. J Wildl Dis 28:80–84.

Tsai SS, Chang TC, Kuo M, Itakura C. 1997. Respiratory and intestinal trichomoniasis in mule ducks. Avian Pathol 26:651–656.

Walsh MT. 1984. Clinical manifestations of cervicocephalic air sacs of psittacines. Comp Cont Educ 6:170–176.

Weissengruber G, Loupal G. 1999. Osteochondroma of the tracheal wall in a Fischer's lovebird (*Agapornis fischeri*, Reichenow 1887). Avian Dis 43:155–159.

Wells RE, Slocombe R, Trapp AL. 1982. Acute toxicosis of budgerigars (*Melopsittacus undulatus*) caused by pyrolysis products from heated polytetrafluoroethylene: Clinical study. Am J Vet Res 43:1238–1242.

Wells RE, Slocombe RF. 1982. Acute toxicosis of budgerigars (*Melopsittacus undulatus*) caused by pyrolysis products from heated polytetrafluoroethylene: Microscopic study. Am J Vet Res 43:1243–1248.

Wilson H, Brown CA, Greenacre CB, et al. 2001. Suspected sodium hypochlorite toxicosis in a group of psittacine birds. J Avian Med Surg 15:209–215.

Wobeser G, Kost W. 1992. Starvation, staphylococcosis, & vitamin A deficiency among mallards overwintering in Saskatchewan. J Wildl Dis 28:215–222.

Woods LW, Chin RP, Barr BC, Galvin C. 1987. Summary and review of diagnostic observations of pet/exotic bird cases at the veterinary laboratory services facility in Petaluma (1/1/86–12/3/86). In: Proceedings of the 36th Western Poultry Disease Conference, Davis, CA, pp 124–127.

3 Gastrointestinal System and Pancreas

NORMAL STRUCTURE

The Beak

The anatomy of the beak in many respects resembles the anatomy of the hoof of a horse. A dense cornified epidermis—the rhinotheca (maxilla) and gnathotheca (mandible)—grows over the dermis and bones of the maxilla and mandible from a germinal layer at the junction of the beak with the skin. Damage to the germinal layer at the base of the beak will result in a defect extending the length of the beak.

Oral Cavity and Pharynx

Birds do not have a soft palate. The hard palate is divided caudally by the longitudinal V-shaped choanal fissure, which connects the oral and nasal cavities. Small, caudally projecting papillae line the oral margins of the choanal fissure. Caudal to the choana on the roof of the oral cavity is the infundibular fissure that connects the oral cavity with the middle ear.

The shape of the tongue varies extensively according to the feeding habits of the bird. The tongue of the finches, canaries, and most commonly kept passerine birds is long, slender, flat and cornified. Psittacine birds have a thick, round, and muscular tongue that is used for manipulating food. The tongue of lories and lorikeets is densely covered with fimbria that evert when the tongue is protruded. These fimbria are used to gather pollen and nectar. At the base of the tongue are the laryngeal mound and the glottis. Birds do not have an epiglottis. Birds also do not have large salivary glands. Instead, in most avian species, a diffuse layer of small compound tubular salivary glands is present beneath the epithelium of the oropharynx. The oral cavity is lined by a stratified squamous epithelium. The rostral portion of the oral cavity, including the tongue and the epithelium adjacent to the tongue, may be heavily cornified, depending on the species of bird.

Esophagus

This can be divided into the cervical esophagus, ingluvies (crop), and thoracic esophagus. Not all birds have a crop. The cervical and thoracic esophagus is lined by a relatively thick stratified squamous epithelium. Beneath the epithelium are mucus-producing glands that resemble salivary glands. These are internal, surrounded by layers of the muscularis externa. The crop is similarly structured but does contain mucous glands. The cervical esophagus is on the right side of the neck. In birds that have a crop, it dilates to become a saclike, highly distensible structure. When fully distended, the crop is nearly transparent. It varies in size and shape according to the species of bird. The crop of the parrot first bulges to the right and then to the left across the midline and fills most of the space between the bones of the clavicle. The crop of nestling parrots is proportionately larger than that of the adult bird.

Proventriculus and Ventriculus

The anatomy of the proventriculus and ventriculus varies considerably between species of birds. The following description applies to most psittacine birds and the commonly kept passerines. Grossly the proventriculus is a thick, spindle-shaped organ. The wall is composed predominantly of compound tubular glands. These glands contain a single round to cuboidal cell that produces both pepsinogen and hydrochloric acid. The glands connect to the lumen of the proventriculus through primary, secondary, and tertiary ducts. The cells lining the tertiary ducts and the mucosal epithelium are tall columnar. The proventricular glands are surrounded by a thin muscularis.

The ventriculus has a thick external muscularis that is necessary for grinding ingested pieces of food. It is widest in vertical cross section and thinner in the horizontal cross section. A tendon covers it caudally. The muscle layer of the caudal ventral aspect of the muscle coat thins, creating a slight outpouching of the ventriculus that grossly appears to be surrounded by the aponeurosis of this tendon alone. Histologically the muscularis contains three layers of smooth muscle, of which the middle layer is the thickest. The ventricular glands are tall, slender columns of cells surrounding a thin lamina propria. At the base of the crypts formed by these glands are simple tubular glands. The ventricular glands secrete a carbohydrate-protein complex called the koilin. Secreted koilin produces a dense, thick, serrated layer that completely lines the ventriculus. Microscopically the koilin emanating from the crypts of the ventricular glands stains more deeply eosinophilic than the koilin produced by the tips of the glands, giving the koilin a laminated appearance. The koilin from the crypts also appears to be softer and wears faster than the koilin from the gland tips, causing the surface of the koilin to be serrated.

The junction between the ventriculus and the proventriculus is the isthmus. This is a very short junction where there is a transition between the proventricular and ventricular glands. Koilin production is not present in the orad portion of this junction. Caudally a thin layer of koilin-like secretions is present at the transition to the ventriculus.

The need for a grinding stomach diminishes in species that feed predominantly on liquid or easily digested food, or in birds that eat whole prey. As a result, the ventriculus will either be thin walled, relatively small, or both in birds such a lories and lorikeets, hummingbirds, some insectivorous birds, and raptors. The size of the ventriculus not only varies with species but also can be altered in any bird by increasing the content of nondigestible fiber in the diet, with increasing amounts leading to a larger organ. This must be considered when determining the significance of ventricular size at necropsy.

Intestines

The intestines of passerine and psittacine birds are relatively simple. The intestines of the budgerigar contain five loops before becoming the colon, which itself is relatively short. The first loop of the intestine is the duodenal loop. Two shorter loops follow. In the middle of the second is the remnant of the yolk sac: the vitelline diverticulum. This is considered the junction between the jejunum and ileum, although this is of little physiologic significance. The ileum is then comprised of two loops of similar length. Psittacine birds do not have ceca, which are poorly developed in commonly kept passerine birds. They are, however, important sites of disease in other species of birds. The microscopic structure of the intestines is very similar to that of mammals. One significant difference is that Brunner's glands are not found in the duodenum. Submucosal lymphoid tissue is found normally in many species of birds, particularly in the distal ileum and in the tips of the ceca. This tissue can significantly alter the shape of the villi.

Cloaca

This is the combined outflow tract of the digestive, urinary, and reproductive tract. The colorectum enters into the coprodeum, the ventral aspect of the cloaca. Dorsally and separated by a horizontal fold from coprodeum is the urodeum, into which the ureters empty. The oviduct in the female enters the urodeum from the left lateral wall. The deferent ducts enter the urodeum in the male. The urodeum and coprodeum open into the common chamber of the proctodeum. The cloaca is lined by a tall colum-

nar epithelium. The villi of the coprodeum resemble those of the colon. Folds, but not villi, are present in the urodeum. Villi in the proctodeum diminish in height and contain few mucus-producing cells. At the skin-mucosal junction, the lining of the proctodeum becomes a stratified squamous epithelium.

Pancreas

The largest portion of the pancreas lies within the loop of the duodenum. This portion extends cranially and may come in contact with the spleen. A portion of the pancreas, in psittacine birds, parallels the abaxial side of the right duodenal loop. The normal pancreas is yellow to yellowish pink, with a finely lobulated surface. Histologically it contains both exocrine and endocrine tissues that resemble its mammalian counterparts. Islets are not uniformly distributed in the pancreas of all birds, and multiple sections from different portions of the pancreas must be made if the islets are to be seen and evaluated.

GASTROINTESTINAL DISEASE
Beak
Anomalies. Deformities can be congenital or acquired. Genetically induced congenital deformities have been reported in budgerigars. Variations in curvature and size are seen (Fig. 3.1). Congenital deformities of uncertain cause are also described. A normal structure at hatching is the egg tooth. This enlargement at the dorsal aspect of the end of the beak is normal and is lost in the few days after hatching.

A lateral deviation of the maxilla is a relatively common lesion in hand-fed nestling macaws. Beak deformities of hand-fed nestling cockatoos are also relatively common. In these birds, the curvature of the maxilla is increased, causing the tip of the maxilla to rest on the oral surface of the mandible. Some of these birds appear to have an overly long mandible or possibly a foreshortened maxilla that may result in a decreased wear on the maxilla

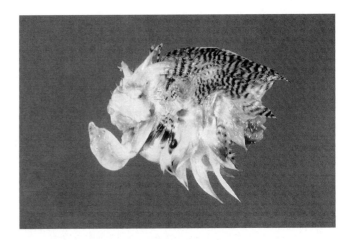

3.1. *Beak malformation of unknown cause. Such malformations may be congenital or acquired.*

and may allow its increased curvature. The cause of these lesions in macaws and cockatoos is not known.

Trauma. Beak trauma is common and most often the result of a bite wound from another bird. Male cockatoos are aggressive during the breeding season, and mate aggression is a common cause of crushed beaks and even more extensive injury to the face and head. If the underlying bone is ripped free, the beak will still heal but will only grow out to the point that it has bone to support it or will grow in bizarre shapes. Psittacine birds are remarkable and can tolerate a considerable loss of much of their beak as long as their tongue remains uninjured.

Nutrition. Malnutrition may cause softening and flaking of the beak. A report of the complete absence of vitamin A in the diet of nestling African grey parrots described transverse ridges in the rhinotheca of these birds. The beak grew out normally when the diet was replaced with one with adequate vitamin A.

Metabolic Disease. Clinical observations suggest that one cause of overgrowth of the beak of parrots is liver disease.

The lesions associated with beak deformities are usually obvious grossly and not examined histologically.

Infectious Disease. The beak is a common target for a number of infectious disease processes.

Psittacine beak and feather disease virus (PBFDV) can affect a wide range of psittacine birds. There are many manifestations of this disease that vary with the species of bird. Beak lesions are common in sulfur-crested and Moluccan cockatoos, galahs, and the little corella. Gross lesions include hyperkeratosis, elongation, ulceration, necrosis, and fracturing of the keratin (Fig. 3.2). Separation of the palatine mucosa from the rhinotheca may occur, and eventually the distal beak may fracture, exposing the underlying bone.

Histologically there is necrosis of the epithelial cells in the basal and intermediate layers, the cornified layer may separate from the dermis, and there can be secondary bacterial or fungal infection with a pleocellular inflammatory infiltrate and organisms present. Intracytoplasmic inclusion bodies may be seen in macrophages infiltrating the epithelium, and intranuclear inclusions are occasionally present in epithelial cells.

Poxviruses can also affect the beak. Beak lesions are most common in nonpsittacine birds but are occasionally seen in psittacine birds. Classically, poxvirus infection cause raised proliferative lesions that may or may not be necrotic and secondarily infected. These lesions are seen on the beak or at the beak-skin margin (Fig. 3.3). Occasionally there may be infection of the basal layers of the beak epidermis, with sloughing of the keratinized layers leading to the gross presentation of a beak with no keratinized structure. Histologically the diagnostic feature of poxvirus infection is swelling of epithelial cells and the formation of intracytoplasmic eosinophilic inclusion bodies (Bollinger bodies). These inclusions are so large as to cause the nucleus to be compressed into a crescent on the side of the cell.

There have been a few reports of polyomavirus infection of the beak germinal epithelium. Inflammation and necrosis were noted, as well as intranuclear inclusion bodies.

Primary bacterial and fungal infections of the beak may be associated with trauma. These lesions present as variable areas of necrosis, inflammation, and hemorrhage. The beak will often soften and become discolored. There may be hyperkeratosis and accumulation of necrotic debris. Histologically heterophils and macrophages predominate, and organisms may be found. Infections of the sinuses, pneumatized bone, or adjacent soft tissues can also result in beak disease that may first be noticed as an expansile lesion resulting in distortion and discoloration of the rhinotheca.

Mites such as *Knemidokoptes* sp. can cause inflammation and proliferation of the beak. The base of the affected beak is typically soft, and the surface has a fine honeycomb texture. In live birds, mites are abundant and can be readily found with a beak scraping. Histologically there is a pleocellular inflammatory reaction, proliferation of keratin, and intralesional fragments of mites.

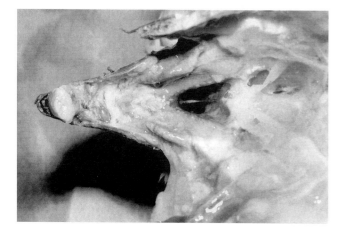

3.2. Beak necrosis due to circovirus infection.

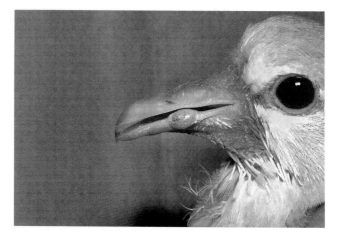

3.3. Poxvirus-induced lesion on a beak.

Neoplastic Disease. Several types of neoplasia have been reported to metastasize to the beak, but squamous cell carcinomas (SCCs) and malignant melanomas are the most common. Fibrosarcoma is considered the most common primary beak tumor. Malignant melanoma may also have the beak area as a primary site.

Grossly all tumors are proliferative masses that distort the beak and surrounding soft tissue. There may be bone lysis (Fig. 3.4). SCCs are typical, with moderately undifferentiated squamous cells forming infiltrative nests and cords. There is often secondary inflammation. Fibrosarcomas are most common in budgerigars and cockatiels, and histologically are comprised of interlacing bundles of neoplastic cells with vesicular nuclei and fibrillar cytoplasm. Mitotic figures are usually abundant. Malignant melanoma is comprised of pleomorphic cells that vary from epithelioid to fusiform. Most cells are pigmented, and there is a high mitotic index.

Oral Cavity

Noninfectious Disease. Noninfectious oral lesions include various types of trauma. Acute lesions present as lacerations or abrasions with variable hemorrhage. With chronicity, there may be an inflammatory response, fibroplasia, and the formation of irregular thickenings in the affected area. Foreign bodies may penetrate the mucosa of the oral cavity and tongue and serve as a nidus for severe chronic inflammation and granuloma formation. These lesions must be differentiated from neoplasia histologically.

Vitamin A deficiency is a common disease in cage birds. Historically birds with vitamin A deficiency have been on an unsupplemented, all-seed diet for many years. Vitamin A is essential for the integrity of mucous membranes and the epithelium. The absence of vitamin A results in squamous metaplasia of mucous glands and the epithelium in several organ systems. The small mucous glands in the oral cavity then fill with keratin and expand to form submucosal nodules that are filled with yellow-white and friable material (Fig. 3.5). These lesions can be

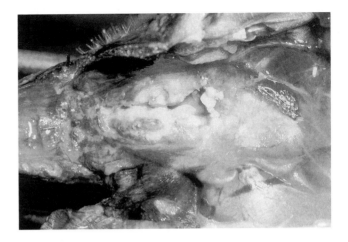

3.5. *Swelling of oral glands and mucosa associated with vitamin A deficiency.*

severe, resulting in obstruction of the choanal slit. Histologically there is squamous metaplasia of oral glands, with subsequent hyperkeratosis (Figs. 3.6 and 3.7). There may be secondary bacterial infections leading to necrosis and an inflammatory infiltrate that is primarily heterophilic. Blunting of the choanal papillae is a subtler lesion that is seen in birds with the early stages of vitamin A deficiency. Other diseases can cause similar changes.

Infectious Disease. Infectious agents causing oral disease in psittacine birds include viruses, bacteria, fungi, flagellates, and nematodes.

Poxvirus infection results in mucosal proliferation and the formation of masses that may be partially necrotic. Grossly the oral mucosa is usually ulcerated and covered with caseous debris. Histologically mucosal epithelial cells are swollen with ballooning degeneration and typically contain eosinophilic cytoplasmic inclusion bodies. Differential diagnoses for this lesion includes vitamin A deficiency, bacterial infection (particularly with *Pseudomonas* sp.), candidiasis, and trichomoniasis. Amazon parrots, particularly blue-fronted Amazon parrots, have histori-

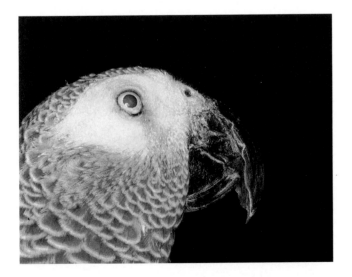

3.4. *Destruction of the beak and surrounding area due to malignant melanoma.*

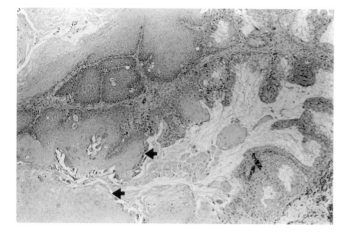

3.6. *Vitamin A deficiency. Note the areas of glandular epithelial metaplasia (arrows) and hyperplasia.*

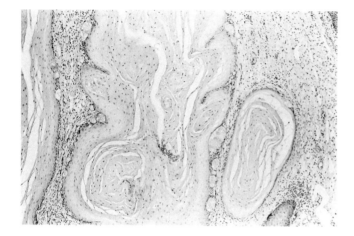

3.7. *Advanced metaplasia of the oral glands in vitamin A deficiency.*

cally had a high incidence of poxvirus infection. Disease in these birds was confined to imported nestling parrots that were being hand fed in quarantine. With the cessation of importation of wild-caught blue-fronted Amazon parrots, this disease is no longer seen in aviculture in North America.

Herpesvirus infections can cause acute necrosis and ulceration of the oral cavity. The gross change is not specific, and diagnosis is made histologically by finding intranuclear inclusion bodies in epithelial cells adjacent to the necrotic foci. These lesions are often overlooked at necropsy, due to the severity of the generalized disease process.

Polyomavirus infection can lead to oral hemorrhage and necrosis. The histologic lesion is characterized by finding karyomegalic nuclei and intranuclear inclusion bodies in epithelial or endothelial cells.

Bacterial infections cause necrosis of the oral mucosa and glands. These infections must be differentiated from poxvirus lesions and may be secondary to vitamin A deficiency. Acute infections may be hemorrhagic, but chronic infections with gram-negative bacteria or mycobacteria

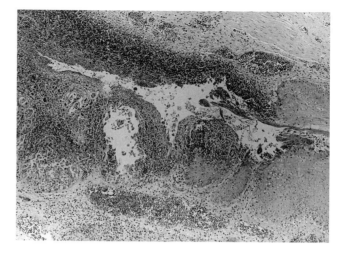

3.8. *Bacterial stomatitis. Severe mucosal necrosis and a pleocellular infiltrate are seen.*

will lead to granuloma formation. Histologically, in bacterial infections, there is necrosis and an infiltrate of heterophils, macrophages, and plasma cells (Fig. 3.8). With chronicity, a central necrotic core surrounded by macrophages and some giant cells is noted. Organisms may be seen, but special stains are necessary in some cases to demonstrate the organisms. Heterophils and macrophages characterize early mycobacterial infections. As the condition becomes chronic, macrophages with abundant cytoplasm form clumps and sheets. Acid-fast organisms are present in the cytoplasm. In some, but not all, cases, necrotic foci and giant cells may be present.

The primary mycotic infection of the oral cavity is *Candida albicans*. Primary infections can occur, but the disease is usually secondary, and a complete necropsy is usually necessary to determine the underlying cause. Grossly the mucosa is thickened, and there may be gray-white plaques (Fig. 3.9). Histologically there may be excessive keratinization, and numerous organisms are present in the mucosa and keratin. Mucosal and submucosal inflammation is variable and primarily comprised of lymphocytes, plasma cells, and macrophages.

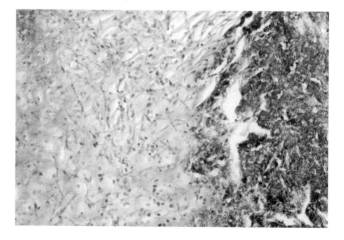

3.9. *Proliferative stomatitis due to* Candida *sp.*

Trichomoniasis is most common in pigeons and wild birds. The oral form of the disease is rare in captive-raised psittacine and passerine species. Grossly, yellow-white nodules and plaques characterize oral trichomoniasis. The gross lesion may be similar to lesions seen with vitamin A deficiency, poxvirus infections, candidiasis, and bacterial infections. Histologically the mucosa may be moderately proliferative, and there is some superficial necrosis. Macrophages and plasma cells are the predominant inflammatory response. Organisms are present and must be distinguished from large pleomorphic macrophages (Fig. 3.10). They stain readily with silver stains. In live birds, the organisms are readily seen on a wet mount. They die rapidly after the bird's death.

Capillaria sp. may cause inflammation with hemorrhage and variable necrosis. Histologically, nematode fragments are found in the mucosa. In some cases, gross changes are minimal or absent, and the nematodes are an incidental finding at necropsy. Infections with this parasite are relatively rare in cage birds, although they are more common in Australian grass parakeets and seen occasionally in other parrot species housed outdoors.

Neoplastic Disease. Tumors of the oral cavity can be either of epithelial or mesenchymal origin. The most common neoplasm of the oral cavity is oral papillomatosis (Fig. 3.11), which is most common in New World psittacines. Macaws, conures, Amazon parrots, and hawk-headed parrots are most susceptible to this disease. Oral lesions are particularly common in the larger macaws but relatively rare in Amazon parrots. Papillomas are most commonly located along the margins of the choanal fissure, at the base of the tongue, and on the glottis. Rarely they may become large enough to obstruct the airways. The papillomatous lesions are white to pink, raised, and focal to locally extensive. Most have a typical cauliflower-like appearance. These lesions wax and wane, however, and smaller, slightly raised, discolored lesions that also represent this disease may be overlooked. Thickening of

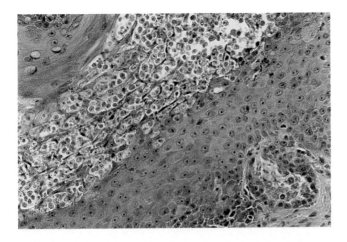

3.10. Oral trichomoniasis. There is mucosal proliferation and scattered necrosis, and numerous organisms are seen.

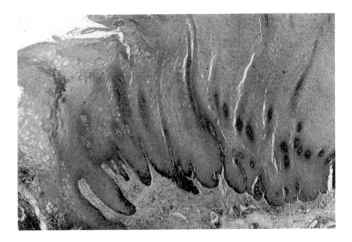

3.11. Typical appearance of oral papilloma.

the choanal margin, discoloration of the choanal mucosa, and blunting of the choanal mucosa are also subtle changes that may be caused by this disease. Grossly the lesions are best observed in live birds and are more difficult to see after death. Papillomas vary in size and may become secondarily infected, with hemorrhage and necrosis noted.

Histologically the papillary structures have a highly vascular connective tissue core and are covered by a proliferative mucosal epithelium. Lymphoplasmacytic infiltration into the connective tissue core is a variable feature of this disease. The etiology of the mucosal papillomas of New World parrots is not known. These lesions are seen to develop in survivors of outbreaks of Pacheco's disease, and herpesviruses are commonly present within papillomas. A protein that is cross-reactive to antibodies made to the L1 protein of a human papillomavirus were found to cross-react with proteins in cutaneous and oral papillomas of two African grey parrots but not in the mucosal papillomas of other parrot species. This finding suggests that the papillomas of the face and oral cavity of African grey parrots are caused by a papillomavirus, but additional research is necessary to confirm this.

SCCs will present as masses of the oral mucosa or tongue. In some cases, necrosis and hemorrhage are seen. The tumors are typical histologically. Salivary gland carcinomas may also be found. Grossly they occur as masses within the mucosa that also may be necrotic and hemorrhagic. Histologically they are comprised of infiltrative nests, acini, and cords of moderately undifferentiated to poorly differentiated epithelial cells with indistinct cytoplasmic boundaries and vesicular nuclei. There is moderate mitotic activity.

Sarcomas reported in the oral cavity include fibrosarcoma and lymphosarcoma. Gross differentiation of these lesions from each other or from granulomas is difficult. Histologically fibrosarcomas are similar to those seen in the beak. Lymphosarcoma is usually lymphoblastic and comprised as a sheet of somewhat pleomorphic immature lymphoid cells (Fig. 3.12). There is usually moderate mitotic activity and mild multifocal necrosis.

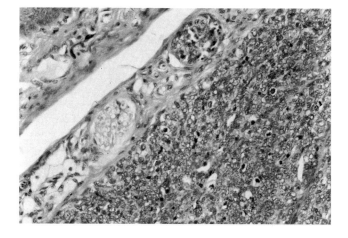

3.12. *Lymphosarcoma. A sheet of poorly differentiated lymphoid cells is effacing the oral submucosa.*

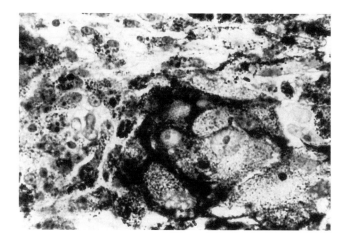

3.13. *Oral malignant melanoma comprised of poorly differentiated cells with abundant cytoplasmic pigment.*

Oral malignant melanoma is unusual unless associated with melanoma of the beak. It is similar grossly and histologically to the tumors of the beak (Fig. 3.13).

Esophagus and Crop

Noninfectious Disease. Primary noninfectious lesions of the crop include crop burns, foreign-body penetration, and vitamin A deficiency. Burns are secondary to hand feeding of overheated food and are usually found in the cranial-ventral portion of the crop. Grossly there may be reddening and edema. Blistering or necrosis occurs in severe cases. Histologically, coagulative necrosis of the crop wall is present and associated with a peripheral inflammatory reaction comprised of heterophils and macrophages.

Foreign bodies may penetrate the wall of the crop, leading to necrosis and loss of food that migrates in the subcutis of the neck, resulting in widespread inflammation and necrosis. Crop perforation is most common in birds that are being tube fed as nestlings or in the hospital. In these birds, the instrument being used for tubing may accidentally perforate the crop or the esophagus, and

large boluses of food may then be injected subcutaneously. Histologically there is a pyogranulomatous reaction, comprised primarily of heterophils, initially. Subsequently macrophages and giant cells are seen if the lesion becomes chronic. There may be a secondary bacterial infection resulting in septicemia.

Vitamin A deficiency results in squamous metaplasia of esophageal glands and proliferation of crop mucosa, often with secondary infections. Histologic changes are similar to those seen in the oral cavity.

Thickening of the crop epithelium is a common finding in birds that are not eating.

An ingluvolith has been reported in one budgerigar. It was primarily uric acid rather than calcium or struvite.

Lymphangiectasis leading to grossly noted fluid-filled spaces in the submucosa is occasionally seen, but the cause is usually not determined.

Infectious disease. Poxvirus infection can lead to proliferative and necrotic lesions similar to those described in

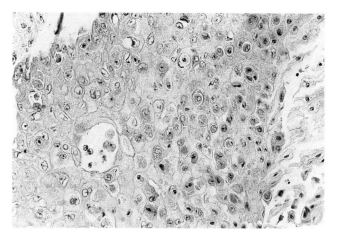

3.14. *Poxvirus infection of the crop. A proliferative epithelium with ballooning degeneration and intracytoplasmic inclusion bodies are seen.*

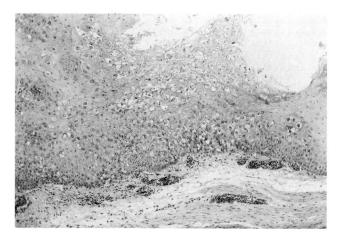

3.15. *Esophageal lesion in herpesvirus infection. There are mucosal hyperplasia, focal necrosis, and intranuclear inclusion body formation.*

the oral cavity (Fig. 3.14). Herpesvirus infection results in mucosal necrosis and hemorrhage. Histologically, intranuclear inclusion bodies are present in mucosal epithelial cells (Fig. 3.15).

In cases of proventricular dilatation disease (PDD), myenteric ganglia may have lymphoplasmacytic inflammatory infiltrates. Biopsy of the crop is a commonly used antemortem morphologic diagnostic tool for PDD because of the ease of access of the crop. Histologic lesions, however, are not as consistently found in the crop as they are in the proventriculus and ventriculus. Therefore the absence of lesions in the myenteric ganglia of the crop does not rule out PDD.

Bacterial infections of the crop and esophagus can be primary or secondary. In immunosuppressed birds, there may be bacterial colonization and overgrowth in the mucosa. This overgrowth is not observable grossly, and little or no inflammatory response is seen histologically. Bacterial and yeast overgrowth of the crop are also common in nestling birds with crop stasis. Failure of the crop to empty is a nonspecific sign and may be secondary to many digestive and systemic disorders. In severe infections of the crop, yellow-white nodules and plaques, hemorrhage, necrosis, and a variable fibrinopurulent exudate affect the mucosal surface. Histologically the presence of bacteria associated with necrosis and a predominantly heterophilic infiltrate is diagnostic. In chronic infection, heterophils, macrophages, and giant cells surround bacterial colonies and necrotic debris.

Yeast infection of the crop can also be a primary problem in some birds, particularly cockatiels, lovebirds, and finches. Gross changes are similar to those seen in the oral cavity, with necrosis and a gray to yellow-white exudate on the mucosal surface. Often the crop wall appears significantly thickened and is thrown into broad folds. Histologically there is proliferation of mucosal epithelium and variable hyperkeratosis. A mononuclear inflamma-

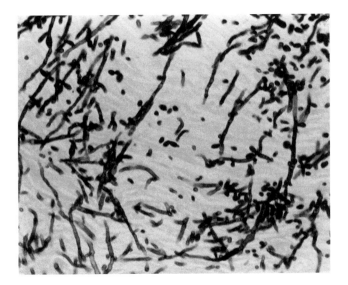

3.17.   *Silver stain illustrating the* Candida *organisms in the crop mucosa.*

tory response may be seen, and organisms are present in the mucosal epithelium (Figs. 3.16 and 3.17).

Mixed bacterial and yeast infections are occasionally found with the organisms noted histologically.

Trichomoniasis causes lesions of the crop in budgerigars and thoracic esophagus in the cockatiels. The disease affects adult birds primarily and causes a proliferative lesion that can be caseous. Histologically the lesion is similar to that seen in the oral cavity. Differential gross diagnoses include poxvirus and bacterial infections, as well as vitamin A deficiency. Finding the organism in the lesion is necessary for a positive etiologic diagnosis. Pigeons, doves, and mockingbirds occasionally develop a form of trichomoniasis resulting in invasion of the tissues of the face, throat, and neck. Grossly the lesions are soft swellings that are red and highly vascular. Histologically the trichomonads induce a marked heterophilic response and locally extensive necrosis.

As in the oral cavity, intraepithelial nematodes or nematode eggs may be found, usually as an incidental his-

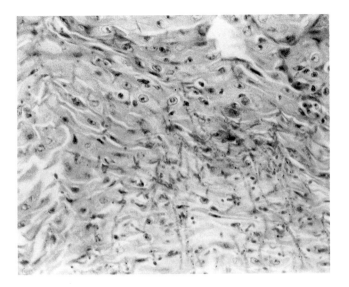

3.16.   *Candidiasis of the crop. There is marked mucosal proliferation associated with pseudohyphae.*

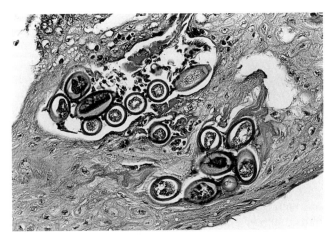

3.18.   *Eggs of* Capillaria *sp. within the crop mucosa.*

tologic lesion (Fig. 3.18). Capillariasis of the esophagus is common in pheasants and of particular concern in the vulturine guinea fowl, where it is associated with a high mortality rate.

Neoplastic Disease. Neoplasms of the esophagus and crop include papillomas and carcinomas. Papillomas are proliferative masses that project into the lumen of the esophagus or crop. Mucosal papillomas of the crop and the esophagus are most common in green-winged, scarlet, military, blue and gold, and great green macaws. These birds typically also have oral and cloacal lesions. Amazon parrots can also have esophageal or crop papillomas but far less commonly than macaws. Histologically there are numerous papillary projections covered by large epithelial cells (Fig. 3.19).

SCCs are also found in the esophagus and crop. Carcinomas are both proliferative and invasive. Secondary infections of the diseased tissue are common and present as variably sized masses that may contain areas of necrosis and hemorrhage. Histologically they are comprised of nests and cords of neoplastic epithelial cells and variable stroma.

Carcinomas of the submucosal glands occur but do not appear to have been previously reported. These lesions are often large and involve much of the wall of the esophagus/crop with extension into surrounding tissue. They can be necrotic and hemorrhagic. Histologically they are comprised of moderately undifferentiated to poorly differentiated epithelial cells forming nests, acini, and trabeculae that infiltrate into surrounding tissue. There is usually minimal to moderate stroma.

Tumors of smooth muscle origin result in large space-occupying masses that may become necrotic and hemorrhage, although they can be asymptomatic when small. Microscopically they are characterized by interlacing bundles of fusiform cells with moderate amounts of cytoplasm. Differentiation between leiomyomas and leiomyosarcomas is done histologically based on characteristics such as degree of anaplasia, mitotic index, and other typical parameters.

Proventriculus

Noninfectious Disease. Gastric impactions that sometimes result in perforation are most common in young psittacines that ingest foreign material. Affected birds have proventricular dilatation, and the proventricular wall is flaccid. Perforation or rupture is characterized by hemorrhage and accumulation of ingesta in and around the affected area.

Birds with severe vitamin A deficiency may have metaplasia of the proventricular glands, leading to gross thickening and accumulation of excessive keratin, which must be differentiated from caseous material due to inflammation/infection.

Severe mineralization of the proventricular mucosa is seen in birds and is believed to be secondary to excessive dietary calcium and may possibly occur in birds ingesting excessive vitamin D_3. The lesion may not be noticeable grossly, but histologically proventricular glands are variably affected (Fig. 3.20). This lesion seems to be more common in macaws, particularly the blue and gold macaw and cockatiels.

Infectious Disease. Infectious diseases affecting the proventriculus include viral, bacterial, mycobacterial, fungal, and parasitic.

The primary problem of suspected viral origin is PDD, which is a disease of the central and peripheral nervous systems. It is discussed in this section because one of the most common lesions associated with this disease occurs in the proventriculus. The disease has also been called neuropathic gastric dilatation, myenteric ganglioneuritis, and splanchnic neuropathy. It is reported in many species of psittacine birds and may occur in other species of birds, ranging from red-tailed hawks to Canada geese. African grey parrots, macaws, Amazon parrots, and cockatoos are the most commonly affected psittacine species.

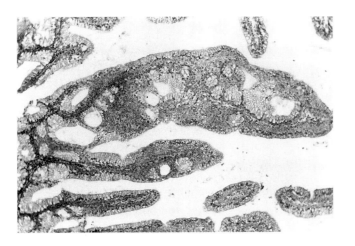

3.19. Papilloma of the crop. Multiple papillary projections are seen.

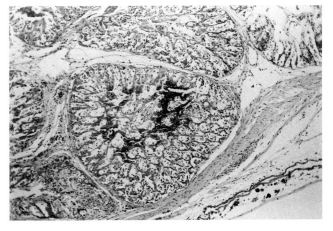

3.20. Mineralization of proventricular glands. Note the diffuse involvement of basement membranes.

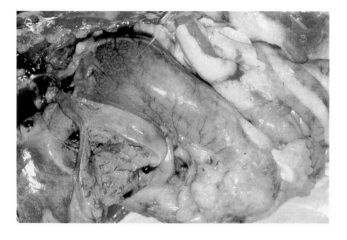

3.21.   Grossly dilated and flaccid proventriculus typical of severe proventricular dilatation disease.

Many birds develop a complete ileus of the digestive tract and, as a result, are severely wasted and have no body fat by the time they die. The primary gross lesions seen in PDD are flaccidity and dilatation of any portion of the gastrointestinal tract, with the proventriculus, ventriculus, and crop being most commonly affected (Fig. 3.21). The proventriculus may be so dilated as to fill much of the left side of the coelomic cavity and to displace the ventriculus to the right and cranially. If the bird has been on a seed diet, the proventriculus and ventriculus will be packed with seeds. Atrophy of the muscles of the ventriculus and thinning of the proventriculus mucosa are common. Multifocal ulceration of the proventricular mucosa also occurs. At necropsy, some birds will not show a gross change in the digestive system.

Histologic lesions are characterized by a lymphoplasmacytic infiltrate of the myenteric plexus of any part of the esophagus, crop, or gastrointestinal tract (Fig. 3.22). The inflammatory infiltrate may also affect the smooth muscle. Crop biopsy has been reported to be an effective method of antemortem diagnosis in 76% of affected birds,

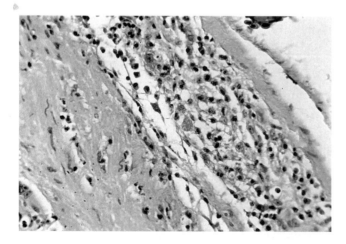

3.22.   Lymphoplasmacytic infiltrate typical of proventricular dilatation disease in nerves and nerve ganglia of the proventriculus.

provided a large biopsy sample and a visible blood vessel are included in the sample. Routine sampling in a diagnostic pathology practice has been less effective (30% to 35% positive).

Proventricular dilation is not pathognomonic for PDD. Any disease that causes partial or complete obstruction of the intestines will result in proventricular dilation. Proventricular dilation is also a common lesion in geese that are poisoned by lead.

Although infrequently seen, internal poxvirus infection and Pacheco's disease can lead to proventricular lesions grossly and histologically similar to those previously described.

Bacterial infections of the proventriculus can be primary or secondary. Gram-negative bacterial infections will present grossly as focal to diffuse hyperemia, with variable necrosis and hemorrhage of the mucosa. Fibrin may be present. In severe cases, the proventriculus can be perforated. Histologically the reaction is primarily heterophilic, with variable numbers of macrophages and plasma cells. Finding the organism is necessary for confirmation of the etiology.

Mycobacteriosis has been reported in the proventriculus of passerine birds and is also seen in psittacine birds. Mycobacterial disease of the small intestine, which is far more common, is discussed in detail in the section on small and large intestine.

An organism that is frequently referred to as "megabacteria" is commonly found on the mucosal surface of the isthmus of budgerigars, canaries, finches, parrotlets, ostriches and, less frequently, poultry. Recent work shows that this organism is actually previously undescribed yeast. The organisms are relatively large (2×20–40 μm), gram positive, periodic acid-Schiff positive, and stain strongly with Calcaflour White MR2 (a chitin stain). They are found densely packed, resembling a logjam, on the surface of the isthmus and often penetrate down between the glands of the isthmus. They may also extend into the ventriculus and penetrate deeply into the koilin.

It is widely accepted by clinicians that this organism is pathogenic and associated with a chronic wasting disease. It must be noted, however, that many birds infected with this organism do not have clinical signs or histologic lesions. Therefore, the presence of this organism in a necropsy specimen without concurrent gross or histologic disease is not conclusive evidence that it contributed to the bird's death.

The primary gross lesion associated with this infection is excessive mucus production. Histologically there is goblet cell hyperplasia and a variable mononuclear inflammatory infiltrate in the mucosa (Figs. 3.23 and 3.24). Although some underlying stress may be necessary for the infection to become clinical, proventriculitis associated with megabacteria is often the only postmortem change in chronically ill birds with severe weight loss. Mild to moderate lymphoplasmacytic infiltrates have also been observed in the lamina propria of the proventriculus of budgerigars that were raised in isolation and were free of

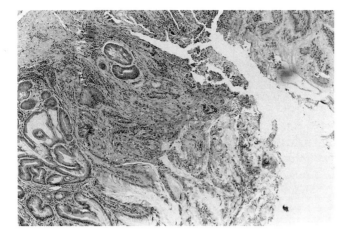

3.23. Megabacterial infection of the proventriculus. *Note the goblet cell hypertrophy/hyperplasia and excessive surface mucus. Minimal necrotic debris is present.*

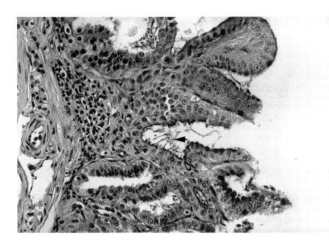

3.24. Megabacterial infection of the proventriculus (arrowhead).

this organism (D. Phalen 2001, unpublished observation); therefore, these changes may not always be attributable to the organism.

Zygomycete fungi cause proventriculitis in several avian species. Gross lesions are similar to bacterial infections, and erosions or ulcers are common. Histologically there is necrosis and hemorrhage, with a pleocellular inflammatory response and intralesional fungal hyphae, which are seen throughout the proventricular wall and within blood vessels.

Cryptosporidiosis of the proventriculus is seen in a variety of psittacine and small passerine birds. Often no gross lesion is reported, but there may be excessive mucus production and variable mucosal hypertrophy. Histologically the organisms are present within the striated border of mucosal epithelial cells. A variable mononuclear inflammatory response and mucosal hyperplasia may occur. Crytosporidiosis is a possible complication of PBFDV infection of cockatoos.

Spiruids, including *Spiroptera* sp. and *Dyspharynx* sp., can colonize the proventriculus. They require an interme-

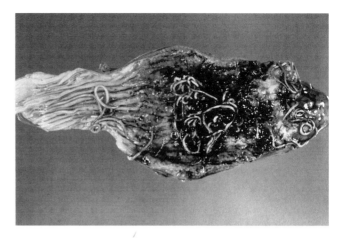

3.25. Proventricular nematodes (Contracecum *sp.*). *Note the thickened mucosa.*

diate arthropod host and thus are primarily seen in birds kept outdoors. In minimal infections, there is no gross change, and the parasites are seen histologically. In severe chronic infections, the wall of the proventriculus, particularly the mucosa, will be thickened, and the proventriculus may be distended. Hemorrhage is seen in severe cases, and nematodes may be found in the lumen (Fig. 3.25). Histologically there is mucosal hyperplasia, excess mucus production, and an inflammatory infiltrate of varying severity that includes heterophils, lymphocytes, and macrophages. Parasite fragments may be present in the mucosa and the lumen (Fig. 3.26). Perforation of the proventriculus may occur, but it is uncommon. Doves and pigeons are commonly infected with *Tetrameres* sp. These large roundworms cause the wall of the proventriculus to have a red, beaded appearance.

Neoplastic Disease. Proventricular papillomas are morphologically similar to those previously described. They are an uncommon lesion and most likely to occur in macaws, particularly the green-winged macaw. These

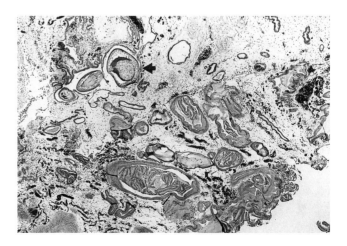

3.26. Proliferative proventricular glands with edema and inflammation. Nematode fragments (arrow) are seen in the deep mucosa.

birds generally have lesions of the esophagus and crop and often are chronically debilitated. Proventricular carcinomas are reported in several species of birds, but in pet birds they are most common in budgerigars, gray-cheeked parakeets, and Amazon parrots. Proventricular carcinomas are often found at the proventricular-ventricular junction and may be difficult to distinguish grossly in some cases. These lesions are generally flat rather than nodular. If they extend to the serosal surface, there may be peritonitis, fibrin deposition, and adhesion to the liver or other organs (Fig. 3.27). If nodular proliferation is noted in the lumen, there may be lumenal hemorrhage associated with ulceration of the tumor.

Histologically carcinomas are comprised of poorly differentiated cells, including goblet cells, and there may be mucin production. Tumor cells are moderately undifferentiated and tend to form infiltrative nests, tubules, and cords, but may be individualized. There is moderate mitotic activity and stromal proliferation. They extend through the muscularis and may proliferate laterally into the ventricular wall and through the serosa. Stromal production is variable (Fig. 3.28). These tumors metastasize infrequently.

Smooth muscle tumors are rare. Grossly and histologically they are similar to those previously described.

Ventriculus

Noninfectious Disease. Trauma to the ventricular koilin and mucosa may be secondary to ingested foreign bodies. Depending on the species and thickness of the ventricular wall, there may be associated perforation. Grossly erosions, ulcers, and hemorrhage are noted, and foreign material may be identifiable in the lesion. Histologically there is also a pleocellular inflammatory response, and the lesion may become secondarily infected by bacteria or fungi.

Grit is small stones that are intentionally fed to birds for the stated purpose of assisting in digestion. Most cage birds do not need grit. When birds are fed grit, they occasionally consume too much, and it will interfere with digestion, causing erosion of the ventriculus and may result in starvation.

Mineralization, possibly associated with excessive dietary calcium, is usually not noted grossly. Histologically the mineral is deposited in the superficial mucosa and the koilin (Fig. 3.29).

A common manifestation of zinc poisoning is an erosive ventriculitis. Histologically the koilin layer is disrupted; there is ulceration of the underlying mucosa and dysplasia of the ventricular glands.

Xanthomatosis is a rare finding in the ventricular musculature. If the lesion is large enough, there is a nodular irregularity to the ventricular wall. Microscopically the xanthoma is similar to that seen in the skin and subcutis,

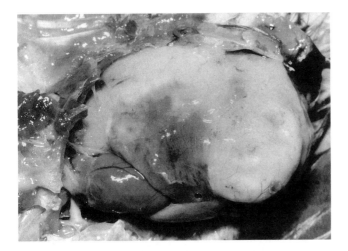

3.27. Thickened, irregular proventricular wall with adhesions secondary to proventricular carcinoma.

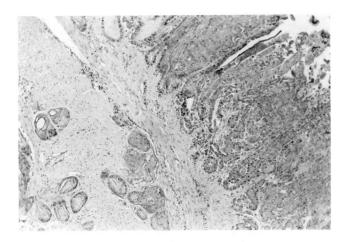

3.28. Infiltrative nests of cells in the muscularis of a bird with proventricular carcinoma. Note the loss of polarity and disorganization of the mucosa.

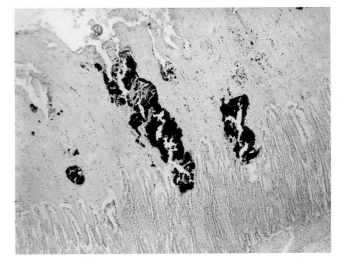

3.29. Multiple foci of mineralization in the superficial mucosa and koilin of the ventriculus.

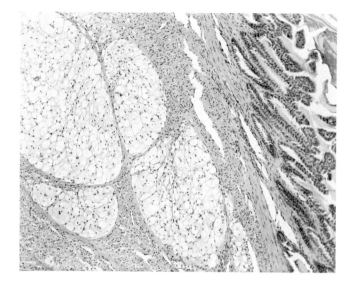

3.30. Xanthoma within the wall of the ventriculus. Multiple expansile masses are seen.

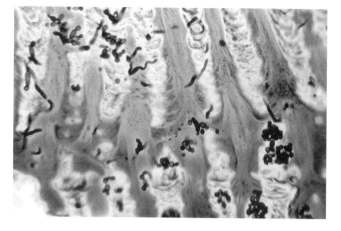

3.32. Ventricular candidiasis. Organisms are present throughout the koilin. There is usually no inflammatory response.

with numerous large, foamy macrophages surrounding cholesterol clefts (Fig. 3.30).

Infectious Disease. PDD commonly affects the ventriculus. Typically the ventriculus is dilated and has a thin wall. Nerves on the serosal surface of the ventriculus may be enlarged. Histologic lesions for PDD of the ventriculus are similar to those described for the proventriculus.

Adenovirus infections are typically multisystemic, but ventricular lesions are the only lesions noted in some birds. Grossly, small areas of necrosis and ulceration of the koilin and mucosa are noted. Histologically, necrosis, hemorrhage, and a mononuclear inflammatory infiltrate are noted. Intranuclear inclusion bodies are seen in mucosal epithelial cells (Fig. 3.31).

Bacterial infections may be primary or secondary and result in loss of koilin, necrosis, and ulceration of the underlying mucosa and hemorrhage. A fibrinous exudate

may cover an underlying ulcer. Histologically a pleocellular inflammatory response is seen, and organisms must be present to make a positive etiologic diagnosis. Immunosuppressed birds may have bacterial colonization of the ventricular koilin, with no associated inflammation.

Ventricular mycosis is seen in a variety of pet birds and is especially common in finches. Fungal organisms (usually *Candida* sp.) are found in the koilin layer and occasionally in the mucosa (Fig. 3.32). Inflammation is usually mild, and gross changes are rarely seen. Destruction of the koilin and ulceration of the underlying mucosa is an uncommon manifestation of yeast infections of the ventriculus. These lesions, like those of bacterial infections of the koilin, may bleed, causing anemia or rarely a fatal blood loss. Occasionally, severe infections by zygomycete fungi occur. In these cases, there is usually gross hemorrhage and necrosis. Histologically there is a marked pleocellular inflammatory infiltrate and numerous organisms, the lesion being similar to that described in the proventriculus (Fig. 3.33).

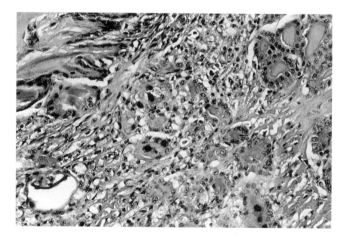

3.31. Adenoviral infection of the ventriculus. Note the large intranuclear inclusion bodies.

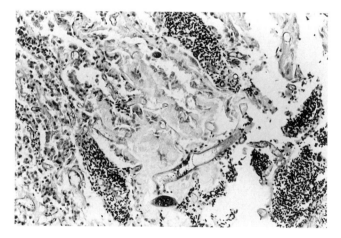

3.33. Ventricular infection by zygomycete fungi. Large, irregular hyphae are seen in an area of necrosis and hemorrhage.

Metazoan infections of the ventriculus can lead to necrosis of the mucosa and koilin or be essentially incidental with little or no gross change, and small nematodes may not be seen at necropsy. Histologically fragments of nematodes are noted in the lumen and mucosa.

Neoplastic Disease. Papillomas and carcinomas are reported and are morphologically similar to those of the proventriculus. Carcinomas are usually at the proventricular junction, and the exact site of origin may be difficult to determine in extensive tumors. These neoplasms may infiltrate into the ventricular muscle and extend laterally some distance from the primary site.

Small and Large Intestine

Noninfectious Disease. Noninfectious diseases of the intestinal tract of pet birds include trauma secondary to foreign bodies, ingested toxins and, infrequently, torsion or intussusception. Trauma and torsion are usually obvious at necropsy, but histologic examination of affected tissue may be necessary to rule out underlying disease. Torsion leads to distension of a portion of the intestine, and edema fluid may be present in the lumen. The intestinal wall is edematous and congested, and histologically there is an infiltrate of heterophils and macrophages. True intussusception must be differentiated from agonal telescoping of a portion of the intestine. In true intussusception, there is edema and congestion, with subsequent inflammation and fibrin deposition and adhesion formation.

Impaction of the intestines is usually the result of improper diet, ingestion of foreign material, and, in some cases, dehydration. The impacted section is dilated and firm, and foreign material and ingesta are present in the lumen. Because the ventriculus is designed to hold ingested items until they are small enough to be digested by the intestines, intestinal foreign bodies are rare in pet birds.

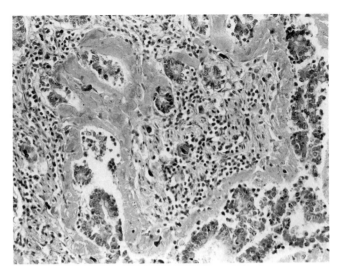

3.35. Amyloid deposition in the basement membranes of the small intestine.

Amyloidosis and mineralization may occur in the intestinal tract, usually with no gross change noted. Mineral is found most frequently in vascular walls and amyloid in vessel walls and the lamina propria (Figs. 3.34 and 3.35).

Hyperplasia of all layers of the smooth muscle of the small intestine is rarely seen in birds, and the cause is not known. The intestinal wall is thickened and intestinal villi are enlarged due to proliferation of smooth muscle in the lamina propria.

Infectious Disease. Numerous infectious agents affect the large and small intestines. Enteritis, to some degree, occurs in approximately 30% of birds, with disease caused by psittacid herpesvirus (Pacheco's disease virus). The lesions are generally mild, but severe enteric necrosis and hemorrhage that is seen grossly on the mucosal and

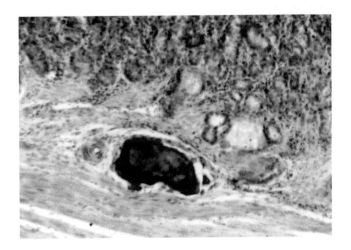

3.34. Focal mineralization in blood vessels of the small intestine. This is usually a part of a generalized problem.

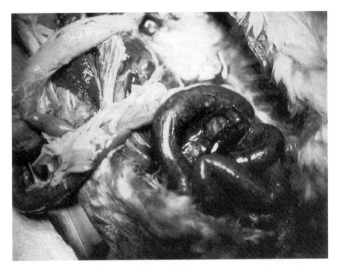

3.36. Severe intestinal hemorrhage due to herpesvirus infection. Both mucosal hemorrhage and serosal hemorrhage are seen.

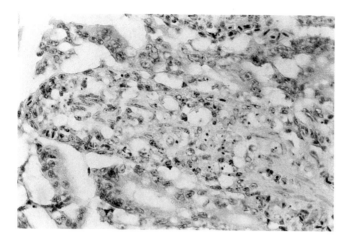

3.37. *Herpesvirus-induced necrosis in the small intestine. There is early syncytial cell formation.*

serosal surfaces may occur (Fig. 3.36). Enterocyte necrosis, variable mononuclear inflammatory infiltrates, and intranuclear inclusion bodies are seen in the mucosa (Fig. 3.37).

Gross dilation of the intestines is an uncommon finding in birds with PDD. Histologically, segmental inflammation of intestinal smooth muscle, nerves, and ganglia is seen in PDD. The degree of gross dilatation will be variable, and histologic changes are similar to those previously described.

Paramyxovirus 1 (exotic Newcastle disease) can potentially infect many species of pet birds. Lesions are variable, but gross hemorrhage and necrosis are present in the intestines of some birds. Histologically the lesions are due to a vasculitis of the intestinal wall and necrosis of submucosal lymphoid tissue. Fibrinoid degeneration and a mononuclear inflammatory infiltrate characterize the vasculitis.

Adenovirus also causes hemorrhagic enteritis in pet birds. Gross necrosis and hemorrhage are noted. Histologically there is variable inflammation, thrombi in intestinal capillaries, and large basophilic intranuclear inclusion bodies in enterocytes.

Reovirus, coronavirus, and rotavirus have been implicated as causes of avian viral enteritis, but their occurrence in pet birds is poorly documented. Gross lesions are nonspecific, with edema and possible mucosal necrosis seen. Blunting and fusion of villi are described in cases of coronavirus infection and, in cases of suspected rotavirus, there is atrophy of villi (Fig. 3.38).

A variety of bacteria cause enteritis in psittacine birds. Gram-negative pathogens can be primary or secondary invaders. Historically, in psittacine birds, any finding of a gram-negative bacteria has been considered by some to indicate disease; however, organisms such as *Escherichia coli* have been found in surveys of psittacine birds without clinical signs or lesions indicative of intestinal disease. Therefore the culture of *E. coli* from the intestine without associated gross and microscopic evidence of disease is insufficient proof that the organism was associated with the bird's death. Salmonellosis is a problem in all bird species. The disease in pet birds was a significant problem among wild-caught birds that were closely confined in quarantine stations. Currently it is more likely to be seen in birds from aviaries that have a significant rodent infestation. *Salmonella* sp. and most pathogenic enteric bacteria generally are invasive, resulting in significant lesions outside of the intestinal tract.

The gross lesions of a bacterial enteritis include redness, exudation and, in some cases, ulceration of the mucosa. Gas or fluid may distend the intestine. Generally there is fecal soiling of the feathers of the vent, a lesion consistent with diarrhea. Histologically necrosis, fibrin deposition, and an infiltrate that is primarily heterophilic characterize the lesion. There may be extension into the submucosa muscularis, and crypt dilatation and abscess formation can be seen. Bacteria may not be present in all lesions (Figs. 3.39, 3.40, and 3.41).

Gram-positive bacteria also cause enteric disease. Enteritis and septicemia due to *Enterococcus hirae* have been reported in 10 psittacine species. This organism, however, is found in the feces of normal birds and may be a part of the normal flora.

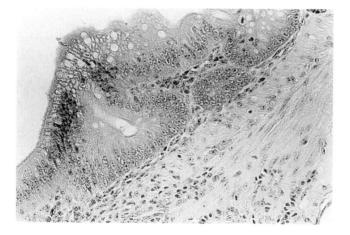

3.38. *Intestinal mucosal atrophy that could be due to rotavirus infection.*

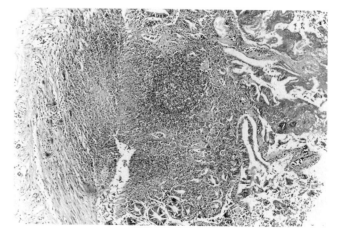

3.39. *Bacterial enteritis. There is severe focal necrosis and inflammation extending into the muscularis.*

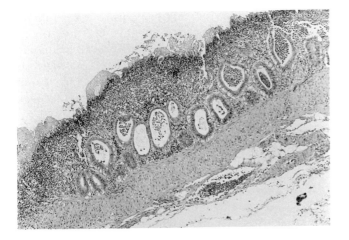

3.40.   *Diffuse necrotizing enteritis due to gram-negative bacteria.*

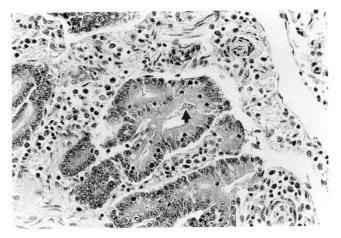

3.42.   *Enterotoxemia. Note the mild inflammatory infiltrate and clumps of large, spore-bearing, rod-shaped bacteria in the mucosa (arrow). This may be the only microscopic change in some cases.*

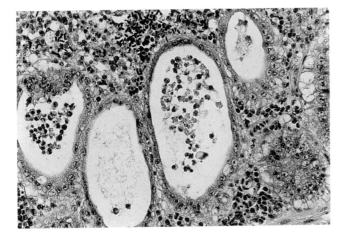

3.41.   *Higher magnification of Figure 3.40. Note the crypt dilatation and infiltration by the heterophils and macrophages.*

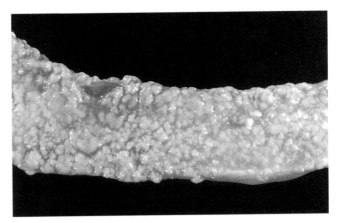

3.43.   *Intestinal mycobacterial infection. There are variably sized thickened areas as the result of infiltration and distortion of the intestinal villi.*

Clostridial overgrowth of the intestines may result in fatal enteritis. Lesions are most severe in the small intestine and vary from focal to diffuse hemorrhage, necrosis, and fibrin deposition. Although severe hemorrhage may be present, no other histologic changes are noted in some cases. Numerous large, gram-positive, spore-forming, rod-shaped bacteria are seen in the lumen and mucosa of affected birds (Fig. 3.42). The lack of histologic lesions may be due to acute death from systemic enterotoxemia. *Clostridium tertium* has been reported in a cockatoo with megacolon. At necropsy, there was severe dilatation of the colon, and a severe lymphoplasmacytic inflammatory reaction was noted histologically.

Mycobacterial infections, which occur sporadically in many species of pet birds, are especially common in gray-cheeked parakeets and red siskins. The primary site of infection for the *Mycobacterium avium-intracellulare* complex and *M. genavense,* the two most common causes of mycobacteriosis in birds, is the intestinal tract. Gross lesions include diffuse and/or nodular thickening and opacification of the intestinal wall (Fig. 3.43).

Histologically the common pattern is a diffuse infiltration of the lamina propria by large macrophages that have abundant amphophilic cytoplasm. These cells contain acid-fast bacteria; however, the abundance of the organism will vary from case to case. In severe cases, the infiltrate may extend through the intestinal wall to the serosa. A variable amount of necrosis and scattered accumulations of small macrophages, lymphoid cells, and heterophils may also be present (Figs. 3.44–3.46). In some birds, multiple granulomas are seen in the submucosa and muscularis (Fig. 3.47).

Chlamydial infections can lead to diffuse mucosal necrosis and a moderate mixed mononuclear inflammatory infiltrate.

Primary mycotic infections of the intestines are rarely reported. Secondary infections, particularly by *Candida* sp. or zygomycete fungi, are occasionally seen, and the lesions are similar to those described in the upper gastrointestinal tract. Finding the organism histologically is necessary for a definitive diagnosis.

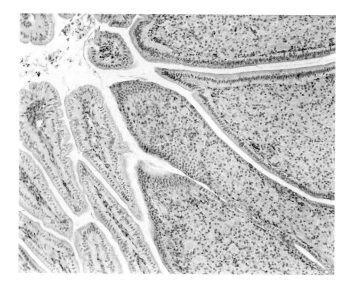

3.44.   Intestinal mycobacteriosis. There is diffuse thickening of the villi due to infiltration of large macrophages with abundant, pale cytoplasm.

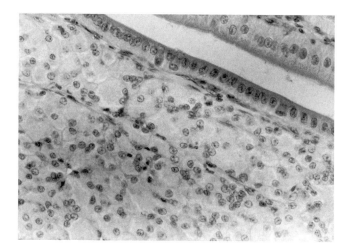

3.45.   Detail of Figure 3.44 illustrating diffuse macrophage infiltration.

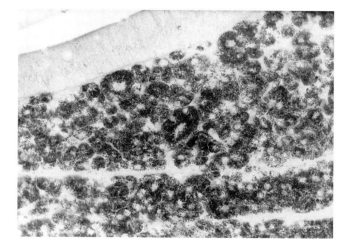

3.46.   Mycobacterial organisms in macrophages demonstrated by acid-fast staining.

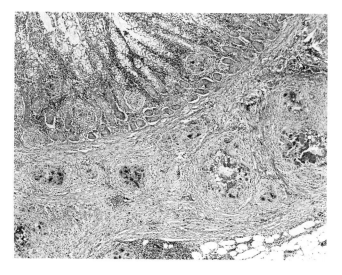

3.47.   Multiple intestinal submucosal granulomas due to mycobacterial infection.

Giardia and *Hexamita* are two flagellates that are considered to cause intestinal disease. These organisms may cause minimal gross change. Excessive fluid and mucus as well as mucosal hyperemia are seen in some birds. Histologically there may be villar atrophy and a mononuclear inflammatory infiltrate or no lesions at all. Organisms are usually found in intestinal crypts but, at least in the case of *Giardia*, will extend the entire length of the villi. Histologically these organisms can be differentiated morphologically in some cases. *Hexamita* is a rod-shaped organism, whereas *Giardia* is a flattened, pear-shaped organism (Fig. 3.48). Flagellates disappear from the intestine rapidly if the intestines are not immediately preserved. Therefore, wet mounts of intestinal, particularly duodenal, scrapings from a bird that has just died are the most sensitive means of finding these organisms. Each of these organisms has characteristic shapes and movements, making the wet mount an excellent means of differentiating them. It is also important to note that giardiasis is extremely common in budgerigars, yet most

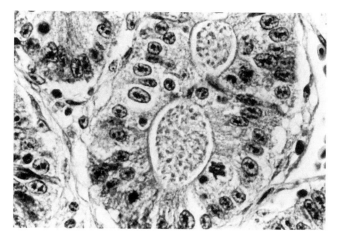

3.48.   Giardia in intestinal crypts. No inflammatory reaction is seen.

infected budgerigars are asymptomatic. Infection is also common in cockatiels, although disease is confined predominantly to nestlings that are near weaning age.

Two species of *Eimeria* (*E. dunsingi* and *E. haematodi*) and one species of *Isospora* (*I. psittaculae*) have been described in psittacine birds. The coccidium of canaries is *I. canaria*. These four organisms complete their life cycle in the intestine. Coccidia also infect many other species of birds, including cranes, waterfowl, and poultry. Coccidiosis in psittacine birds is rarely seen because current avicultural practices interrupt the infection cycle.

Coccidial infections may be inapparent or result in disease. When disease occurs, gross lesions varying from excessive fluid in the intestinal lumen to dilation of the intestine and gray-yellow foci are visible on the serosal surface. A fibrinonecrotic enteritis occurs in severe cases. Histologically organisms will be present in enterocytes. Different species of coccidia have different trophisms for different portions of the intestinal tracts. In some cases, finding organisms in the enterocytes may be the only change (Fig. 3.49). In more severe infections, there is a variable nonsuppurative inflammatory response and there may be necrosis.

Cryptosporidiosis is reported in a wide range of birds, including ducks, chickens, psittacine birds, and ostriches. Infection is not always associated with disease. Disease, in companion birds, is often secondary to another immunosuppressive disorder, but *Cryptosporidia* may also be the primary pathogen. Cryptosporidiosis is characterized grossly by mucosal thickening and excessive mucus production. Histologically, variable mucosal hyperplasia, mucus production, and a lymphoplasmacytic and histiocytic inflammatory response are seen. Villi may be misshapen and thickened. Atrophic villi are also seen in some cases. Small organisms are found in the microvillus border of enterocytes and in the surface mucus (Fig. 3.50).

Toxoplasmosis, which is uncommon in pet birds, has been reported in passerine birds, including canaries, and in lories, a regent parrot, a superb parrot, and a crimson rosella. It causes a systemic disease. Intestinal lesions may or may not occur. The intestines may be dilated, and there

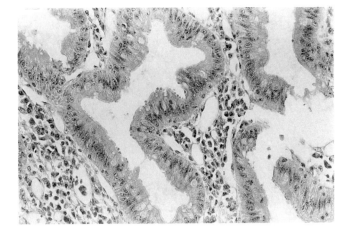

3.50. Intestinal cryptosporidiosis. The mucosa is variably proliferative and irregular. Organisms are present on the apical surfaces of enterocytes.

may be pasting of the vent, suggesting diarrhea. Multifocal to locally extensive necrohemorrhagic enteritis, with intralesional organisms, that may result in a transmural lesion and peritonitis is reported, but is not a consistent lesion.

Although not seen in common pet species, *Histomonas* is a cause of typhlitis, particularly in Galliformes. Gross lesions are similar to those in turkeys, with enlargement of the ceca, mottling of the cecal wall, and a caseous exudate in the lumen. Histologically, diffuse severe transmural necrosis extends is seen (Fig. 3.51). Organisms may be difficult to see unless special stains are used (Fig. 3.52).

Encephalitozoon hellem is an obligate intracellular single-celled parasite that may be found incidentally in the intestine or be associated with serosal and mucosal hemorrhage. Histologically the organisms are most commonly present in the mucosal epithelial cells but are occasionally

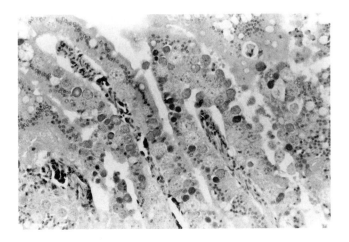

3.49. Coccidial organisms in enterocytes. Minimal necrosis is seen, but there is essentially no inflammation.

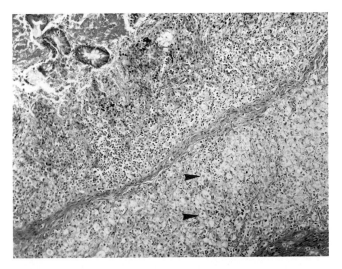

3.51. Severe transmural necrosis and inflammation of the cecum in histomoniasis. A few organisms are present (arrowheads).

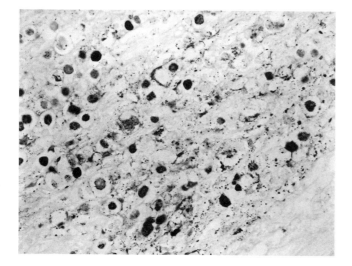

3.52. *Silver-stained section to demonstrate* **Histomonas** *in necrotic tissue.*

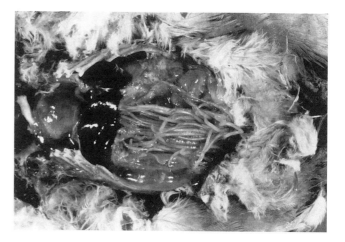

3.54. *Ascarid infestation of the small intestine. The intestinal lumen was occluded, and numerous worms are seen.*

seen in the macrophages within the lamina propria. Mucosal hyperplasia and a lymphoplasmacytic and heterophilic inflammatory response may accompany the organisms. *Encephalitozoon hellem* is seen most commonly in lovebirds, but many lovebirds shed the parasite and show no signs of disease. Parasite shedding is threefold more likely in lovebirds that are concurrently infected with PBFDV. Disease is also appears more likely to occur in other parrots with PBFDV infection.

Metazoan parasites are infrequent causes of clinical disease in well-managed aviaries or in household pets. Cestodes are occasionally diagnosed at necropsy. There is usually no associated gross or histologic lesion (Fig. 3.53). Cestodes are particularly common in Australian finches and wild-caught African grey parrots and cockatoos. These parasites will survive in their hosts for many years and have the potential for causing intestinal obstruction in rare cases.

Birds with schistosomiasis may have scattered granulomas in the submucosa and muscularis. Egg fragments are usually seen in the lesions.

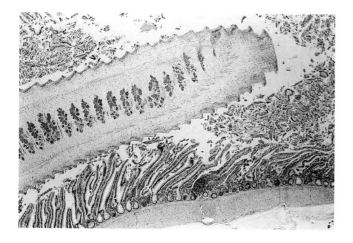

3.53. *Cestode found incidentally at necropsy. No reaction is seen.*

A number of nematodes have been reported in cage birds. Numerous parasites may be found in the intestinal lumen in severe cases, and the intestine may be blocked (Fig. 3.54). Of particular concern are roundworms, which are particularly common in Australian grass parakeets (*Neophema* sp.) and cockatiels that are raised in cages that reach the ground. Recently roundworms of wild-bird origin have been observed to cause intestinal disease in a macaw, an Amazon, and cockatoos housed outdoors. Worms obstructed the intestinal tract of these birds and were also present in the bile and pancreatic ducts. Histologic lesions may be minimal and are usually characterized by an excessive accumulation of mononuclear inflammatory cells within the lamina propria of the intestine. Fragments of adults, larvae, and eggs can be found in the mucosa and the lumen. In some cases, invasion of the mucosa results in necrosis, severe inflammation and, occasionally, perforation of the intestinal wall.

Acanthocephalids are rarely found in birds. As in mammals, they penetrate into the intestinal wall, and gross nodules are seen on the serosal surface. In addition to necrosis, there is a pleocellular inflammatory response.

Neoplastic Disease. Primary neoplasms of the intestine include carcinoma and several types of sarcoma. Carcinomas are infrequent. They present as variably sized masses that may be ulcerated on the mucosal surface. Histologically they are comprised of poorly differentiated epithelial cells that form infiltrative nests and cords separated by minimal to moderate amounts of stroma (Fig. 3.55).

Sarcomas present as masses within the intestinal wall that vary from firm and red-brown to gray-white or yellow. Myxosarcoma will have a shiny myxoid appearance grossly and is comprised of anaplastic cells with fibrillar cytoplasm surrounded by myxoid ground substance.

Leiomyomas and leiomyosarcomas are comprised of interlacing bundles of cells with fibrillar cytoplasm and vesicular nuclei. Differentiation between leiomyoma and leiomyosarcoma depends on mitotic activity and the

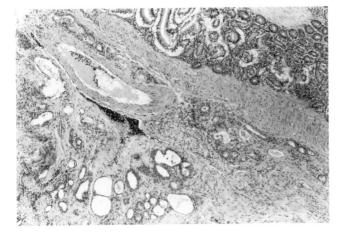

3.55. *Infiltrative tubular structures in intestinal carcinoma. Neoplastic structures extend through the wall and elicit a variable amount of stromal proliferation.*

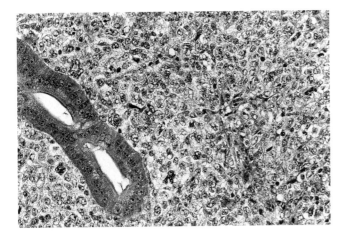

3.56. *Effacement of the intestinal mucosa by a sheet of neoplastic histiocytic cells.*

degree of cellular anaplasia. Fibrosarcoma with myxoid degeneration also is seen in pet birds and may have a similar gross and histologic appearance.

Lymphosarcoma and histiocytic sarcoma of the intestinal tract usually presents as a diffuse or nodular thickening that must be differentiated from conditions such as mycobacteriosis. Neoplastic cells may extend from the mucosa to the serosa, usually effacing the normal architecture of the intestinal wall (Fig. 3.56).

Cloaca

Noninfectious Disease. Impaction of the cloaca can result from a variety of causes, including failure to pass an egg, intrinsic disease of the cloacal wall, and loss of muscle tone due to virus-induced ganglioneuritis (PDD). Grossly there is dilatation of the cloacal wall, and it may be irregularly thickened (Fig. 3.57). The lumen may contain an egg, impacted fecal material, or products of inflammatory disease. Abscesses of the cloacal wall may partially obstruct the cloaca or rupture into the lumen of the cloaca.

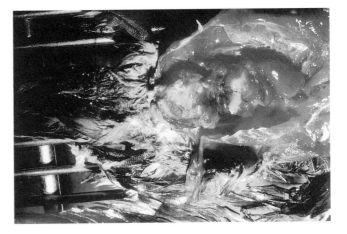

3.57. *Dilated impacted cloaca. This appearance can be the end result of a variety of causes.*

There are a variety of causes of cloacal prolapse. The prolapsed mucosa will appear nodular or proliferative, and there may be areas of necrosis and hemorrhage. Histologic examination may be necessary to differentiate prolapse and associated inflammation from cloacal papillomatosis. The prolapsed mucosa will be somewhat thickened and inflamed, but mucosal epithelial cells will not be markedly hypertrophied, and papillary structures are not seen. A variable pleomorphic inflammatory infiltrate is usually present, and, if there is a primary or secondary infection, microorganisms may be seen. Cloacal prolapse is especially common in tame umbrella cockatoos. It is speculated that behavioral factors rather than disease cause the prolapse.

The use of barium in radiologic diagnosis can lead to a lesion that is occasionally encountered at necropsy. The barium will be taken up by the mucosa of the large intestine and cloaca and is seen diffusely in the submucosa and muscularis. A slight discoloration of the cloacal wall may be seen grossly. Microscopically, free and phagocytosed barium are present as a brown crystalline material (Fig. 3.58), and there may be mild fibroplasia.

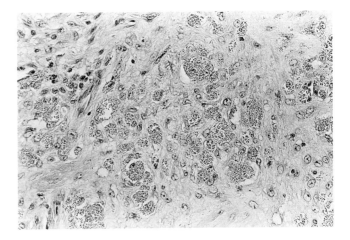

3.58. *Phagocytosed barium being taken into the wall of the cloaca. Note the accompanying fibroplasia.*

Infectious Disease. Infections affecting the cloaca are the same as those seen in the upper intestinal tract, and the gross and histologic features are similar

Neoplastic Disease. Papilloma is the most common cloacal neoplasm. They are more common in New World parrots, particularly Amazon parrots and macaws, and occur in the cloacal mucosa near the junction with the skin but may extend into the cloaca for some distance (Fig. 3.59). Lesions may be focal or diffuse. When the papillomas are large, they prolapse and ulcerate. Chronic soiling of the surrounding skin leads to inflammation, fibrosis, and stricture of the vent. If repeated surgical removal of the cloacal papillomas is performed, strictures of the cloaca develop.

Histologically they are typical papillomas covered by a layer of stratified cuboidal to pseudostratified columnar epithelial cells (Fig. 3.60). The thickness of the epithelial layer can vary considerably, depending on where in the cloacal mucosa the lesion originates. A fibrovascular core supports the epithelium. Lymphoplasmacytic infiltration of the fibrovascular core is a common, but inconsistent,

finding. In some birds, there is an apparent correlation between the occurrence of cloacal papillomas and proliferative biliary, pancreatic, or upper intestinal lesions, and these changes should be ruled out in affected birds. The etiology of this lesion is still under investigation. An infectious agent is suspected, given the apparent infectious nature of this disease. Evidence of papillomaviruses in these lesions has not been found, but a high percentage of these lesions contain psittacid herpesviruses identical or closely related to those that cause Pacheco's disease.

Cloacal carcinoma is an infiltrative tumor that leads to thickening of the cloacal wall. Carcinomas are usually firm and gray-white. They are comprised of moderately undifferentiated to poorly differentiated epithelial cells that form infiltrative cords and nests. There is usually moderate to abundant scirrhous stroma, and necrosis and hemorrhage are seen (Fig. 3.61).

Smooth muscle tumors, which are infrequently reported, present as thickened lesions of the cloacal wall or may protrude from the vent. Histologically they are typical, and differentiation between benign and malignant varieties must be done by established cytologic criteria.

Exocrine Pancreas

Diseases affecting the exocrine pancreas may also affect the islets of Langerhans. Specific diseases of the endocrine pancreas are covered in chapter 10.

Noninfectious Disease. Prolonged caloric deficiency in birds will lead to pancreatic atrophy. Grossly the change may not be visible, but histologically there is acinar epithelial atrophy associated with a normal islets of Langerhans.

The pancreas is the target organ in cases of zinc toxicity. Gross lesions may not be noticeable, but slight parenchymal mottling is occasionally seen. The primary microscopic lesion is vacuolation and degranulation of acinar cells (Fig. 3.62). Necrosis of individual cells may also be present. Minimal mononuclear inflammatory infiltrates may be seen.

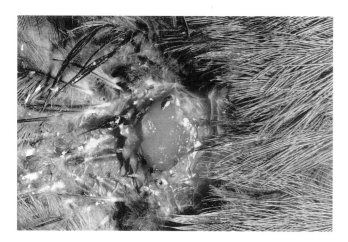

3.59. Typical appearance of cloacal papillomatosis.

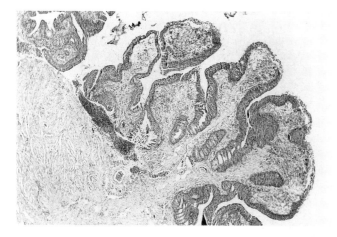

3.60. Multiple papillary structures in cloacal papillomatosis. Vascular stroma are covered by hypertrophied epithelial cells.

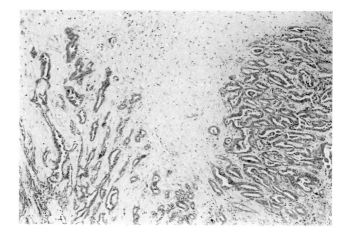

3.61. Cloacal carcinoma. Tubular and trabecular structures are infiltrative into a dense fibrous stroma.

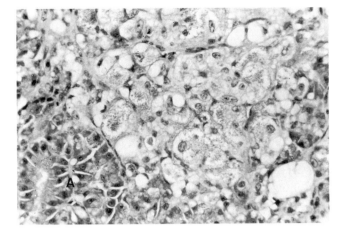

3.62.   Pancreatic acinar degeneration and vacuolation consistent with zinc toxicity. More normal cells are at the lower left (A).

Acute pancreatic necrosis is seen in psittacine birds, particularly Quaker parakeets. Many of these birds die suddenly. Gross lesions include a firm pale pancreas, variable hemorrhage, and adjacent fat necrosis characterized by firm yellow-white foci. A marked serous and serosanguineous effusion has been reported in one cockatoo. Gross changes are due to acute coagulation necrosis of pancreatic acini, hemorrhage within the pancreatic lobules, and multifocal necrosis of mesenteric adipose tissue (Fig. 3.63). One of the causes of the lesions maybe a high-fat diet, but the exact cause has not been determined

Fat accumulation in the pancreatic acinar cells sometimes accompanies severe fatty liver disease, as is sometimes seen in Amazon parrots. This change is usually not grossly visible.

Pancreatic fibrosis of undetermined cause is also seen infrequently. Grossly the pancreas is firm and irregular, and microscopically interstitial fibrosis replaces normal acini (Fig. 3.64).

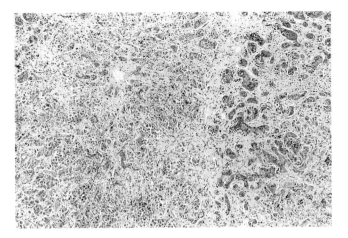

3.64.   Severe pancreatic fibrosis. Acinar remnants are scattered throughout the section.

Infectious Disease.   Viral and bacterial agents reported to cause pancreatitis include herpesvirus, polyomavirus, adenovirus, paramyxovirus (PMV-3), poxvirus, a variety of gram-negative bacteria, and chlamydiophila. Gross lesions vary from none to hemorrhage and necrosis, and there may be a purulent exudate in cases of bacterial pancreatitis.

Paramyxovirus can cause chronic pancreatitis, particularly in *Neophema* sp. and small passerine birds. Affected pancreases are firm and irregular. A variable lymphoplasmacytic and histiocytic inflammatory response and lymphoid follicle formation characterize the lesion (Fig. 3.65). Fibrosis is seen in some cases.

Herpesvirus, polyomavirus, poxvirus, and adenovirus usually induce pancreatic necrosis and variable inflammation as part of a systemic disease process. Etiologic specificity is determined by finding characteristic intranuclear inclusion bodies (Figs. 3.66 and 3.67).

Bacterial infection is histologically characterized by necrosis, fibrin deposition, and a primarily heterophilic response, whereas infection with *C. psittaci* results in a nonsuppurative pancreatitis.

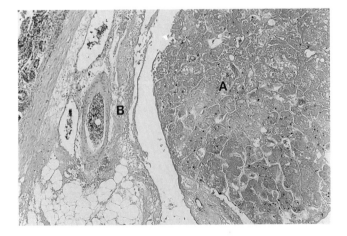

3.63.   Acute pancreatic necrosis. There is total coagulation of pancreas (A), and minimal edema of peripancreatic fat (B) and fibrin deposition.

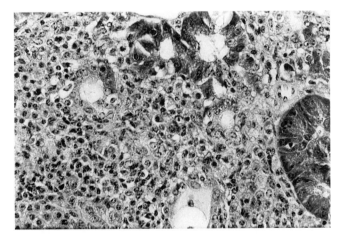

3.65.   Chronic lymphohistiocytic inflammation in the pancreas of a bird with chronic paramyxovirus-3 infection.

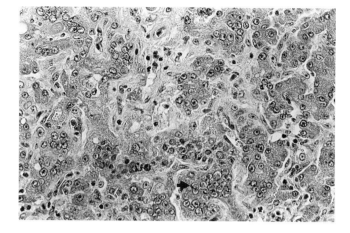

3.66. *Herpesvirus infection of the pancreas. Necrosis, syncytial cell formation, and intranuclear inclusion bodies are seen (arrow).*

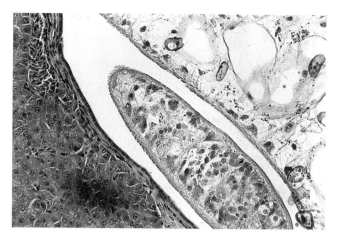

3.68. *Trematode in pancreatic ducts. Variable periductal cellular swelling and edema are seen.*

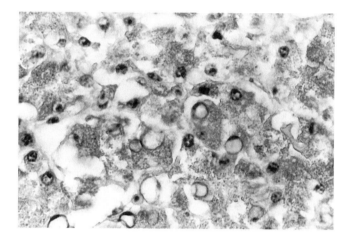

3.67. *Polyomavirus infection. There is karyomegaly and inclusion body formation in pancreatic acinar cells.*

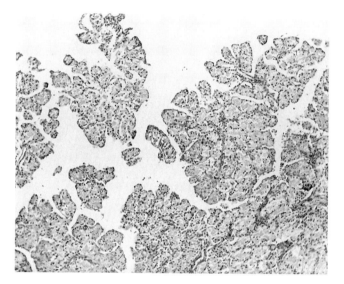

3.69. *Low-grade papillary adenocarcinoma of the pancreas. This type of tumor is unusual in birds.*

Parasitic pancreatitis can follow the plugging of pancreatic ducts by nematodes or trematodes. Grossly pancreatic ducts are thickened and prominent. Trematodiasis may result in brown-black pigmentation. Histologically the pancreatic ducts are dilated and contain the parasites in the duct. Inflammatory changes are minimal to mild (Fig. 3.68). Pancreatic trematodiasis is seen almost exclusively in Amboina king parrots.

Proliferative and Neoplastic Disease. Bile duct hyperplasia and papilloma formation is seen in some birds with internal papillomatosis. They may accompany bile duct changes or occur independently of them.

Low-grade papillary adenocarcinoma is occasionally seen. These tumors are comprised of moderately undifferentiated cells within acinar-like structures. Groups of these structures form papillary projections (Fig. 3.69).

Carcinomas are usually infiltrative, with poorly defined borders. Grossly there may be obvious infiltration of the adjacent small intestine, and, in severe cases, most of the normal pancreatic architecture is lost. There may be

severe adhesion formation binding the intestines and other organs into a solid mass. These tumors occur most commonly in cockatiels. Abdominal effusion is another common manifestation of this disease. Carcinomas are comprised of poorly differentiated epithelial cells that form acini, nests, and trabeculae that efface normal pancreatic tissue and extend into surrounding tissue (Figs. 3.70 and Figs. 3.71).

ADDITIONAL READING

Anderson NJ. 1997. Recurrent deep foreign body granuloma in the tongue of an African grey parrot (*Psittacus erithacus erithacus timneh*). J Avian Med Surg 11:105–109.

Antinoff N, Hoefer H, Rosenthal KL, et al. 1997. Smooth muscle neoplasia of suspected oviductal origin in the cloaca of a blue-fronted Amazon parrot (*Amazona aestiva*). J Avian Med Surg 11:268–272.

Bauck L. 1992. A clinical approach to neoplasia in the pet bird. Semin Avian Exotic Pet Med 1:65–72.

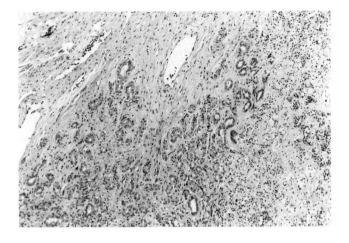

3.70.   Infiltrative pancreatic carcinoma with abundant stromal proliferation and effacement of normal tissue.

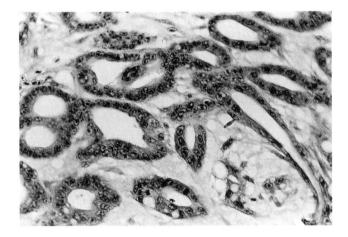

3.71.   Detail of pancreatic carcinoma. Poorly defined acini and tubules are characteristic of the lesion.

Campbell TW. 1986. Neoplasia. In: Harrison GJ, Harrison LR, eds. Clinical avian medicine and surgery. Philadelphia: WB Saunders, pp 500–508.

Cannon C. 1992. Proventricular and ventricular obstruction with bedding materials. J Assoc Avian Vet 6:40.

Cheesman MT, Riddel C. 1995. Esophagitis due to a herpesvirus associated with mortality in a psittacine aviary. Avian Dis 39:3.

Clark FD. 1984. Proventricular dilatation syndrome in large psittacine birds. Avian Dis 28:813–815.

Clipsham R. 1993. Noninfectious diseases of pediatric psittacines. Semin Avian Exotic Pet Med 1:22–23.

Clipsham R. 1995. Avian pathogenic flagellated enteric protozoa. Semin Avian Exotic Pet Med 4:112–123.

Clyde VL, Patton S. 1996. Diagnosis, treatment and control of common parasites in companion and aviary birds. Semin Avian Exotic Pet Med 5:75–84.

Cooper JE, Lawton MPC, Greenwood AG. 1988. Papillomas in psittacine birds. Vet Rec 119:535.

Deriese LA, Chiens K, Dehedt P, et al. 1995. *Enterococcus hirae* infections in psittacine birds: Epidemiologic, pathological and bacteriological observations. Avian Pathol 24:523–531.

Dhillon AS. 1988. An outbreak of enteritis in a psittacine flock. In: Proceedings of the Association of Avian Veterinarians, Houston, TX, pp 185–188.

Gerlach H. 1954. Bacteria. In: Ritchie BW, Harrison GJ, Harrison LR, eds. Avian medicine: Principles and application. Lake Worth, FL: Wingers, pp 949–989.

Gerlach H. 1994. Viruses. In: Ritchie BW, Harrison GJ, Harrison LR, eds. Avian medicine: Principles and application. Lake Worth, FL: Wingers, pp 863–948.

Gomezvillamanlos JC, Delasmulas JMM, Hervas S, et al. 1995. Splenoenteritis caused by adenovirus in psittacine birds: A pathological study. Avian Pathol 24:553–563.

Goodwin MA, Krabill VA. 1989. Cryptosporidiosis in birds: A review. Avian Pathol 18:365–384.

Graham DL. 1988. Internal papillomatous disease. In: Proceedings of the Association of Avian Veterinarians, Houston, TX, p 31.

Graham DL. 1994. Acute pancreatic necrosis in Quaker parrots (*Myiopsitta monachus*). In: Proceedings of the Association of Avian Veterinarians, Reno, NV, pp 87–88.

Gregory CR, Latimer KS, Campagnoli RP, et al. 1996. Histologic evaluation of the crop for diagnosis of proventricular dilatation syndrome in psittacine birds. J Vet Diagn Invest 8:76–80.

Gregory CR, Ritchie BW, Latimer KS, et al. 1997. Proventricular dilatation disease: A viral epornitic. In: Proceedings of the Association of Avian Veterinarians, Reno, NV, pp 43–52.

Hess L, Bartick T, Hoefer H. 1998. *Clostridium tertium* infection in a Moluccan cockatoo (*Cacatua moluccensis*) with megacolon. J Avian Med Surg 12:30–35.

Hillyer EV, Moroff S, Hoefer H, et al. 1991. Bile duct carcinoma in two out of ten Amazon parrots with cloacal papillomas. J Assoc Avian Vet 5:91–95.

Hoefer HL. 1997. Diseases of the gastrointestinal tract. In: Altman R, Clubb S, Dorrestein GM, Quesenberry K, eds. Avian medicine and surgery. Philadelphia: WB Saunders, pp 419–453.

Hubbard GB, Schmidt RE, Eisenbrandt DL. 1985. Fungal infections of venriculi in captive birds. J Wildl Dis 21:25–28.

Latimer KS, Rakich PM, Niagro FD, et al. 1991. An updated review of psittacine beak and feather disease. J Assoc Avian Vet 5:211–220.

Latimer KS, Niagro FD, Rakich PM, et al. 1997. Investigation of parrot papilloma virus in cloacal and oral papillomas of psittacine birds. Vet Clin Pathol 26:158–163.

Leach MW. 1992. A survey of neoplasia in pet birds. Semin Avian Exotic Pet Med 1:52–64.

Ley DH. 1987. Avian cryptosporidiosis: An emerging disease. In: Proceedings of the First International Congress on Zoologic Avian Medicine, Oahu, HI, pp 299–303.

Mannl A, Gerlach H, Leipold R. 1987. Neurotrophic gastric dilatation in Psittaciformes. Avian Dis 31:214–221.

McDonald S, Lowenstine L, Ardans A. 1981. Avian pox in blue fronted Amazon parrots. J Am Vet Med Assoc 179:1218–1222.

Murphy J. 1992. Psittacine trichomoniasis. In: Proceedings of the Association of Avian Veterinarians, New Orleans, LA, pp 21–24.

Murtaugh RJ, Ringler DS, Petrak ML. 1986. Squamous cell carcinoma of the esophagus in an Amazon parrot. J Am Vet Med Assoc 188:872–873.

Page CD, Haddad K. 1995. Coccidial infections in birds. Semin Avian Exotic Pet Med 4:138–144.

Pass DA, Perry RA. 1984. The pathogenesis of psittacine beak and feather disease. In: Proceedings of the Association of Avian Veterinarians, Toronto, pp 113–119.

Pass DA, Perry RA. 1984. The pathology of psittacine beak and feather disease. Aust Vet J 61:69–74.

Perry RA, Gill J, Cross GM. 1992. Disorders of the avian integument. Vet Clin North Am (Small Anim Pract) 21:1302–1327.

Petrak ML, Gilmore CE. 1982. Neoplasms. In: Petrak ML, ed. Diseases of cage and aviary birds, 2nd edition. Philadelphia: Lea and Febiger, pp 606–637.

Rae MA, Rosskopf WJ. 1992. Mycobacteriosis in passerines. In: Proceedings of the Association of Avian Veterinarians, New Orleans, LA, pp 234–242.

Ritchie BW, Niagro FD, Kyjert PD, et al. 1985. A review of psittacine beak and feather disease. J Assoc Avian Vet 3:143–150.

Rosskopf W. 1996. Digestive system disorders. In: Rosskopf W, Woerpel R, eds. Diseases of caged and aviary birds, 3rd edition. Baltimore: Williams and Wilkins, pp 436–448.

Roudybush T. 1986. Growth, signs of deficiency and weaning in cockatiels fed deficient diets. In: Proceedings of the Association of Avian Veterinarians, Miami, FL, pp 333–340.

Rupiper DJ. 1993. Hemorrhagic enteritis in a group of great-billed parrots (*Tanygnathus megalorynchos*). J Assoc Avian Vet 7:209–211.

Schmidt RE. 1992. Morphologic diagnosis of avian neoplasms. Semin Avian Exotic Pet Med 1:73–79.

Schmidt RE. 1996. Pathology of caged birds. In: Rosskopf W, Woerpel R, eds. Diseases of caged and aviary birds, 3rd edition. Baltimore: Williams and Wilkins, pp 857–879.

Spear BL. 1998. A clinical look at the avian pancreas in health and disease. In: Proceedings of the Association of Avian Veterinarians, St. Paul, MN, pp 57–64.

Steinberg H. 1988. Leiomyosarcoma of the jejunum in a budgerigar. Avian Dis 32:166–168.

Sundberg JP, Junge RE, O'Banian MK, et al. 1988. Cloacal papillomas in psittacines. Am J Vet Res 47:928–932.

Tsai SS, Park JH, Hirai K, et al. 1992. Aspergillus and candidiasis in psittacine and passerine birds with particular reference to nasal conditions. Avian Pathol 21:699–709.

Tsai SS, Hirai K, Itakura C. 1992. Histopathological survey of protozoa, helminths and acarids of imported and local psittacine and passerine birds in Japan. Jpn J Vet Res 40:161–174.

Van Zant F. 1991. Zinc toxicosis in a hyacinth macaw. In: Proceedings of the Association of Avian Veterinarians, Chicago, IL, pp 255–259.

Wolfe P, Lazaz B, Landes E, et al. 1995. An ingluvolith in a budgerigar (*Melopsittacus undulatus*). Klientierpraxis 40:301.

4 Liver

NORMAL STRUCTURE

The avian liver is comprised of right and left lobes that fuse on the midline in the dorsal middle to cranial third. Cranially and caudally the lobes are completely separated by cranial and caudal incisures. The incisures incompletely penetrate the middle third of the liver as they cross its ventral surface and join. Additional subdivision into dorsal and ventral sections may occur in right or left lobes. The right lobe is usually larger than the left lobe in the majority of species of birds. However, lobes can be of equal size, and rarely the left lobe of the liver is larger than the right in some species. The cranial aspect of both liver lobes surrounds the ventral surface of the heart apex. The ventral surface of the liver is in direct contact with the sternum, and, in the majority of birds, the normal liver does not extend beyond the caudal edge of the sternum. The gallbladder, when present, is located on the visceral surface of the right lobe. It may be pear shaped or long and cylindrical. The gallbladder may extend caudally to the level of the cloaca in some species. Although present in the rock dove, the gallbladder is absent in most species of pigeons and doves, in psittacine birds, and in the ostrich. The proventriculus, ventriculus, and spleen are in contact with, and leave impressions on, the visceral surface of the liver. The right and left hepatic peritoneal cavities are completely enclosed by the posthepatic septum, parietal peritoneum, dorsal and ventral mesenteries, and left hepatic ligaments. Fluid leaking from the liver capsule is trapped within the hepatic peritoneal spaces and does not enter the intestinal peritoneal space.

The liver has two sources of blood: the hepatic arteries and the hepatic portal veins. The right and left portal veins drain the intestines. The right and left hepatic arteries originate from a bifurcation of the celiac artery. Both hepatic arteries and portal veins enter the liver through the hilus. From the hilus, the hepatic arteries and portal veins branch to form a network that extends to the periphery of the liver. As they branch into the liver, branches of the biliary system, which drain the liver, accompany them. The combination of portal vein, hepatic artery, and bile ducts are called the portal triad. The hepatic portal veins drain into the hepatic sinusoids. The hepatic arteries also connect with the sinusoids by arterioles or through a capillary plexus. Hepatocytes are polygonal cells with a large spherical, oval, centrally located nucleus. The cytoplasm of the hepatocytes contains many mitochondria and an extensive system of smooth and rough endoplasmic reticulum. Branching laminae of hepatocytes, one to two cells thick, make up the parenchyma of the liver. The sheets of hepatocytes are separated by sinusoids that are lined by fenestrated endothelial cells and phagocytic Kupffer's cells. Between the endothelial cells and the hepatocytes is a space (the space of Disse) that surrounds the hepatocytes with plasma. Bile drains from the hepatocytes into bile canaliculi that are on the opposite side of the hepatocytes from the space of Disse. The bile canaliculi drain into intralobular bile ducts.

Structurally the liver is divided into lobules. Each lobule has a central hepatic vein (central vein) that receives the drainage of the sinusoids. The portal triads are present at the periphery of the lobules. The lobules of some mammals (e.g., pigs) are well defined by connective tissue. The lobules of birds, however, are not defined, and the hepatic parenchyma appears continuous. The central veins drain into the right and left hepatic veins that fuse in the liver to form the caudal vena cava that exits the cranial aspect of the liver on its dorsal surface. The canaliculi drain the lobules into the interlobular ducts of the portal triads. These come together to form the lobar bile ducts, which fuse to form the right and left hepatic ducts and ultimately the hepatoenteric duct, which enters the duodenum. If a gallbladder is present, it is connected to the hepatoenteric duct by the hepatocystic duct. Bile ducts are lined by simple cuboidal or columnar epithelium and surrounded by loose connective tissue. There may be elastic fibers or smooth muscle around larger ducts. The gallbladder has the same layers as the hepatoenteric bile duct.

Microscopically the capsule of liver is comprised of a thin layer of collagen and elastic fibers. It is continuous with the interstitial connective tissue. Intrahepatic loose connective tissue is most prominent in portal areas.

Normal variations in the gross and microscopic anatomy of the liver are seen in embryos and recently hatched chicks. The liver of precocial species is yellow at hatch and remains that way for 8 to 14 days before becoming the red-purple of the adult liver. The yellow is due to pigment carried with lipids that arrive from the yolk sac in the late stages of incubation. Microscopically the hepatocytes will have a foamy appearance due to their large content of glycogen and lipid that is being reabsorbed from the yolk. In altricial species, the liver is usually red-purple from the time of hatching. Extramedullary hematopoiesis occurs in the embryonic liver. Some hematopoietic activity remains for varying times after the hatching.

Hepatic extramedullary erthyropoiesis is a common finding in birds with chronic blood loss. Likewise, hepatic extramedullary granulopoiesis occurs in some birds with chronic inflammatory diseases. The nutritional status of a bird may have an impact on the liver. Birds that have been in a negative calorie balance prior to death will tend to have a smaller liver than well-nourished birds. If a bird has recently eaten, hepatocytes increase their glycogen and lipid causing them to enlarge and develop a foamy cytoplasm.

HEPATIC DISEASE

Congenital Disease
Extrahepatic biliary cysts are occasionally seen in birds. Other anomalous lesions are not reported.

Infectious Disease
Viruses

Psittacid Herpesviruses (PsHVs). The PsHVs are a heterogeneous group of avian herpesviruses. Serologically three to five serotypes are recognized. Genetically there is even more variation. One serotype and its corresponding genotype are most commonly associated with an acute fatal disease (Pacheco's disease) seen in many species of parrots. Other serotypes and genotypes have also been isolated from birds with Pacheco's disease but less frequently. An identical disease caused by a herpesvirus that is reported to have occurred in toucans is assumed to have been caused by a PsHV. PsHVs are maintained in nature in birds that are persistently infected with the virus. Amazon parrots and certain species of conures and macaws have been shown to shed virus continuously in oral secretions and feces. Ingestion, inhalation, and conjunctival exposure have experimentally been shown to result in infection and disease. Parent-fed offspring of adult birds infected with the PsHVs can become infected with PsHVs and not develop signs of disease. Horizontal transmission rather than vertical transmission is suspected in these birds.

Pacheco's disease may occur in an individual bird or as an explosive outbreak. Signs of disease are often minimal or entirely absent prior to death. Necropsy specimens are typically well muscled and have adequate body fat. Uncommonly, there will be some degree of atrophy of the pectoral muscle mass. Grossly, the liver may be enlarged and friable. Often, however, the disease progresses so quickly that the liver is not enlarged. In these cases, the

liver may appear normal or contain focal areas of discoloration that represent foci of necrosis. Whether the liver is enlarged or not, it often has a variable yellow-gray mottling, with or without hemorrhage (Figs. 4.1 and 4.2). Diffuse color changes in the liver may be mistaken for hepatic lipidosis. Histologically, acute hepatic necrosis is a nearly consistent finding. Necrosis is multifocal and moderate to massive without a specific anatomic distribution. When the necrosis is massive, only the hepatocytes adjacent to the portal triads do not die. The amount of inflammation present is generally minimal and often completely absent. Syncytial cell formation may occur but is uncommon. Intranuclear inclusion bodies are typically abundant but may be rare or absent. When there is massive necrosis, inclusion bodies are often found only in the nuclei of the biliary epithelium. The inclusion bodies may fill the nucleus, or there may be a clear zone between the inclusion and marginated chromatin (Figs. 4.3 to 4.5). Inclu-

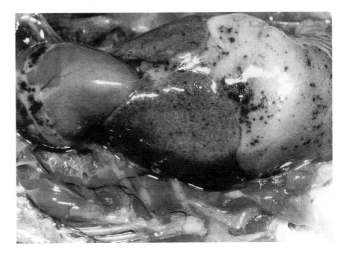

4.1. *Enlarged, mottled liver due to Pacheco's disease. Hemorrhages are seen in the liver and other tissues.*

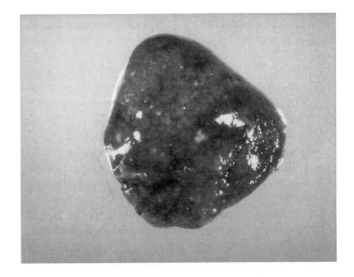

4.2. *Severe necrosis leading to the "scotch grain" appearance of the liver in Pacheco's disease.*

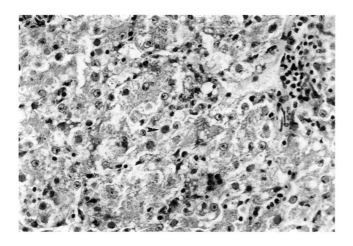

4.3. Pacheco's disease. There is an area of diffuse necrosis and inclusion body formation, and many dark intranuclear inclusions fill the nucleus (arrowhead).

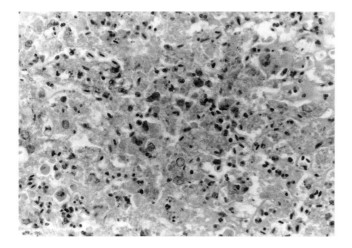

4.4. Almost complete loss of cellular detail in a herpesvirus-infected liver. Intranuclear inclusion bodies can be seen.

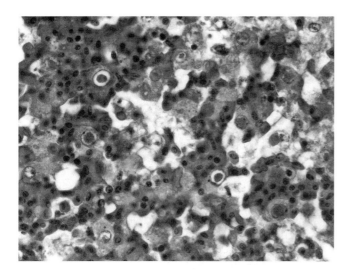

4.5. Minimal necrosis and well-defined intranuclear inclusion bodies due to herpesvirus infection. A definite halo is seen between the inclusion and the thickened nuclear membrane.

sion bodies are typically deeply eosinophilic but may be lightly basophilic.

Extrahepatic lesions occur with a fair degree of frequency in PsHV disease. Splenic necrosis with the presence of viral inclusion bodies is common but is less consistent than hepatic necrosis (chapter 8). Multifocal necrosis and viral inclusion bodies within the pancreas are also relatively common findings. The amount of necrosis is generally mild but may be locally extensive in rare cases. The crop is another commonly affected organ. The crop epithelium is affected by multifocal ballooning degeneration of the basal cell layer, causing erosions, ulcers and, rarely, vesicles. Inclusion bodies are also present in these lesions. Intestinal lesions are relatively uncommon and generally mild, often being confined to the presence of inclusion bodies in the nuclei of crypt epithelial cells (chapter 3). Rarely a severe necrotizing tracheitis will also be observed (chapter 2). Extrahepatic lesions may occur in the absence of hepatic necrosis in unusual cases.

Avian polyomavirus and adenoviruses also cause intranuclear inclusions and hepatic necrosis. Both of these viruses typically cause some degree of nuclear enlargement and generally have lightly basophilic to clear (avian polyomavirus) or deeply basophilic (adenovirus) inclusion bodies. Additional diagnostic tools available for differentiating these viruses include DNA in situ hybridization, immunofluorescent staining, polymerase chain reaction (PCR) using herpesvirus-specific primers, electron microscopy of fixed tissues (Fig. 4.6) or the supernatant of homogenized tissues, and virus isolation in primary chicken embryo fibroblasts or embryonated eggs. PsHVs are typical herpesviruses and under the electron microscope are enveloped and approximately 180 to 220 nm in diameter. At the time of death, birds are viremic, and virus can be isolated from lung, liver, kidney, spleen, and brain. All of these organs would also be positive by

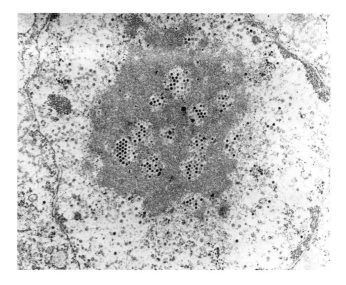

4.6. Herpesviral particles in an intranuclear inclusion body.

PCR. PsHVs are found in the liver of some birds that do not have Pacheco's disease. Therefore a positive PCR assay in the absence of characteristic lesions of Pacheco's disease implies that the virus was not the cause of death.

Herpesvirus infections also occur in a number of other species of birds that are kept in captivity. These infections include duck virus enteritis, crane herpesvirus, and pigeon/falcon herpesvirus. Hepatic necrosis with inclusion bodies is a common finding in birds with these infections.

Cytomegalovirus. Cytomegalic herpesvirus has been a cause of systemic disease in finches. The primary clinical signs and lesions are seen in the respiratory tract (chapter 2), but the liver also may be affected. Gross changes include yellow-white foci typical of necrosis. Histologically there is necrosis and distortion of intact hepatocytes, many of which have karyomegalic nuclei and large basophilic intranuclear inclusion bodies.

Avian Polyomavirus (APV). Disease due to APV occurs predominantly in psittacine birds. However, a disease with similar histologic features has been also reported in a green aracaris and in passerine species, including several species of finch. Genetic analysis of the virus that killed the green aracaris strongly suggests that it was of psittacine origin. The virus or viruses causing disease in passerines remain to be genetically characterized. Although the histologic lesions vary between budgerigars and nonbudgerigar parrots, the virus that causes disease in these birds is the same.

Infected birds shed virus in droppings, oral secretions, and feather and skin dander. The most likely route of infection is by inhalation of the virus. It has been speculated that vertical transmission occurs in budgerigars. Proof of this, however, is lacking. Once birds are infected, they become viremic, and virus can be found in nearly all organs of both symptomatic and asymptomatic birds. Virus shedding in the droppings follows soon after the onset of viremia.

Infection and disease are not synonymous; in fact, the vast majority of APV infections are asymptomatic. Disease and death are predominantly confined to nestling parrots less than 14 weeks old. Macaws, conures, caiques, eclectus, and ring-necked parrots are most likely to die of APV disease. Small outbreaks of APV disease in adult birds have been reported but are rare. Disease in adult birds is most common in eclectus parrots, caiques, lovebirds, and finches. Psittacine beak and feather disease virus (PBFDV) infection is thought to be immunosuppressive and may predispose some adult birds to APV disease.

Gross lesions vary with the species affected. Affected budgerigars are typically 10 to 20 days old. Grossly, stunting, abnormal or delayed feather development, skin discoloration, abdominal distension, perihepatic effusion and ascites, hydropericardium, hepatomegaly, with focal areas of necrosis, and widely scattered petechial hemorrhages are common lesions. Budgerigars that survive the acute infection will often fail to develop their primary wing and tail feathers, or these feathers will be dystrophic.

Nonbudgerigar parrots with APV disease are typically well grown, are well muscled, and have substantial body fat. Historically they are being hand fed and not parent fed. Conure nestlings are typically 2 to 4 weeks of age, macaws 4.8 weeks of age, and eclectus parrots 4.14 weeks of age. Gross lesions are striking and include a generalized pallor of all tissues, with subcutaneous and subserosal hemorrhages. The spleen and liver are typically enlarged and friable, and the liver may exhibit varying degrees of mottling (Figs. 4.7 to 4.9). Less commonly, ascites and pericardial effusion are present. Similar lesions are also seen in adult birds with APV disease. Disease in nestling cockatoos, Amazon parrots, and African grey parrots is relatively uncommon. Liver lesions in these birds are less prominent or may be absent. In finches, the liver may be enlarged with mottling and hemorrhage seen in some cases.

Histologically, in budgerigars, the nuclei of virally infected cells are enlarged, have marginated chromatin, and centrally contain a finely granular basophilic to amphophilic inclusion. Inclusions occur in multiple

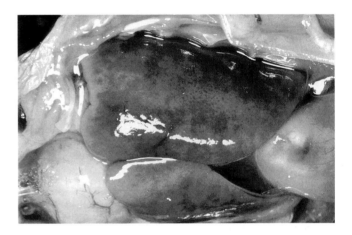

4.7. Foci of severe hepatic hemorrhage due to polyomavirus infection.

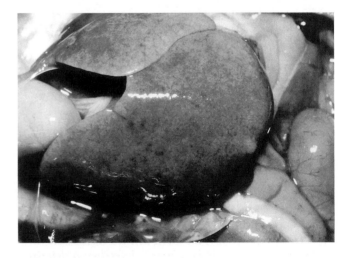

4.8. Diffuse hepatic discoloration due to polyomavirus-associated necrosis.

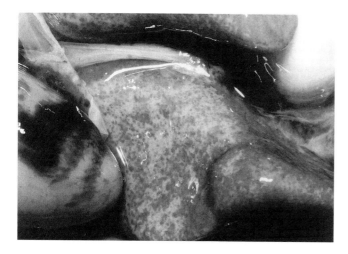

4.9.   Severe polyomavirus-induced hepatic necrosis. The darker areas are foci of intact hepatocytes. There is also severe epicardial hemorrhage.

4.10.   Multifocal to confluent hepatic necrosis and hemorrhage due to polyomavirus infection.

organs and tissue types including, but not limited to, liver, spleen, kidney (mesangial and tubule cells), feather follicles, skin, esophagus, brain, and heart. (See the relevant chapters.) A moderate, multifocal, apparently random, hepatic necrosis is common. Inclusion bodies are often abundant in the spleen and are accompanied by necrosis of the perivascular histiocytes and other phagocytic cells. Massive infection of the germinal epithelium of the feather follicle is also common in APV infections of budgerigars. Inflammatory changes accompanying the aforementioned lesions are generally minimal. A nonsuppurative encephalitis targeting the Purkinje cells in the cerebellum is a variable manifestation of APV disease in the budgerigar and is seen in some outbreaks but not in others.

Histologically, in nonbudgerigar parrots, hepatic necrosis to some degree is present in nearly all cases. Liver necrosis is multifocal to coalescing and, when severe, spares only the periportal hepatocytes. The spaces left by the necrotic hepatocytes fill with blood (Figs. 4.10 and 4.11). Characteristic inclusion bodies as described in the budgerigar (Fig. 4.12) may be seen in Kupffer's cells. The amount and severity of necrosis and hemorrhage and the occurrence of inclusion bodies are variable, depending on the species affected. Cockatoos may have no histologic changes. Cockatiels often have multifocal necrosis and few, if any, inclusion bodies. Typical moderate to severe midzonal to massive necrosis is seen in other psittacine birds. Lesions in passerines species and the aracaris are similar to those of psittacine birds (Fig. 4.13). Splenic and renal lesions are also common in birds with APV disease. Occasionally APV can be superimposed on birds with chronic-active hepatitis, leading to acute necrosis and inclusion body formation as well as the typical chronic lesions described later in this chapter (Fig. 4.14).

APV disease in lovebirds is somewhat unique. Disease does occur in nestling lovebirds. Hepatic necrosis is a common finding in these birds, but inclusion bodies are

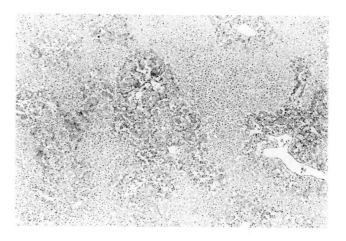

4.11.   Severe midzonal to massive polyomavirus-associated necrosis.

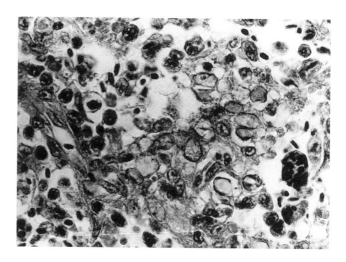

4.12.   Detail of karyomegaly and intranuclear inclusion body formation in polyomavirus infection. The number of inclusions present is typical of the infection in budgerigars.

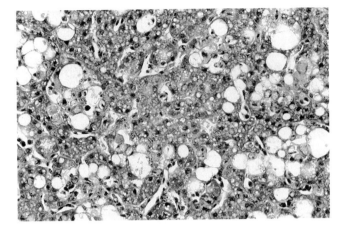

4.13. Necrosis and inclusion body formation in a finch with polyomavirus infection.

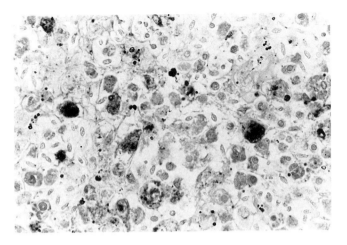

4.15. Polyomavirus DNA demonstrated by in situ hybridization.

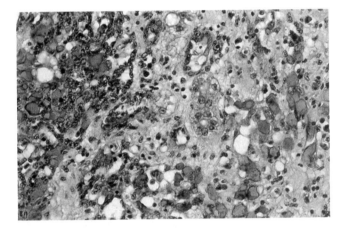

4.14. Polyomavirus inclusions in a bird with chronic hepatic disease and fibrosis.

commonly found in other organs as well. Fledgling and young adult lovebirds are also susceptible to APV disease. This may also be a manifestation of immunosuppression from a concurrent PBFDV, as this disease is extremely common in this species.

Birds that die of APV disease are viremic. Virus can be found in large concentrations in all tissues and the blood by PCR assays. In situ hybridization of paraffin-embedded sections of the spleen or liver (Fig. 4.15) or immuno-fluorescent staining of impression smears of these organs are assays that can be used to confirm infection. Electron microscopy of fixed sections of tissues or the supernatant of homogenized tissue can also be used to demonstrate the virus. APV is a naked icosahedral virus with a diameter of 42 to 48 nm. It is considerably smaller than the adenoviruses.

Adenovirus. Adenovirus infections are most commonly recognized as incidental lesions in parrots that died of other causes. This is particularly true in lovebirds and budgerigars where characteristic inclusion bodies are sporadically found in renal tubular cells. Historically, adenovirus disease is reported predominantly in lovebirds. In

white-masked lovebirds (*Agapornis personata*) with conjunctivitis, 30% mortality is reported. Inclusion bodies are seen in the conjunctival epithelium and renal tubules. Acute necrotizing pancreatitis, a multisystemic disease, and hepatic necrosis all are attributed to adenovirus infections in lovebirds.

Recently a fatal adenovirus infection causing hepatitis has been described in nestlings of Senegal parrots and related genera. The disease occurs sporadically within aviaries. In one collection, the disease occurred in 3 of 4 years in offspring from a single pair of Senegal parrots. Affected parrots typically present acutely ill or are found dead. Grossly the liver is discolored red-black, and scattered yellow-gray areas may be present (Fig. 4.16).

Histologically there is multifocal necrosis with no particular lobular pattern, hemorrhage, nonsuppurative cholangitis, and large, darkly basophilic, intranuclear inclusion bodies within hepatocytes (Fig. 4.17). The inclusion bodies usually are characteristic, but in a few cases there has been minimal nuclear enlargement, and the inclusions have been pale (Fig. 4.18). Infection can be further verified by DNA in situ hybridization on paraffin-embedded tissues. Electron microscopy of thin sections or

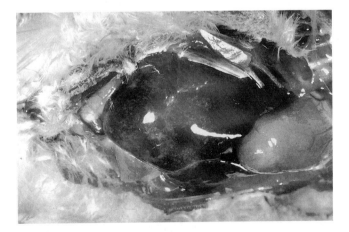

4.16. Swollen, mottled liver in adenovirus infection.

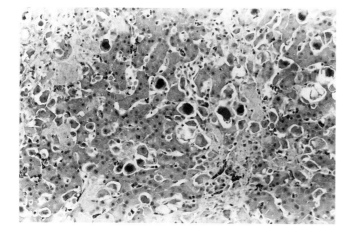

4.17. Adenovirus infection. Note the necrosis and karyomegaly and typical intranuclear inclusion bodies in the hepatocytes.

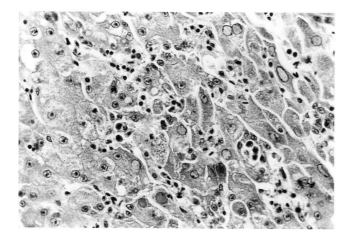

4.18. Somewhat atypical appearance of adenovirus infection with minimal necrosis and clear, rather than dark, inclusion bodies.

supernatants from homogenized tissues can also be used to identify adenovirus virions. Adenoviruses are naked icosahedral viruses with a diameter of 65 to 80 nm. They are abundant in the nuclei of infected cells.

Paramyxovirus (PMV). There are five serotypes of avian PMVs. PMV-1, 2, 3, and 5 are known to cause disease in cage birds. PMV-3 is most common in pet species. The liver is usually a secondarily affected organ, with primary infections seen in the respiratory tract or gastrointestinal tract. The organ systems affected may be dependent on the particular strain of virus. Grossly the liver may be enlarged. Histologically a lymphoplasmacytic infiltrate is present within portal areas. Inclusion bodies are not seen.

Circovirus (Psittacine Beak and Feather Disease Virus). Circovirus infections can involve the liver, but it is not a common extracutaneous site. Liver lesions are usually present only in young birds with systemic disease but can be seen in some older birds that die with severe feather dam-

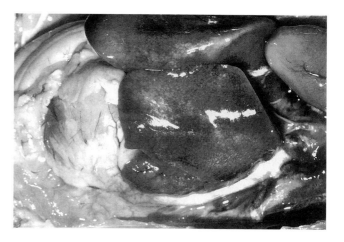

4.19. Slightly discolored liver in circovirus infection.

age. Usually the liver appears normal, but there may be a few scattered discolored foci (Fig. 4.19).

Histologically there is multifocal necrosis and congestion. Infrequently inclusion bodies are seen in Kupffer's cells. A lymphoplasmacytic infiltrate may be present in portal areas (Figs. 4.20 and 4.21). In birds that are

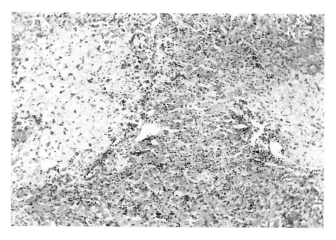

4.20. Multifocal hepatic necrosis in circovirus infection.

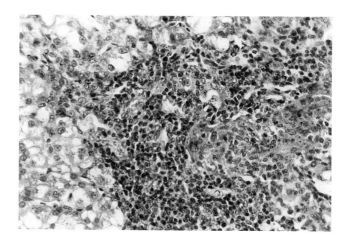

4.21. Nonsuppurative cholangiohepatitis that is occasionally seen in circovirus infection.

immunosuppressed, there may be severe secondary bacterial hepatitis with a minimal inflammatory response.

Reovirus. The vast majority of cases of reovirus disease in parrots are reported in birds that were either in quarantine or had been recently released from quarantine. Disease outbreaks were initially described in imported lots of African grey parrots, but epornitics of this disease have subsequently been documented in other African, Indian, and Australian parrots. Disease in New World species of parrots is rare. Naturally occurring reovirus disease is often complicated by the presence of multiple concurrent infections, including salmonellosis, aspergillosis, and PMV-3 infections.

Gross lesions are not specific. Hepatomegaly and splenomegaly with focal depressed discolored areas of the hepatic capsular and cut surfaces are the most common lesions described. Enteritis and petechial and ecchymotic hemorrhages are also seen. Multifocal hepatic necrosis with lymphoreticular infiltration is a consistent, but nonspecific, lesion. Necrosis of the spleen, intestinal lamina propria, and the bone marrow is also described. Inclusion bodies are not seen with light microscopy, but intracytoplasmic viral particles can be seen with electron microscopy. Reoviruses are nonenveloped but have a double capsid and are 75 to 80 nm in diameter. They are readily isolated in chicken embryo fibroblasts and chicken embryo kidney cells. Immunofluorescent antibody staining is another means of confirming infection.

Hepadnavirus. This DNA virus (duck hepatitis B) is one of several viral agents causing hepatitis in ducks. The disease is often subclinical, but there can be persistent infections and vertical transmission. The host range is limited to Pekin ducks and close taxonomic relatives, but it has been experimentally transmitted to geese.

The virus causes hepatic necrosis and periportal inflammatory infiltrates. The virus receptors (gp180) are concentrated in the Golgi apparatus of hepatocytes.

Other Viral Disease. A number of viruses can occasionally cause hepatic lesions in birds. These include togavirus, rotavirus, parvovirus, orbivirus, and coronavirus. In cases of hepatic disease that have lesions consistent with a viral infection but no change specific to one of the common causes of pet bird hepatitis and necrosis, these viruses can be considered as differential etiologic possibilities.

Gross and histologic changes are usually not specific, and electron microscopy, viral isolation, or DNA probes are necessary for an exact etiologic diagnosis.

Bacteria. The liver is commonly targeted by systemic bacterial infections in birds. Both gram-positive and gram-negative bacteria cause hepatitis. *Staphylococcus* and *Streptococcus* species are the most common gram-positive organisms isolated from the liver. They generally disseminate through the blood from chronic necrotizing skin lesions or may reach the liver by extension from adjacent

air sacs. Infections with these bacteria are more common in finches and canaries than in parrots. Clostridia are gram-positive rods of intestinal origin that cause hepatitis. Another gram-positive rod is *Listeria monocytogenes*, which causes a systemic disease commonly involving the liver. It is a relatively rare pathogen of cage birds.

Gram-negative bacteria cause most systemic bacterial infections of psittacine birds. Members of the Enterobacteriaceae, including *Escherichia coli*, *Klebsiella* sp., *Proteus* sp., *Enterobacter* sp., *Salmonella* sp., and *Yersinia pseudotuberculosis*, are common isolates. *Pseudomonas* sp. is also a common isolate. Systemic infections with these organisms usually result from invasion from the gut and, less frequently, by extension up the biliary tree. Infected wounds and respiratory and urinary infections with these organisms may also result in systemic infections involving the liver. *Yersinia pseudotuberculosis* is commonly reported in passerine species, ramphastids, turacos (Cuculiformes), and doves in Europe but is rarely recovered as a pathogen in the United States. *Pasteurella multocida* is an another gram-negative bacterium that causes septicemia. This organism is usually introduced into a cage bird by a cat bite. The organism grows so rapidly that it may be seen histologically in huge numbers in all organs and the blood.

Gross lesions caused by *Staphylococci* and *Streptococci* include variable hepatic swelling and multifocal to confluent yellow-white foci within the parenchyma. There may be abscess formation in chronic cases. Varying degrees of hemorrhage may be present in cases of clostridial hepatitis. Histologically, multifocal to confluent necrosis and an inflammatory reaction comprised primarily of heterophils and macrophages are seen. Bacteria are sometimes found in the lesion.

Hepatitis caused by gram-negative bacteria results in a grossly swollen and congested liver. The liver may be markedly enlarged and meaty in subacute to chronic infections. Gray-white-yellow foci are seen throughout the parenchyma. Their size and number are variable (Fig. 4.22). Histologic changes are characterized by multifocal

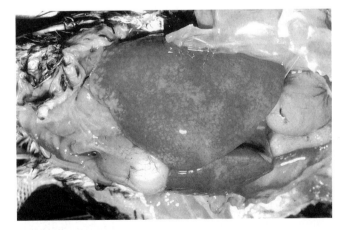

4.22.   *Enlarged, pale liver with a gram-negative bacterial infection.*

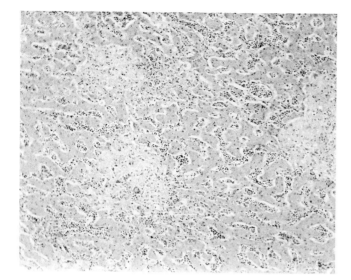

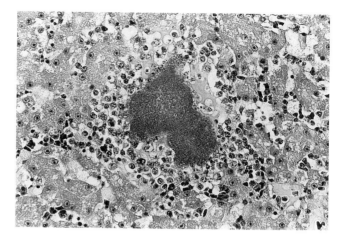

4.25.   Bacterial hepatitis. A bacterial colony is surrounded by a pleocellular inflammatory infiltrate.

4.23.   Multifocal necrosis and variable inflammation in bacterial hepatitis.

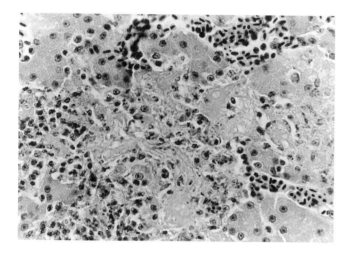

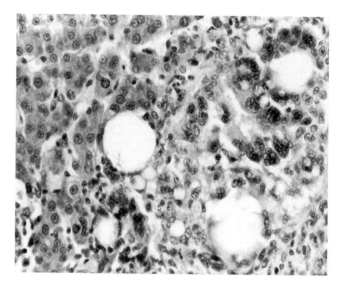

4.24.   Hepatitis due to Salmonella sp. Note the pleocellular inflammation, necrosis, and fibrin deposition.

4.26.   Chronic bacterial hepatitis with early granuloma formation.

necrosis and fibrin deposition, with an inflammatory response that includes primarily heterophils and macrophages (Figs. 4.23 and 4.24). Rod-shaped, gram-negative bacteria can be found free in the lesions. They are most frequently seen at the edges of necrotic foci and in the cytoplasm of Kupffer's cells and macrophages (Fig. 4.25). With chronicity, granulomas may form (Fig. 4.26). Colonies of *Yersinia* (Fig. 4.27) have a characteristic appearance. Other gram-negative bacteria cannot be identified by their histologic appearance or the lesions that they cause.

PBFDV infections of young psittacine birds often are accompanied by secondary bacterial infections. Grossly affected livers are usually markedly enlarged and mottled. The liver lesion may be the most striking lesion seen at necropsy. If the possibility of circovirus infection is not considered and the bursa of Fabricius not examined histologically, the primary problem may be overlooked. Histo-

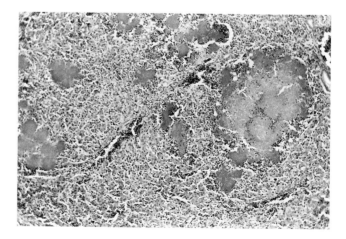

4.27.   Typical appearance of hepatitis due to Yersinia sp. Large bacterial colonies are usually found throughout the affected tissue.

logically the hepatic lesion is characterized by a variable degree of necrosis and an inflammatory response that is made up primarily of macrophages, many of which contain bacteria (Fig. 4.28). Free bacteria may also be found in the hepatic sinusoids. The normal heterophil response is lacking, possibly due to the virus's effect on the immune system (chapter 8).

Systemic bacterial disease is often seen in nestling parrots that are being hand fed. In these cases, it is very easy to blame the pathogen for the bird's death and not take into consideration the husbandry conditions in which the bird was raised. Incubator temperature, ventilation, and humidity have a strong impact on the health of a chick at hatch. Weak chicks often fail to thrive and are at increased risk for bacterial diseases. Calorie intake, nutrient content of the diet, the chick's hydration, and the temperature of the brooder can all have a significant impact on the chick's growth rate and immune status. Again, problems in any of these areas may result in immune suppression and a subsequent bacterial disease.

The liver is an excellent site for culturing bacteria that can be grown by traditional methods. Often bacteria will be cultured from a liver that has the histologic appearance of a bacterial hepatitis but in which organisms cannot be seen. Heart blood and spleen are other excellent sources to culture if a bacterial infection is suspected. Postmortem bacterial invasion of the liver and other organs is common in birds that have undergone decomposition prior to necropsy. These organisms may be seen histologically in the liver but are never intracellular and are not associated with an inflammatory reaction.

Mycobacteria. *Mycobacterium avium* (MA), serotypes 1, 2, 3, and 8, and *Mycobacterium genavense* (MGE) are the most common mycobacteria that infect birds. *Mycobacterium tuberculosis* (MTB) has also been documented in psittacine birds but is uncommon. Probably all species of birds are susceptible to mycobacterial infection. However, infec-

tions are relatively uncommon in most species of birds. When outbreaks do occur, they are most frequent in collections of captive waterfowl, zoo birds, gray-cheeked (*Brotogeris pyrrhopterus*) and canary-winged parakeets (*B. versicolorus*), certain species of tropical doves, and Australian finches. Once the environment is contaminated with the organism, infections of other birds in the collection and new birds introduced to the collection are likely. The route of exposure depends on the organism. Birds contract MTB directly from people by inhalation of aerosolized bacteria. By contrast, MA and MGE are contracted by ingestion of the organisms. MA appears to be ubiquitous in the environment. The factors that determine whether a bird will contract MA and MG are not known but probably include a bird's genetic susceptibility and the number of organisms to which a bird is exposed.

Mycobacteriosis is a chronic disease, so birds that die with this disease are typically thin or emaciated. Mycobacterial disease can be localized or diffuse. Localized lesions are uncommon and are generally found on the face, skin, or leg and are generally caused by MTB. MA and MGE typically cause a widely disseminated disease. Following ingestion, they first colonize cells in the intestines. Here changes may be so severe as to interfere with digestion. From the intestines, mycobacteria spread widely. Any organ system can be affected, but the liver, spleen, lung, air sac, skin, and bone marrow are most commonly involved.

Affected livers may contain yellow to gray-tan, soft nodules or be diffusely enlarged (Figs. 4.29 and 4.30). Amyloidosis of the kidney and liver is a common complication of MA infections and may contribute to the clinical signs. Microscopically, mycobacterial infections take on two primary forms but may contain elements of both. In the first, classic tubercles contain a central necrotic (caseous) area surrounded by macrophages, multinucleated giant cells, histiocytes, and plasma cells (Fig. 4.31). Bacteria may be scarce in these lesions. More commonly in pet species, early hepatic lesions are comprised of heterophils and small macrophages within portal areas and

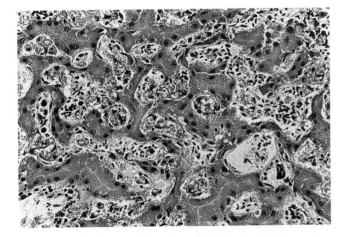

4.28. Bacteremia and bacterial hepatitis secondary to circovirus infection that led to severe immunosuppression. Numerous macrophages containing bacteria are seen in the sinusoids.

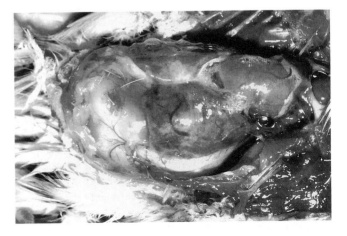

4.29. Hepatic mycobacteriosis with a slight mottling noted grossly.

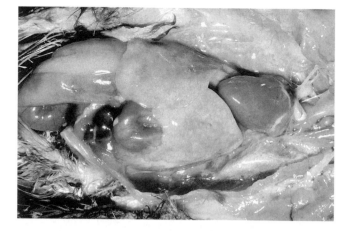

4.30.   Severe hepatic mycobacteriosis with diffuse pale-ness and irregular nodules in the parenchyma.

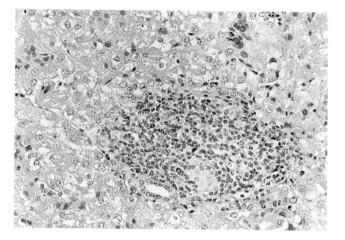

4.32.   Early hepatic mycobacteriosis. Lymphocytes and a few small macrophages are present in the lesion. Organ-isms may not always be seen at this stage.

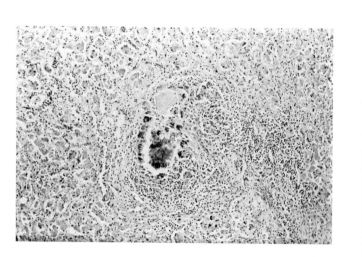

4.31.   Hepatic mycobacteriosis with a focus of caseation and giant cell formation. This type of lesion is not always seen.

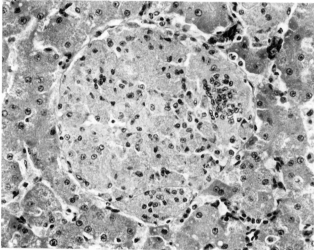

4.33.   Mycobacterial hepatitis with the formation of a granuloma comprised of large macrophages containing acid-fast bacteria.

scattered in the parenchyma (Fig. 4.32). As these lesions develop, they are comprised of small foci and eventually extensive sheets of bacteria-laden histiocytes (Figs. 4.33). The specific organism, the species of the host infected, the host's immune response, and the stage of infection all contribute to the nature of the lesion. The amount of necrosis and caseation varies. It may be more severe in waterfowl than in psittacine birds. In hematoxylin-eosin (H&E)-stained sections, the cytoplasm of macrophages infected with mycobacteria are blue-gray and have a finely granular appearance suggestive of the presence of numerous small organisms (Fig. 4.34). Proof that the organisms are there requires acid-fast staining.

Obligate Intracellular Bacteria. Psittacosis or ornithosis is a disease caused by an obligate intracellular bacterium—*Chlamydophila psittaci*—formally *Chlamydia psittaci*. There are eight serovars within this species. Serovars A and E are found in cage birds. Serovar B is enzootic in pigeons. All avian serovars are potentially zoonotic, and psittacosis is a reportable disease. Pathologists should take precautions to

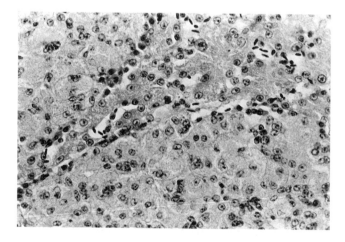

4.34.   Detail of hepatic mycobacteriosis. The granules in the macrophages are acid-fast bacteria that are mini-mally visible on routine hematoxylin-eosin-stained sec-tions.

keep from exposing themselves to this organism. Infections can occur by ingestion, inhalation, or conjunctival exposure to the organism. Organisms propagate in epithelial cells of the respiratory tract and then generalize to other organs. The disease in psittacine birds has variable manifestations. Subclinical infections are common, especially in cockatiels. A mild form of the disease manifesting as a chronic conjunctivitis and sinusitis is also common in cockatiels. New World parrots are often affected with a severe multisystemic disease. Multisystemic disease is also seen in cockatiels and other species of parrots.

Hepatic and splenic enlargement is a common finding in birds with psittacosis. Concurrent air sacculitis is another common manifestation of psittacosis and should alert pathologists that they may be dealing with this disease. Affected livers may have minimal gross changes, but many are enlarged and discolored and may contain numerous gray-yellow foci of necrosis (Fig. 4.35). Histologically there is an inflammatory reaction that is primarily mononuclear and may be diffuse within sinusoids. Many of the macrophages contain green-brown pigment consistent with bile pigment and/or hemosiderin (Figs. 4.36 and 4.37). Multifocal to confluent necrosis can also

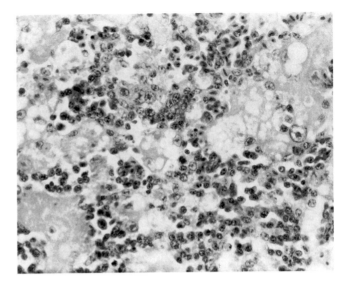

4.37.   Typical inflammatory response in hepatic Chlamydophila infection.

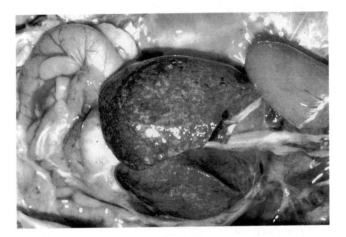

4.35.   Hepatic enlargement and severe necrosis and inflammation due to Chlamydophila infection.

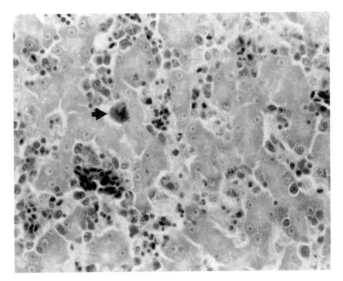

4.38.   Degenerating cell with dark basophilic smudge representing cytoplasmic accumulation of Chlamydophila organisms (arrow). On routine stains, individual organisms are difficult to see.

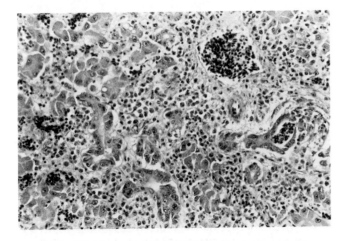

4.36.   Hepatic necrosis and diffuse lymphohistiocytic infiltrate characteristic of Chlamydophila infection.

be seen, and some heterophils may be present as a response to necrosis. In some cases, organisms can be found in macrophages and/or hepatocytes (Fig. 4.38). Although sometimes difficult to find on H&E-stained sections, they can be visualized with Giminez's and other special stains (Fig. 4.39). In chronic disease, portal fibrosis and bile duct hyperplasia occurs.

In many cases of psittacosis, the organisms may be seen in Giminez-stained impression smears of liver, spleen, or air sacs even though not found in fixed tissue. Immunofluorescent staining of impression smears is also a sensitive and rapid method of detecting the organism. PCR with specific primer sets is readily available in many

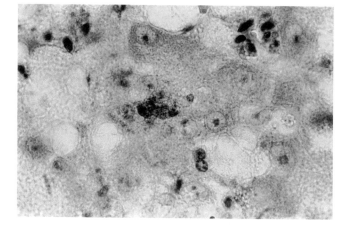

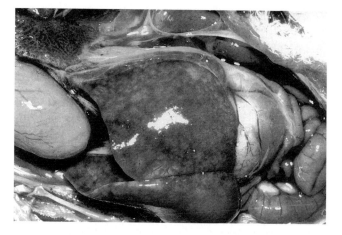

4.39. *Gimenez-stained section demonstrating* **Chlamy-dophila** *organisms. Many appear as large clumps, but a few individual organisms can be seen.*

4.40. *Enlarged, discolored liver seen in* **Sarcocystis** *infection. Both the gross appearance and the inflammatory infiltrate can be similar to Chlamydophila infection.*

diagnostic laboratories and can be used as confirmatory diagnostic assay. *Chlamydophila psittaci* can also be grown in Vero cells, but it may take several days before the organism can be detected

Bacillus piliformis is a rod-shaped, gram-positive bacterium that cannot be grown in cell-free media. It affects a wide variety of mammals and has been reported in a cockatiel. The organism exists in the environment and may spread via the fecal-oral route. Stress probably plays a part in the activation of clinical disease. Grossly the liver is enlarged, pale, and mottled, containing numerous foci of necrosis. Histologically there is multifocal necrosis, a variable pleocellular inflammatory reaction, and intracytoplasmic bacilli in hepatocytes. These may be difficult to see without Giemsa or silver stains.

Fungi. The liver is usually involved in mycotic infections as a result of extension from the lung or air sacs, or as a result of hematologic spread. Several species of *Aspergillus* are the most common organisms affecting the liver, but other fungi are occasionally identified. Systemic *Candida* infections, particularly in immunosuppressed birds, may result in liver invasion.

Gross lesions are similar to those caused by bacteria and viruses. Affected livers are enlarged and contain multifocal gray-white areas of necrosis. Histologic lesions are similar to those seen in bacterial infections, being characterized by necrosis and a pleocellular infiltrate including heterophils and macrophages. With chronicity, abscesses will form. Finding fungal organisms in the lesion is necessary for a specific diagnosis.

Parasites. Both protozoan and metazoan parasites cause avian liver disease. Protozoal pathogens come from several taxonomic groups.

Phylum Apicomplexa. Infections with *Toxoplasma gondii*, *Sarcocystis* sp., and *Atoxoplasma* can all cause significant

liver disease. Affected livers are typically enlarged, have rounded edges, and contain multiple diffuse subcapsular white foci (Fig. 4.40). Acute infections may result in a soft friable liver, whereas, in chronic infections, livers may be firm. Lesions caused by all three organisms are very similar. Necrosis is multifocal and random. It may be mild to severe. The accompanying inflammatory infiltrate is composed of macrophages, lymphocytes, and plasma cells in portal areas and sinusoids (Fig. 4.41). Heterophils may be seen in cases of toxoplasmosis associated with multifocal areas of necrosis. Organisms are usually not seen in *Sarcocystis* infections. When they occur, they are present in vascular endothelial cells. Organisms are also difficult to find when the lesion is caused by atoxoplasmosis. They are typically found in macrophages or Kupffer's cells and have a characteristic comma-shaped appearance and are 1 to 3 μm long. *Toxoplasma gondii* organisms are similar in size but are round and usually are more plentiful and are found in macrophages or in extracellular spaces.

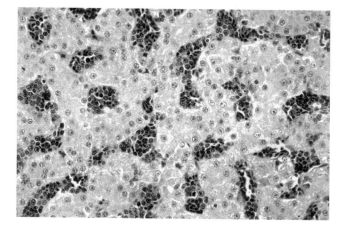

4.41. *Lymphoplasmacytic and histiocytic inflammatory infiltrate seen in sarcosporidial infection.*

Birds affected by hepatic cryptosporidiosis often have no gross hepatic lesions. Cryptosporidia attach to the surface of bile duct epithelial cells. There may be some proliferation of bile duct epithelium, and a mild chronic mononuclear inflammatory response is sometimes seen.

Hemoprotozoa. Organisms from the genera *Plasmodium*, *Leukocytozoon*, and *Hemoproteus* are capable of inducing hepatic disease. Hepatic lesions caused by infection with *Plasmodium* sp. include liver enlargement and, particularly in falcons, a diffuse gray-black discoloration. Histologically, numerous macrophages, plasma cells, and lymphocytes infiltrate affected livers. Organisms (exoerythrocytic schizonts) may be found in some of the inflammatory cells (Fig. 4.42). In falcons, malarial pigment is present in macrophages (Fig. 4.43).

Leukocytozoon schizogony occurs in macrophages and hepatocytes. Grossly affected livers are variably enlarged and pale and contain numerous dark, red-black, raised foci. These foci bleed when incised (Fig. 4.44). Histologically the dark foci are areas of hemorrhage surrounding megaloschizonts and necrotic hepatic tissue. The megaloschizonts vary from 110×40 mm to over 600×400 mm. Some schizonts may be ruptured, and released merozoites may be phagocytosed by macrophages. Hepatocytes are usually slightly swollen and vacuolated (Fig. 4.45).

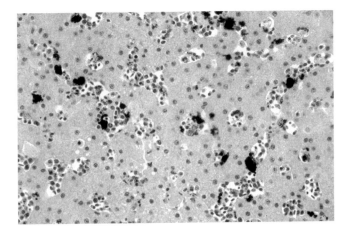

4.43.   Hepatitis in a falcon due to Plasmodium *sp. The reaction is similar to that in the canary, but malaria pigment is seen in raptors.*

Hemoproteus is usually considered nonpathogenic. Gross lesions are not seen, but histologically schizonts can be found in endothelial cells of the liver vasculature.

Phylum Sarcomastigophora

Trichomonas gallinae. Trichomoniasis is generally confined to the oral cavity and esophagus. In squabs,

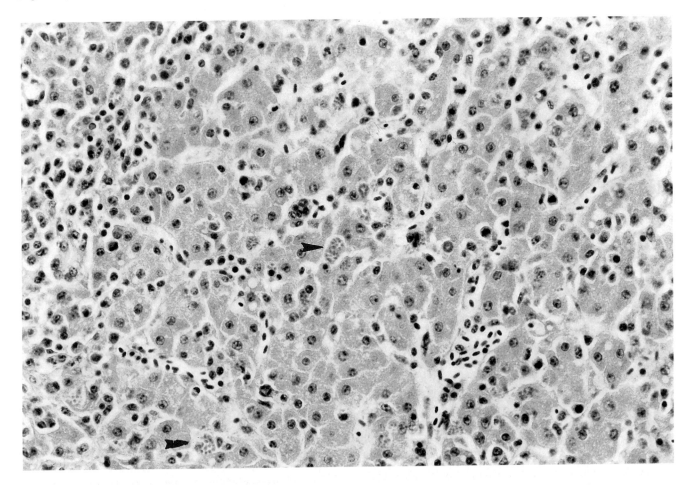

4.42.   Hepatitis associated with malaria in a canary. Exoerythrocytic schizonts can be seen (arrowheads).

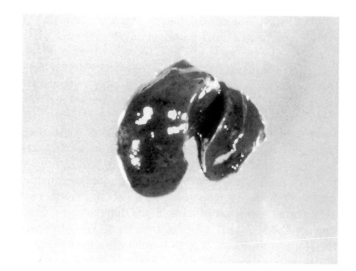

4.44. *Liver from a bird with systemic* **Leukocytozoon** *infection. The numerous small dark foci are areas of hemorrhage surrounding megaloschizonts.*

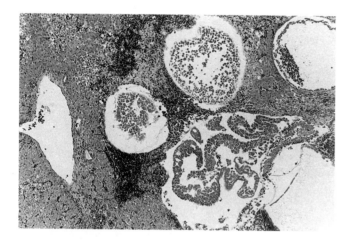

4.45. *Histologic appearance of liver with megaloschizonts of* Leukocytozoon *and surrounding hepatic necrosis and hemorrhage.*

however, trichomoniasis can become generalized, and the liver is commonly involved. Affected livers are enlarged with focal to coalescing areas of caseous necrosis. Fibrinous casts of the liver and, less commonly, ascites are seen in more severe cases. Granulomas are also present in the lung, in the intestinal mesentery, and around the heart. A mixed population of inflammatory cells of which a high proportion is heterophils surrounds necrotic areas. Epithelioid cells and giant cells are occasionally present. Organisms are not visible in H&E-stained sections but are readily visible using a modified silver stain. Extensive perivascular heterophil infiltration in the liver and kidney (possibly extramedullary myelopoiesis) is also reported.

Histomonas meleagridis. Histomoniasis is predominantly a disease of turkeys but also causes significant prob-

lems in quail, ruffed grouse, and chickens. It is transmitted within the eggs of *Heterakis gallinarium* that are ingested by earthworms. Infection occurs when free-ranging birds eat infected earthworms. The disease is characterized by a typhlitis (chapter 3) and hepatitis. Grossly, liver lesions consist of multiple, round, yellow-green, depressed foci. Histologically the gross lesions represent multifocal to locally extensive and, at times, coalescing granulomas. The trophozoites are pale, round, and eosinophilic, varying in size from 5 to 20 m. They are generally abundant and are strongly periodic acid-Schiff positive (Figs. 4.46 and 4.47).

Phylum Microspora. The phylum Microspora contains over 1000 species that infect a huge range of vertebrate and invertebrate hosts. Only a single species—*Encephalitozoon hellem*—is documented to infect birds. For the most

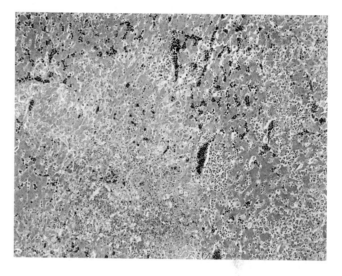

4.46. *Severe hepatic necrosis and inflammation in a bird with histomoniasis.*

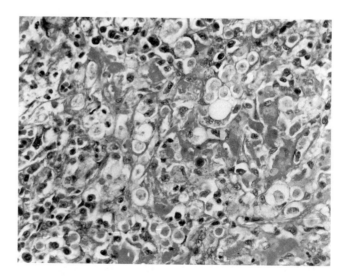

4.47. *Higher magnification of Figure 4.46, illustrating histomonads in the hepatic parenchyma. Most of the organisms are surrounded by a clear zone.*

part, *E. hellem* commonly and asymptomatically infects budgerigars and lovebirds and perhaps other species of birds as well. However, disease does occur in these species and has been also reported in eclectus parrots, lories, a blue-fronted Amazon parrot, ostriches, and hummingbirds. Disease appears most likely to occur in birds that are immunosuppressed. Concurrent infections with the PBFDV are common and may predispose birds to disease. *Encephalitozoon hellem* also causes disease in people who are severely immunocompromised.

Target organs for *E. hellem* are the liver, kidney, spleen, intestine and, less commonly, the eye. (See the relevant chapters.) Disease, when it occurs, has predominated in flocks of budgerigars and flocks of lovebirds. Varying degrees of morbidity and mortality occur. Live birds may have diarrhea and appear unthrifty. Gross necropsy findings include pasted vents, pale voluminous feces, watery intestinal contents, and undigested seeds in the feces. Liver and spleen enlargement are variable findings, as is liver mottling. Histologically there may be mild to moderate hepatic necrosis and an infiltrate of macrophages and lymphocytes. Round, approximately 1.5-m-diameter, lightly basophilic organisms are found in hepatocytes, bile duct epithelium, and free in the areas of necrosis. Although they stain poorly with H&E (Fig. 4.48), they are readily visible with Brown and Brenn and trichrome stains.

When there is substantial hepatic necrosis, infection is often accompanied by a mononuclear cell infiltrate.

Metazoan Parasites: Trematodes. Trematodes have a complicated life cycle that involves one or more intermediate hosts. As a result, infections with these parasites are confined almost exclusively to wild or wild-caught cage birds. Most captive waterfowl are incubator hatched so that, unless these birds are exposed to wild waterfowl, they are not likely to have trematodes either. Flukes, such as *Fasciola hepatica*, damage the liver by migrating through it to the predilection site, the bile ducts. Both cockatoos and emus are reported to be parasitized by flukes that have a predilection for the bile ducts. Once in the bile ducts, trematodes may cause little disease or gross thickening of the bile ducts. Histologically there may be a minimal mononuclear inflammatory reaction in some cases (Fig. 4.49). Fibrosis and bile duct hyperplasia can be seen in chronic disease (Fig. 4.50).

Emus with *F. hepatica* infection have an eosinophilic reaction, as well as infiltration of macrophages and lymphocytes. There may also be granuloma formation with giant cells and variable degrees of fibrosis. Aberrant colonization of the biliary tree by intestinal flukes may also occur, resulting in similar lesions.

Schistosomes are commonly found in waterfowl but are also reported in passerine species. Birds are infected by

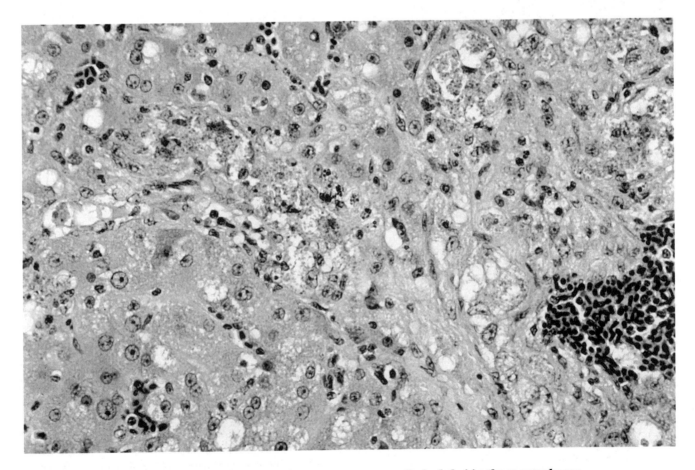

4.48.   *Microsporidial hepatitis. Numerous organisms are seen as small, dark foci in the macrophages.*

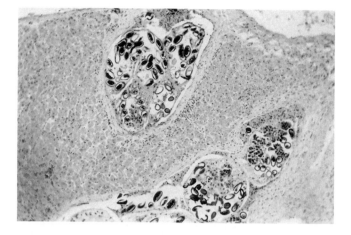

4.49.   Trematode eggs in dilated bile ducts. A minimal inflammatory reaction and mild fibrosis are seen.

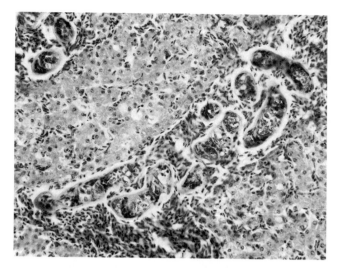

4.51.   Fragments of schistosomes are seen in the hepatic sinusoids.

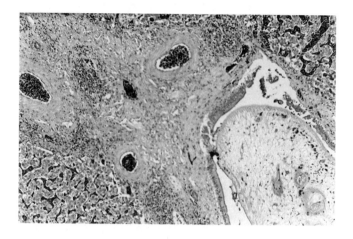

4.50.   A trematode is seen in a dilated bile duct. There is severe fibrosis and inflammation.

cercariae that are found in contaminated bodies of water. The cercariae penetrate the skin and enter the circulatory system, where they develop into adult worms. The adult worms in birds inhabit the portal veins, hepatic sinusoids, the aorta, or the mesenteric arteries, depending on the species of schistosome (Fig. 4.51). Schistosomes release their eggs, which then penetrate small vessels in the intestines and liver. The eggs induce a granulomatous foreign-body reaction.

Noninfectious Disease
Nutritional/Metabolic Disorders

Hepatic Lipidosis. Hepatic lipidosis is a problem in a wide variety of birds. One cause of hepatic lipidosis in chickens is biotin deficiency, but the exact pathogenesis of hepatic lipidosis in pet species is often not known. Excessive calorie intake, inadequate utilization of fat, hepatic enzyme defects, deficiency of dietary lipotrophs, or toxic damage are all possible causes. Hepatic lipidosis, in pet birds, seems to be most common in Amazon parrots, cockatiels, budgerigars, macaws, and rose-breasted cockatoos, as well

as in young cockatoos. The cause in older animals is commonly a dietary excess of fatty food. The disease in cockatoo chicks appears to be related to diets that contain excessive fat and/or excessive hand feeding. These chicks usually present with a swollen abdomen and obviously enlarged liver. Adult birds with hepatic lipidosis often die with no premonitory signs.

Grossly affected livers are enlarged, pale and/or yellow, and friable (Fig. 4.52). Histologically, in uncomplicated cases, hepatocytes are variably vacuolated and swollen (Fig. 4.53), with no other lesion seen. Mild degrees of lipidosis are commonly seen in birds that have been in a negative calorie balance prior to death. In these cases, hepatocytes may contain one or multiple small lipid vacuoles.

Visceral Urate Deposition (Gout). The liver capsule is a common location for urate deposits in birds with visceral gout. The exact pathogenesis may not always be obvious,

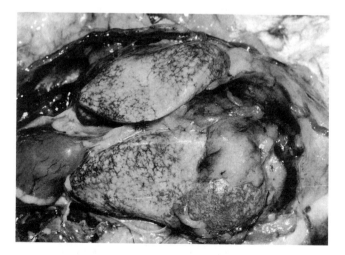

4.52.   Enlarged, pale, friable liver with severe lipidosis.

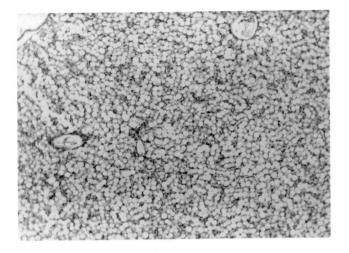

4.53. *Typical histologic appearance of severe fatty liver.*

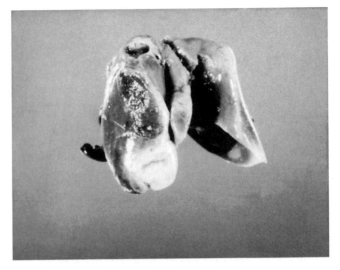

4.54. *Large, pale, irregular liver due to diffuse amyloidosis.*

but the condition is usually secondary to renal disease or inadequate water intake. Any species of bird can be affected. Grossly the hepatic capsule contains gray-white plaques or streaks, and the urate deposits may completely obscure the underlying liver. Parenchymal lesions can also be seen. Urates are water soluble and will dissolve while the tissue is fixed in formalin. Histologically the radially arranged needlelike crystals are gone, but they leave behind empty spaces of the same shape that are surrounded by a pale amorphous eosinophilic material. Capsular urate deposits are often more amorphous than they are crystalline and therefore appear as irregularly round eosinophilic masses. Necrosis and an inflammatory reaction that is primarily heterophilic may accompany the urate deposits.

Amyloidosis. This is the general term applied to several diseases characterized by the deposition of one of several forms of amyloid. Only amyloidosis caused by the deposition of AA amyloid has been described in birds. AA amyloid is the product of the proteolytic cleavage of serum amyloid A, an acute-phase protein. Serum amyloid A is believed to be persistently elevated in birds with chronic granulomatous disease. Amyloidosis is a common lesion in waterfowl. Additionally the white Pekin duck is genetically predisposed to amyloidosis, and lesions are present in these birds by 2 years of age. Amyloidosis is relatively rare lesion in other birds, including doves, finches, and parrots. The distribution of organ involvement varies from bird to bird

Grossly, infiltrated organs may be pale, firm, and waxy or friable. Affected organs are enlarged, sometimes massively (Fig. 4.54). On cut section, they stain with iodine. Amyloidosis grossly may resemble hepatic lipidosis. Histologically amyloid is amorphous, pale eosinophilic or amphophilic, and the amount present is variable. Amyloid deposition occurs in the liver in the space of Disse and in the media of blood vessels, and on basement membranes (Fig. 4.55). In severe cases, the amyloid can efface

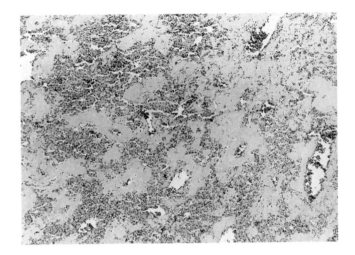

4.55. *Severe hepatic amyloidosis.*

much of the hepatic parenchyma and lead to hepatic failure. Amyloid is differentiated from other acellular eosinophilic material, such as fibrin and immune-complex deposition, by positive staining and birefringence with Congo red stain. Avian amyloid, however, does not consistently stain well with Congo red.

Pigmentary Hepatopathies. Iron pigment in the liver is a common histologic finding. When it is confined to phagocytic cells, the iron is in the form of hemosiderin, a metabolite of hemoglobin. Hemosiderosis results from either a higher than normal rate of red cell destruction or decreased utilization of iron for new hemoglobin production. The most common hemolytic disease of birds is heavy-metal poisoning. *Plasmodium* infections may result in massive hemolysis and hepatic hemosiderosis. Immune-mediated hemolytic anemia is rare in cage birds, being reported only once in a blue-crowned conure. One author (D.N.P.), however, has suspected it in a blue and gold macaw given serum contaminated with hemoglobin from a chicken and in a sun conure with an uncharacterized bleeding disorder. The most common cause of hemosiderosis is reduced red blood cell production. Birds that are in a negative calorie balance or have chronic disease stop producing red blood cells or produce them at a decreased rate. Red blood cell destruction continues, however, at a constant rate, and, as a result, iron accumulates in phagocytic cells in the liver, spleen, and kidney. This is a reversible change and is not associated with liver disease.

Iron accumulation in hepatocytes, iron-storage disease (ISD), is an entirely different entity than hemosiderosis. ISD is predominantly a disease of captive mynahs (*Gracula* sp.), birds of paradise (Paradisaeidae), quetzals (*Pharomachrus* sp.), several species of toucans (Ramphastidae), and fairy bluebirds (*Irena puella*). Infrequently it is seen in other species of birds, including parrots. Work done with mynahs suggests that ISD develops in susceptible species because they are highly efficient at absorbing dietary iron and do not down regulate iron absorption sufficiently when fed iron-rich diets. It is presumed that in the wild these birds feed on diets that contain little iron or iron that is in a form that is not readily absorbed from the digestive tract. It is also assumed that the diet fed these birds in captivity contains either excess iron or iron that is readily digestible, resulting in the accumulation of iron in the liver and other tissues. ISD in lories was traced back to a diet containing a hugely excessive amount of iron, and ISD does not occur in these birds when fed an appropriate diet. ISD has been called hemochromatosis, but this may be inappropriate because hemochromatosis refers to a human disease characterized by a genetic defect in iron metabolism.

Excessive liver iron and ISD are not synonymous. Iron will accumulate in the liver for long periods prior to the onset of disease. Therefore the presence of iron in hepatocytes in the absence of other lesions does not constitute sufficient grounds for a diagnosis of ISD. Birds with ISD may die suddenly and be in good body condition or have chronic muscle wasting. Ascites is a common finding and may be secondary to liver disease or heart failure. The liver in birds with ISD is enlarged and gold-brown. Small, scattered, dark foci may be seen (Fig. 4.56). The histologic appearance varies with the amount of iron deposited. Iron can be seen in hepatocytes and in Kupffer's cells and macrophages. There may be an associated inflammatory process that includes lymphocytes and scattered heterophils. In severe cases, there is variable hepatic necrosis and, with chronicity, fibrosis develops. Prussian blue staining will confirm the pigment as iron but is usually not necessary (Figs. 4.57 to 4.59).

Bile pigments are commonly found in the liver. The pigments may be present in canaliculi or within Kupffer's cells. Bile pigments are seen in the livers of birds that have hepatic diseases that result in bile stasis.

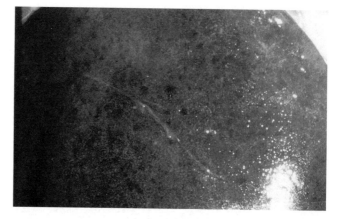

4.56.   Iron-storage disease in a toucan. The liver is discolored, and the multiple dark foci represent collections of Kupffer's cells/macrophages containing pigment.

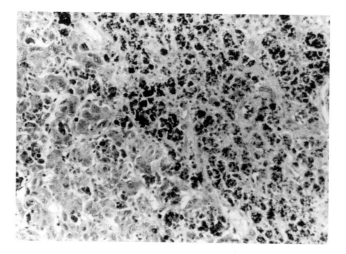

4.57.   Iron-storage disease. The iron can be seen primarily in Kupffer's cells and macrophages, although a small amount is in hepatocytes.

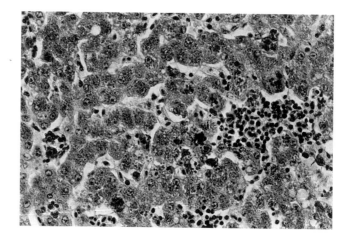

4.58.   Iron-storage disease. In this case, the iron is primarily in the hepatocytes.

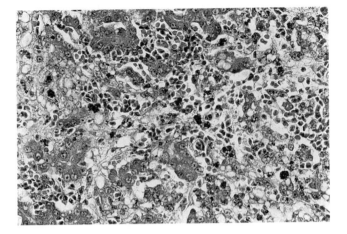

4.59. *Iron-storage disease in a lorikeet. In addition to pigment accumulation in macrophages and hepatocytes, there is variable necrosis.*

Lipofuscin pigment accumulates in hepatocytes secondary to a variety of diseases. It is considered a "wear and tear" pigment and is due to excessive biologic oxidation at the cellular level. Vitamin E deficiency is one possible cause.

Lysosomal Storage Disease. In emus, lysosomal disease is usually considered a nervous system problem (chapter 10), but lesions may also be found in the liver. Grossly there may be minimal mottling due to histologic foci of finely vacuolated cells that may be macrophages (Fig. 4.60).

Xanthomatosis. Internal xanthomas may be found in the liver, where they are comprised of numerous cholesterol clefts that efface normal parenchyma (Fig. 4.61).

Chronic-Active Hepatitis. Chronic-active hepatitis, or cirrhosis, is relatively common in psittacine birds, particularly Amazon parrots, cockatiels, macaws, and budgerigars. Because of the chronicity of the lesion, the

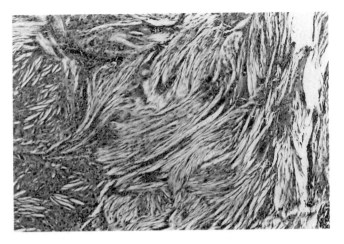

4.61. *Xanthoma within hepatic parenchyma.*

cause of the hepatitis can rarely be determined. Cockatiels are extremely sensitive to aflatoxins, and it has been speculated that chronic-active hepatitis in these birds may result from a previous exposure to aflatoxins. Chronic-active hepatitis, in other species, is seen in cases of chronic infectious diseases, particularly chlamydiosis, and exposure to bile excreted toxins.

Grossly affected livers are variably shrunken, pale, and fibrotic. The capsule is often thickened, and the edges of the liver are rounded. In extreme cases, there may only be small firm nodules in place of the normal liver (Figs. 4.62 to 4.64). Perihepatic effusion is common. The histologic appearance varies with the stage of the disease. Early lesions consist of hepatocyte vacuolation, a pleocellular inflammatory infiltrate primarily in portal areas, bile duct proliferation, and mild fibrosis (Fig. 4.65). The lesion may progress to severe fibrosis and diffuse biliary hyperplasia (Figs. 4.66 to 4.69). In some cases, severe extramedullary hematopoiesis is seen (Fig. 4.70).

Heart Failure. Right-sided heart failure results in the dilation of the hepatic veins and congestion of the hepatic

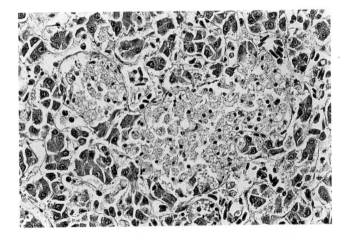

4.60. *Lysosomal storage disease with foci of cells containing finely vacuolated cytoplasm.*

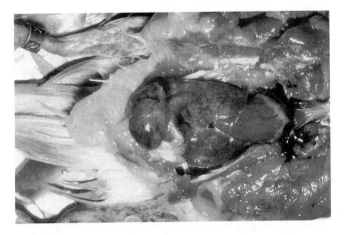

4.62. *Early chronic-active hepatitis. Slight discoloration and irregularity are noted.*

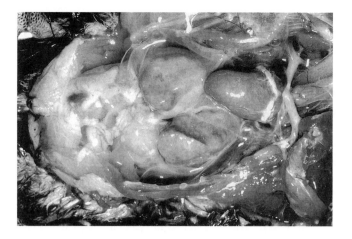

4.63. *Moderate to severe chronic-active hepatitis. The liver is pale, firm, and nodular.*

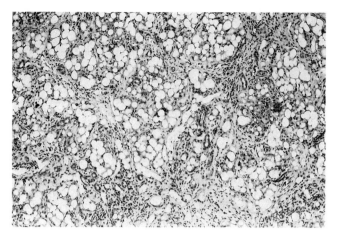

4.66. *Chronic-active hepatitis with moderate fibrosis, bile duct hyperplasia, extramedullary hematopoiesis, and inflammation. The hepatocytes are vacuolated.*

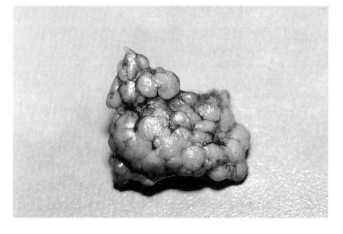

4.64. *End-stage liver as a result of chronic-active hepatitis.*

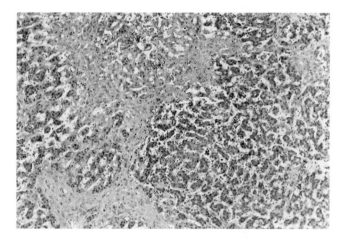

4.67. *Moderate to severe fibrosis with minimal inflammation and hepatocyte atrophy rather than vacuolation and swelling.*

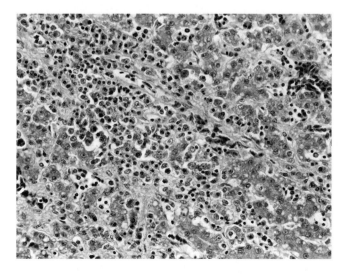

4.65. *Early chronic-active hepatitis with mild fibrosis and diffuse inflammation.*

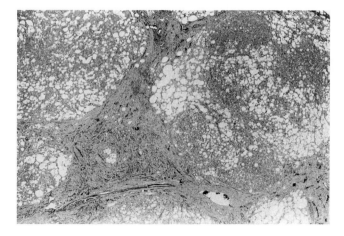

4.68. *Severe chronic-active hepatitis. Marked fibrosis and nodular hyperplasia are seen.*

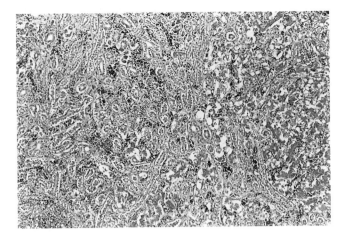

4.69. *Chronic-active hepatitis with fibrosis and severe bile duct hyperplasia.*

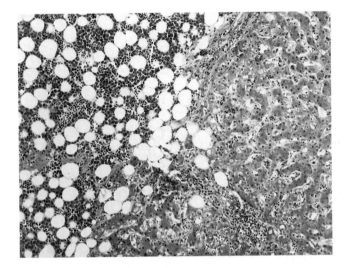

4.70. *Extramedullary hematopoiesis as occasionally seen in chronic-active hepatitis. Nodular hyperplasia is also seen.*

sinusoids. Initially the liver may be enlarged. Chronic right-heart disease results in severe atrophy of the centrolobular hepatocytes, fibrosis, and capsular thickening. Perihepatic effusion may be prominent. Grossly the liver lobes are small, have rounded margins, and have a gray surface caused by the thickened capsule.

Toxins. Many toxins can affect the avian liver. Lesions seen are not specific in most cases, and an etiologic diagnosis usually cannot be made on the basis of morphologic changes. In lead toxicosis, there may be some hepatic enlargement. Histologic lesions noted include hemosiderosis and variable hepatocyte swelling. Zinc toxicity may result in hepatic lesions that include hemosiderosis and erythrophagocytosis. Vitamin D_3 or vitamin D_3 analog rodenticides cause secondary liver lesions comprised of mineralization of basement membranes of sinusoids and blood vessels. Vitamin D_3 toxicity and possibly excessive dietary calcium may also result in metastatic mineral-

ization. Mycotoxins that are bile excreted, such as aflatoxin, can cause periportal necrosis and inflammation. In chronic cases, there is bile duct hyperplasia and fibrosis as described in chronic-active hepatitis.

Neoplastic Disease

Epithelial Tumors. Primary tumors may be of hepatocellular or bile duct origin, but bile duct tumors are more common. Bile duct proliferation, and possibly tumor formation, is reported in association with internal papillomatosis. Affected birds are predominantly macaws, Amazon parrots and, less frequently, conures. Gross lesions consist of variably sized masses that vary in consistency from friable to firm and from gray to yellow-white to red-brown (Fig. 4.71). They may be present in one or more lobes of the liver. They are typically multifocal and grow by expansion, crowding out the normal liver. Birds with these masses may die suddenly and be in good flesh, or they may have had a protracted illness with advanced muscle wasting and be devoid of body fat.

Proliferation of fairly well differentiated ductular structures, accompanied by variable amounts of stroma, characterize bile duct adenomas (Fig. 4.72). Carcinomas are

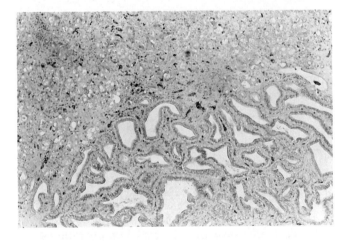

4.71. *Nodular mass typical of bile duct carcinoma.*

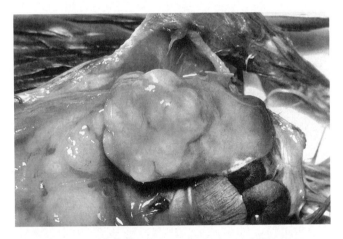

4.72. *Bile duct adenoma comprised of irregular ducts lined by fairly well differentiated epithelium.*

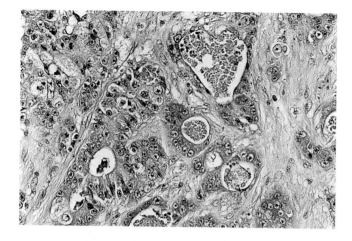

4.73.   Bile duct carcinoma. Infiltrative nests and trabeculae are present, and there is a moderate amount of fibrous stroma.

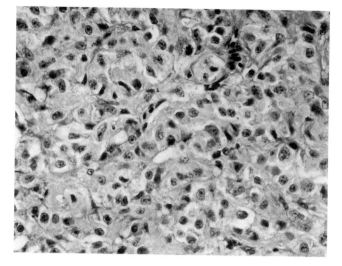

4.75.   Hepatocellular carcinoma. Poorly differentiated hepatocytes form cords separated by minimal amounts of stroma.

comprised of less well differentiated ducts, nests, cords, and individualized cells in some cases (Fig. 4.73). Mitotic figures are usually infrequent. Occasionally carcinomas have cystic spaces. Metastasis is infrequently seen.

Hepatocellular carcinomas tend to be red-brown and friable. Masses may be solitary or multiple. Histologically hepatomas contain well-differentiated cells. Portal triads are absent in hepatomas, which is the only characteristic that differentiates them from hyperplastic nodules (Fig. 4.74). Hepatocellular carcinomas are comprised of moderately undifferentiated to poorly differentiated hepatocytes that form cords and nests. Minimal mitotic activity is noted. There is usually minimal stroma (Fig. 4.75).

Mesenchymal Tumors. Primary mesenchymal tumors of the liver include fibrosarcoma, lymphosarcoma, leiomyosarcoma, hemangioma and hemangiosarcoma, and myelolipoma. There are no specific gross features for these tumors. They present as solitary or multiple nodules or masses and are usually firm, with the exception being

hemangioma/hemangiosarcomas that may be friable and hemorrhagic.

Histologic features of these tumors are similar to those that occur in any other location, though hemangiosarcomas in the liver tend to be more solid than in other tissues, but with a few vascular channels lined by poorly differentiated endothelial cells (Fig. 4.76). Fibrosarcoma and leiomyosarcoma are comprised of interlacing bundles of fusiform cells. Fibrosarcomas usually have a much higher mitotic rate (Fig. 4.77). Occasionally, hepatic sarcomas contain large cells with karyomegalic nuclei (Fig. 4.78). Polyomavirus particles have been seen in these cells by electron microscopy, but their significance has not been determined.

Lymphosarcoma grossly may present with multiple gray-yellow foci that mimic some severe infectious diseases (Fig. 4.79). In severe cases, however, entire lobes may be replaced by the tumor (Fig. 4.80). Histologically

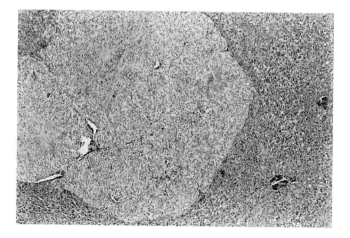

4.74.   Well-demarcated hepatoma growing by expansion.

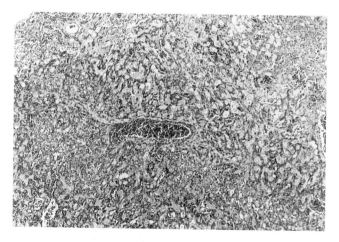

4.76.   Hemangiosarcoma effacing hepatic parenchyma.

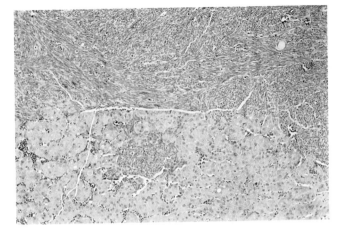

4.77. *Primary hepatic fibrosarcoma comprised of interlacing bundles of neoplastic cells.*

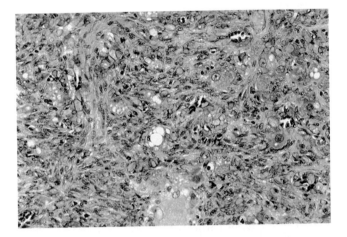

4.78. *Hepatic sarcoma containing scattered cells with karymegalic nuclei and intranuclear inclusion bodies. In many cases, these inclusions contain polyomavirus particles.*

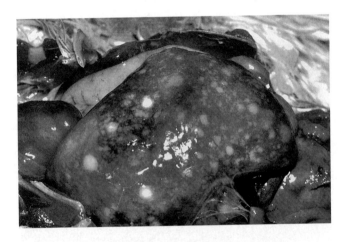

4.79. *Hepatic lymphosarcoma. The gross appearance can be similar to that in severe infectious disease.*

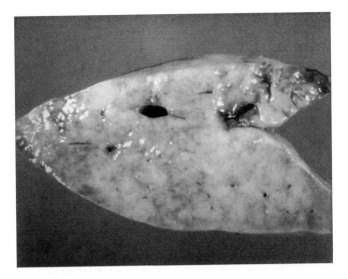

4.80. *Portion of liver lobe almost completely replaced by neoplastic lymphoid cells.*

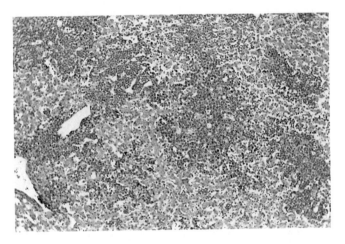

4.81. *Effacement of liver by fairly monomorphic lymphoblasts.*

sheets of immature lymphoid cells are seen replacing normal hepatic architecture (Fig. 4.81). Histiocytic sarcomas are also occasionally seen. The cells are pleomorphic with abundant cytoplasm and are diffusely infiltrative (Fig. 4.82). Malignant myeloproliferative disease may also be seen in the liver.

Myelolipomas are similar to those in mammals, containing well-differentiated adipose cells and bone marrow elements (Fig. 4.83).

Malignant Melanoma. The liver may be the primary site of malignant melanoma. Grossly, multiple, gray-black nodules are seen. Histologically the tumor is comprised of poorly differentiated melanocytic cells with variable cytoplasmic pigment (Fig. 4.84).

Metastatic Tumors. Potentially any carcinoma, sarcoma, or melanoma can metastasize to the liver; however,

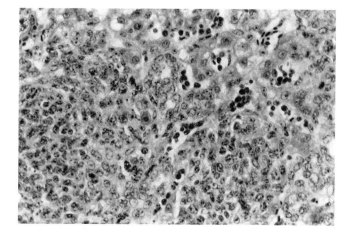

4.82. Infiltration of liver by neoplastic cells consistent with histiocytes.

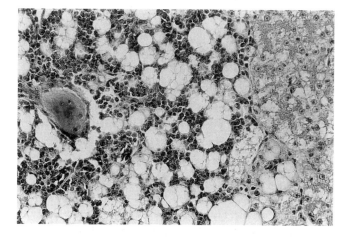

4.83. Hepatic myelolipoma. These tumors histologically resemble normal bone marrow.

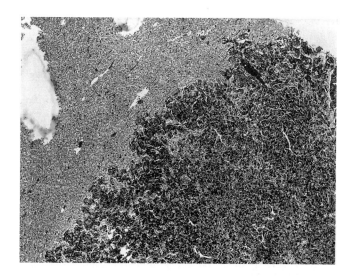

4.84. Malignant melanoma diffusely infiltrative in hepatic parenchyma.

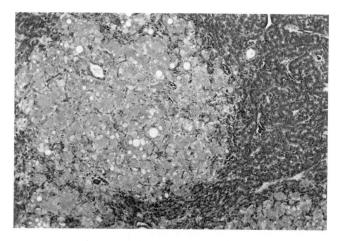

4.85. Pancreatic carcinoma metastatic to the liver. The light areas are foci of remaining hepatocytes.

metastatic liver disease is uncommon. When liver metastasis does occur, it is usually by tumors of renal, pancreatic, or proventricular origin (Fig. 4.85). Extension of Sertoli's cell tumor from the testicle has also been seen (Fig. 4.86). Grossly these tumors present as variably sized nodules, and histologic examination is necessary for differentiation.

Nonneoplastic Epithelial Proliferative Lesions. Hepatocellular hyperplasia and cyst formation is seen in all birds. There may be nodular hepatocellular hyperplasia presenting as single or multiple red-brown or slightly yellow nodules. Histologically these nodules contain enlarged hepatocytes that may have vacuolated cytoplasm. Portal triads are seen in the nodules, differentiating them from adenomas.

Bile duct hyperplasia is more common than hepatocellular hyperplasia. As mentioned previously, this condition has been associated with internal papillomatosis. Grossly the lesion may vary from multiple yellow-white firm nodules to almost diffuse enlargement of a lobe. Histologically there is proliferation of well-differentiated ducts and

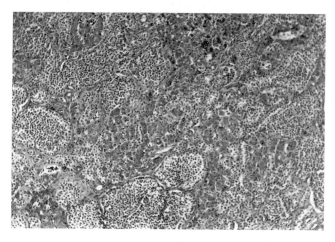

4.86. Extension of Sertoli's cell tumor into the liver.

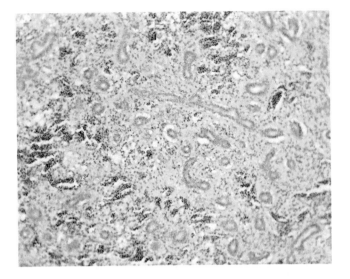

4.87. Marked fibrosis and bile duct hyperplasia of undetermined cause.

moderate to marked amounts of fibrous connective tissue (Fig. 4.87). Bile duct hyperplasia is most common in those psittacine birds that have a high incidence of chronic-active hepatitis but is seen in a wide variety of pet birds. It can be severe enough to compromise hepatic function and be a primary cause of death. A careful histologic examination is necessary to differentiate hyperplasia, particularly when severe, from biliary adenoma.

ADDITIONAL READING

Arey LB. 1957. Developmental anatomy. Philadelphia: WB Saunders, pp 251–256.

Aranaz A, Liebana E, Mateos A, Domingues L. 1997. Laboratory diagnosis of avian mycobacteriosis. Semin Avian Exotic Pet Med 6:9–17.

Barton JT, Bickford AA, Cooper GL, et al. 1992. Avian paramyxovirus type 1 infections in racing pigeons in California. I. Clinical signs, pathology, and serology. Avian Dis 36:463–468.

Battison AL, Machin KL, Archer FJ. 1996. Ascites and hepatic cirrhosis in a cockatiel (Nymphicus hollandicus). J Am Anim Hosp Assoc 32:237–242.

Bauck L. 1995. Nutritional problems in pet birds. Semin Avian Exotic Pet Med 4:3–8.

Bernier G, Morin M, Marsolais G. 1981. A generalized inclusion body disease in the budgerigar (Melopsittacus undulatus) caused by a papovavirus-like agent. Avian Dis 25:1083–1092.

Breiner DM, Urban S, Schaller H. 1998. Carboxypeptidase-D (gp 180) a Golgi-resident protein, functions in the attachment and entry of avian hepatitis-B viruses. J Virol 72:8089–8104.

Clipsham R. 1995. Avian pathogenic flagellated enteric protozoa. Semin Avian Exotic Pet Med 4:112–125.

Clyde VL, Orosz SE, Munson L. 1996. Severe hepatic fibrosis and bile duct hyperplasia in four Amazon parrots. J Avian Med Surg 10:252–257.

Coleman CW. 1991. Bile duct carcinoma and cloacal prolapse in an orange-winged Amazon parrot (Amazona amazonica amazonica). J Assoc Avian Vet 5:87–89.

Degernes LA, Trasti S, Healy LN, et al. 1998. Multicystic biliary adenocarcinoma in a blue and gold macaw (Ara ararauna). J Avian Med Surg 12:100–107.

Desser SS. 1972. The fine structure of Leukocytozoon simondi. VI. Hepatic schizogony. Can J Zool 51:605–609.

Eskens U, Kaleta EF, Unger G. 1994. An enzootic disease caused by a herpesvirus—Pacheco's parrot disease—in a flock of psittacine birds. Tierarztl Prax 22:542–553.

Flammer D, Butterworth H, Whitt DA. 1989. Atoxoplasmosis in canaries. J Am Fed Aviculture 15:24–26.

Garcia A, Latimer KS, Niagro FD, et al. 1993. Avian polyomavirus infection in three black-bellied seed crackers (Pyrenestes ostrinus). J Assoc Avian Vet 7:79–82.

Garcia A, Latimer KS, Niagro FD, et al. 1994. Diagnosis of polyomavirus-induced hepatic necrosis in psittacine birds using DNA probes. J Vet Diagn Invest 6:308–314.

Gaskin JM. 1988. Avian reoviruses: Are they for real? J Am Fed Aviculture 16:24–26.

Graham DL. 1987. Characterization of a reo-like virus and its isolation from and pathogenicity for parrots. Avian Dis 31:411–419.

Greiner EC, Ritchie BW. 1994. Parasites. In: Avian medicine: Principles and application. Lake Worth, FL: Wingers, pp 1007–1029.

Griener LA, Sheridan BW. 1967. Malaria (Plasmodium relictum) in penguins at the San Diego Zoo. Am J Vet Clin Pathol 1:7–17.

Hillyer EV, Moroff S, Hoefer H. 1991. Bile duct carcinoma in two out of ten Amazon parrots with cloacal papillomas. J Assoc Avian Vet 5:91–95.

Jackson MK, Phillips SN. 1996. Necrotizing hepatitis in pet birds associated with Pseudomonas fluorescens. Avian Dis 40:473–476.

King AS, McLelland J. 1984. Birds: Their structure and function. London: Bailliere, Tindall, pp 106–107.

LaBonde J. 1995. Toxicity in pet avian patients. Semin Avian Exotic Pet Med 4:23–31.

Lafferty SL, Fudge AM, Schmidt RE, et al. 1999. Avian polyomavirus infection and disease in a green aracaris (Pteroglossus viridis). Avian Dis 43:577–585.

Latimer KS, Rakich PM, Kircher IM, et al. 1990. Extracutaneous viral inclusions in psittacine beak and feather disease. J Vet Diagn Invest 2:204–207.

Latimer KS, Rakich PM, Niagro FD, et al. 1991. An updated review of psittacine beak and feather disease. J Assoc Avian Vet 5:211–220.

Latimer KS, Niagro FD, Williams OC, et al. 1997. Diagnosis of avian adenovirus infections using DNA in-situ hybridization. Avian Dis 41:773–782.

Lee KP, Henry NW, Rosenberger JK. 1978. Comparative pathogenicity of six avian adenovirus isolates in the liver. Avian Dis 22:610–619.

Leeson S, Diaz G, Summers JD. 1995. Aflatoxins. In: Poultry metabolic disorders and mycotoxins. Guelph: University Books, pp 249–280.

Lenhoff RJ, Luscombe CA, Summers J. 1999. Acute liver injury following infection with a cytopathic strain of duck hepatitis B virus. Hepatology 29:563–571.

Marion PL, Cullen JM, Azcarraga RR, et al. 1987. Experimental transmission of duck hepatitis B virus to Pekin ducks and domestic geese. Hepatology 7:724–731.

McFerran JB, Adair B McC. 1977. Avian adenoviruses: A review. Avian Pathol 6:189–217.

McLelland J. 1991. A color atlas of avian anatomy. Philadelphia: WB Saunders.

Oros J, Rodriquez JL, Fernandez A, Herraez AE. 1998. Simultaneous occurrence of Salmonella arizonae in a sulfur crested cockatoo (Cacatua galerita galerita) and iguanas. Avian Dis 42:813–823.

Page CD, Greiner EC, Schmidt RE. 1987. Leukocytozoonosis in crested oropendolas (Psaracolius decumanus). AAV Today 1:155–157.

Page CD, Haddad K. 1995. Coccidial infections in birds. Semin Avian Exotic Pet Med 4:138–144.

Phalen DN, Wilson VG, Graham DL. 1991. Epidemiology and diagnosis of avian polyomavirus infection. In: Proceedings of the Association of Avian Veterinarians, Chicago, IL, pp 27–31.

Phalen DN, Wilson VG, Graham DL. 1994. A practitioner's, guide to avian polyomavirus testing and disease. In: Proceedings of the Association of Avian Veterinarians, Reno, NV, pp 251–257.

Phalen DN, Wilson VG, Gaskin JM, et al. 1999. Genetic diversity in twenty variants of the avian polyomavirus. Avian Dis 43:207–218.

Poonacha DB, Williams PD, Stamper RD. 1985. Encephalitozoonosis in a parrot. J Am Vet Med Assoc 186:700–702.

Rae M. 1995. Hemoprotozoa of cages and aviary birds. Semin Avian Exotic Pet Med 4:131–137.

Raidal SR. 1995. Viral skin disease of birds. Semin Avian Exotic Pet Med 4:72–82.

Ramis A, Tarres J, Fondevila D, Ferrer L. 1996. Immunocytochemical study of the pathogenesis of Pacheco's parrot disease in budgerigars. Vet Microbiol 52:49–61.

Randall CJ, Lees S, Higgins RJ, Harcourt-Brown NH. 1986. Microsporidian infection in lovebirds (Agapornis spp.). Avian Pathol 15:223–231.

Reavill DR. 1996. Fungal diseases. In: Rosskopf W, Woerpel R, eds. Diseases of cage and aviary birds. Baltimore: Williams and Wilkins, pp 586–595.

Riddle C. 1987. Liver. In: Avian histopathology. Lawrence, KS: Allen, pp 57–65.

Ritchie BW. 1995. Avian viruses: Function and control. Lake Worth, FL: Wingers.

Rossi G. 1998. A poorly differentiated hepatic hemangiosarcoma in an Amazona farinosa parrot. Avian Pathol 27:427–430.

Saunders GK, Sponenberg DP, Marx KL. 1993. Tyzzer's disease in a neonatal cockatiel. Avian Dis 37:891–894.

Schmidt RE, Hubbard GB. 1987. Liver, gallbladder and pancreas. In: Atlas of zoo animal pathology, vol 2. Boca Raton, FL: CRC, pp 61–82.

Schmidt RE. 1992. Morphologic diagnosis of avian neoplasms. Semin Avian Exotic Pet Med 1:73–79.

Shane SM, Camus A, Strain MG, et al. 1993. Avian tuberculosis. Avian Dis 37:1172–1176.

Scaddings S, Ackerley SK. The virtual embryo. Development of the chick. http://www.uoguelph.ca/zoology/devobio/48hrchck/48ck26.htm.

Stephens CP, On SLW, Gibson JA. 1998. An outbreak of infectious hepatitis in commercially reared ostriches associated with Campylobacter coli and Campylobacter jejuni. Vet Microbiol 61:183–190.

Stoll R, Luo D, Kouwenhoven B, et al. 1993. Molecular and biological characteristics of avian polyomaviruses: Isolates from different species within the polyomavirus genus. J Gen Virol 74[Part 2]:229–237.

Sturkie PD. 1986. Avian physiology. New York: Springer-Verlag, pp 269–358.

Tully TN. 1993. Clinical aspects of companion bird chlamydial infections. Semin Avian Exotic Pet Med 2:157–160.

Vanrompay D, Ducatelle R, Haesebrouck F. 1995. Chlamydia psittaci infections: A review with emphasis on avian chlamydiosis. Vet Microbiol 45:93–119.

Vaughan JL, Charles JA, Boray JC. 1997. Fasciola hepatica infection in farmed emus (Dromaius novaehollandiae). Aust Vet J 75:811–813.

Wadsworth PF, Majeed SK, Brancker WM, Jones DM. 1978. Some hepatic neoplasms in non-domesticated birds. Avian Pathol 7:551–555.

Wilson RB, Holscher M, Hodges JR, Thomas S. 1985. Necrotizing hepatitis associated with a reo-like virus infection in a parrot. Avian Dis 29:568–571.

Woods LW, Plumlee KH. 1999. Avian toxicoses: Veterinary diagnostic laboratory perspective. Semin Avian Exotic Pet Med 8:32–35.

Young P. 1997. Selected herpesviral diseases of birds. Semin Avian Exotic Pet Med 4:62–71.

Zinke A, Kahnt K, Kaup FJ, Kummerfeld N. 1999. Chronic-active hepatitis in a blue-fronted Amazon (Amazona aestiva aestiva): Clinical, laboratory and morphological findings. Kleintierpraxis 44:447–451.

5 Urinary System

NORMAL STRUCTURE

Kidney

Avian kidneys are bilaterally symmetrical and lie within ventral depressions of the synsacrum that are known as the renal fossae. They are retroperitoneal and firmly fixed in place. Nerves from the lumbar and sacral plexi pass through the kidney, a feature that can lead to secondary neurologic problems with renal neoplasia or other lesions that impinge on these nerves. The kidneys are divided into the cranial, middle, and caudal divisions. The size and shape of these divisions are fairly consistent in psittacine birds but vary considerably in other species. In most passerine species, the middle division is fused with the caudal division. The caudal divisions are fused on the midline in herons, puffins, and penguins. Attenuation between divisions is reported in Old World Columbidae, Coraciidae, Cuculidae, and Strigidae. Hornbills have distinctly separate cranial and caudal divisions, with no intervening middle division. The kidneys represent approximately 1% of body weight in small birds and somewhat less in large birds.

There are three pairs of renal arteries: the cranial, the middle, and the caudal. The cranial artery is a branch of the aorta, and the middle and caudal arteries originate from the ischiadic arteries. The external iliac artery crosses the kidney at the separation of the cranial and middle divisions. The ischiadic artery crosses the kidney at the junction of the middle and caudal divisions. Each artery supplies its respective division of the kidneys. The caudal renal veins receive drainage from the intralobular veins. The caudal renal vein joins the external iliac vein to form a common trunk that runs across the cranial pole of the kidney. The two iliac veins then join to form the caudal vena cava.

The most unique aspect of the avian kidney vasculature is the renal portal system. The joining of the paired external iliac veins and the caudal renal veins forms this vascular ring. Additionally, blood can flow into or out of the renal portal veins through the caudal mesenteric vein, the internal iliac vein, and the internal vertebral venous sinus. Branches from the portal ring supply the interlobular veins.

Microscopically the avian kidney is divided into independently functioning units called lobules. The unit comprised of all the lobules draining into a common secondary branch of the ureter is the called the lobe. Individual lobes may cross divisions. Lobules are distributed throughout the kidney and may contact the surface of the kidney or are completely embedded within the kidney. Each lobule has a cortex and medullary cone. In cross section, the cortex is defined by a central (intralobular) vein and peripheral interlobular veins. The intralobular veins empty into the capillary sinus that surrounds the cortical tubules. Midway between these veins is a branch of the intralobular renal artery. Afferent arterioles that feed the glomeruli arise from branches of the intralobular renal artery.

Birds have two types of nephrons: the reptilian type and the mammalian type. All of the components of the reptilian-type nephrons remain within the cortex. The reptilian-type proximal convoluted tubules loop out away from the glomerulus toward the interlobular veins and back. Each tubule then comes in contact with its afferent arteriole, forming the juxtaglomerular complex before becoming the distal convoluted tubule. The distal convoluted tubule loops toward the central vein and back, becoming a collecting tubule. The mammalian-type nephron begins with a glomerulus that is located at the junction of the cortex and the medullary cone. Its proximal convoluted tubule extends from the glomerulus and makes a loop in the cortex toward the interlobular vein before descending into the medullary cone to form the nephronal loop. The straight descending section narrows to form a thin segment and then abruptly widens to form the thick ascending segment. The thick limb comes in contact with its afferent artery, forming the juxtaglomerular complex. It then becomes the distal convoluted tubule and follows the same pattern as the reptilian-type nephron. Blood from the efferent arterioles of both the reptilian-type and the mammalian-type glomeruli empties into the capillary sinus, which drains into the intralobar veins. Proximal tubules are lined by cuboidal to columnar epithelium with a well-developed brush border. Cells decrease in size and the cytoplasm becomes basophilic in Henle's loop and distal tubules. Distal tubules also have a narrower lumen and no brush border. Surrounding the lobule are the perilobular collecting ducts, which run parallel to the interlobular veins and drain the collecting tubules. Thus the arrangement of the cortex of a lobule from edge to center is as follows: a surrounding network of interlobular veins and proximal collecting ducts, a peripheral zone composed primarily of proximal convoluted tubules, a zone of glomeruli, and a zone between the glomeruli and the central vein composed primarily of distal convoluted tubules.

The medullary cones are comprised of collecting ducts descending from the cortex and the nephronal loops of the mammalian-type nephrons. In passerine birds, this arrangement is highly structured with a central core of nephronal loops and a peripheral margin of collecting ducts. These elements may intermingle in other species of birds. Avian collecting ducts are dendritic, continuously joining until they become a secondary branch of the ureter.

The appearance of the avian glomerulus is structurally similar to the mammalian glomerulus, but there are several important differences. Mesangial cells, in the avian kidney, are more numerous and are clumped at the vascular pole, instead of the more diffuse distribution seen in the mammalian glomerulus.

Additionally there are fewer capillary loops, and the capillary loops are less convoluted in the avian glomerulus.

Ureter

The ureter begins in the cranial division of the kidney and continues caudally in a groove on the ventral renal surface. It receives multiple primary branches, which in turn are made up of secondary branches, each of which drains the collecting ducts of the renal lobes. The ureter is stellate in cross section and is lined by mucus-secreting, pseudostratified columnar epithelium. Its wall contains fibrous connective tissue and smooth muscle. Each ureter terminates in the urodeum of the cloaca.

SYSTEMIC EFFECTS OF RENAL FAILURE

The predominant nitrogenous waste product produced by birds is uric acid. The majority of uric acid is actively secreted by the proximal tubules. The remaining 10% is filtered by the glomerulus. Severe dehydration, extensive damage to the proximal tubules, lesions that obstruct urine outflow, or congenital malformations of the kidney are necessary for the development of uricemia. Elevations in plasma uric acid levels secondary to kidney failure result in gout, the precipitation of uric acid crystals on mesothelial surfaces and within the kidney. These lesions may be nodular (urate tophi), such as those that are found on synovial surfaces, or they may be diffuse, such as those found in the pericardium, liver capsule, air sacs, and peritoneum. Affected surfaces are chalky white, as are the contents of the urate tophi. Articular gout also occurs, but

this lesion is not necessarily the result of hyperuricemia, and renal lesions may not be present.

RENAL DISEASE

Congenital Disease

Renal hypoplasia or aplasia occurs sporadically in birds. It may be unilateral with no clinical signs and is often diagnosed as an incidental necropsy finding. Divisional aplasia is common in some breeds of chickens. The cranial division is most likely to be absent. The middle and caudal divisions are less commonly affected. Compensatory hypertrophy of the opposite kidney is generally present.

Renal cysts may be solitary or multiple. The condition usually results from failure of fusion of the cortical portions of the tubule with collecting tubules of ureteral origin. If the lesion is severe, the result will be renal failure. Cysts usually have smooth borders grossly, and histologically flattened epithelial cells line the dilated tubules (Fig. 5.1). Glomerular hypervascularity has been reported in canaries. It leads to glomerular deformation but does not result in immediate renal failure.

A normal finding in some recently hatched birds is the persistence of embryonic tissue, which is distributed on the periductal margins of the lobule and consists of densely clustered, newly differentiated glomeruli and undifferentiated tubules.

Infectious Disease

Viral Disease. Adenoviruses and the avian polyomavirus commonly affect the avian kidney. Birds dying of a psittacid herpesvirus infection (Pacheco's disease) will uncommonly have inclusion bodies in the renal tubular epithelium.

Adenovirus infection of the kidney is seen in a variety of psittacine birds. Grossly there may be some nonspecific renal enlargement. Microscopic lesions are usually minimal, varying from mild interstitial mononuclear cell infiltration to tubular epithelial cell vacuolation and necrosis.

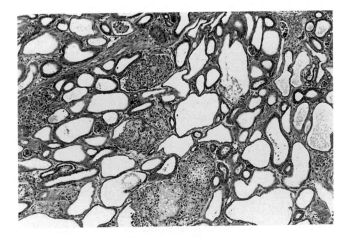

5.1. *Polycystic kidney with multiple cystic tubules.*

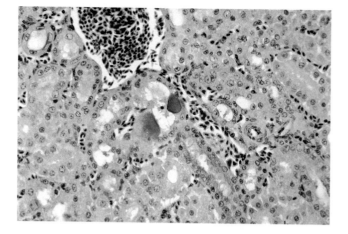

5.2. Large intranuclear inclusion bodies in renal tubular epithelial cells. These bodies are typical of adenovirus infection.

Scattered tubular epithelial cells have karyomegalic nuclei containing large, darkly eosinophilic or basophilic inclusion bodies (Fig. 5.2). In some birds, particularly budgerigars and cockatiels, the only lesion may be large intranuclear inclusion bodies in tubular epithelial cells. Viral particles can be seen by electron microscopy (Fig. 5.3). Adenovirus infections in lovebirds are often found incidentally at necropsy. Most of these birds have only a few widely scattered inclusions.

Polyomavirus infection may cause the kidneys to be slightly swollen. Histologically, in budgerigars, renal tubular epithelial cells may have karyomegaly, with affected nuclei containing clear or amophophilic, slightly granular inclusion bodies. These can be differentiated from those of adenovirus by their tinctorial properties.

Both primary and secondary lesions may occur in nonbudgerigar psittacine birds with avian polyomavirus disease. Intranuclear inclusion bodies and accompanying karyomegaly are commonly seen in mesangial cells (Fig. 5.4). Mesangial cell necrosis is also common. Glomeruli will appear swollen due to capillary endothelial cell swelling. Up to 70% of these birds will develop a secondary glomerulopathy. This lesion is caused by the deposition of dense aggregates of immune complexes. All contain immunoglobulin G and viral antigen. Less commonly they also contain immunoglobulin M. These aggregates, which are strongly periodic acid-Schiff positive, are found predominantly within the capillary lumens and the mesangium (Fig. 5.5). Subendothelial deposits may also occur to a lesser extent. The immune complexes may be so massive as to occlude the capillary lumens completely. Minimal interstitial nonsuppurative inflammation is occasionally seen. The glomerulopathy is consistent with a type III hypersensitivity reaction.

Finches with polyomavirus infection may have both renal tubular epithelial and mesangial karyomegaly with intranuclear inclusion bodies. Chronic renal disease with glomerular sclerosis is seen in Gouldian finches that survived acute polyomavirus infection.

One of us (D.N.P.) has observed a disease characterized by ascites and anasarca that is seen uncommonly in several species of nonbudgerigar parrots. All birds are positive by polymerase chain reaction for avian polyomavirus infection. Renal lesions include a proliferative glomerulopathy and glomerular sclerosis, lesions expected if a bird were to survive the acute form of avian polyomavirus disease. The anasarca and ascites are attributed to a protein-losing nephropathy and/or decreased hepatic production of albumin following avian polyomavirus-induced hepatic necrosis.

Nonsuppurative inflammation may be present in the renal interstitium in other viral infections, including reovirus and paramyxovirus. Paramyxovirus 1 in pigeons may cause an interstitial lymphoplasmacytic nephritis and tubular necrosis with granular and hyaline casts present in the tubules. West Nile virus causes a variable lymphoplasmacytic interstitial nephritis as part of generalized disease (Fig. 5.6).

Bacterial Disease. Bacteria can enter the kidney either by ascending the ureters or by hematogenous spread. In either type of infection, the kidneys may be grossly enlarged, with varying degrees of necrosis. Necrotic areas appear grossly as multifocal white-yellow foci within the renal parenchyma (Fig. 5.7). Initial hematogenous lesions may be present in glomeruli. Organisms may be seen associated with necrosis and a pleocellular inflammatory infiltrate. Fibrin thrombi suggestive of disseminated intravascular coagulation are sometimes noted (Fig. 5.8).

Acute ascending infections that are characterized by abundant bacteria are found in tubules and occasionally in the interstitium. Necrosis of the tubular epithelium is prominent, but inflammation is minimal or nonexistent. Distal collecting tubules and cortical collecting ducts are primarily affected while the medullary areas are spared. Subacute ascending infections have a marked inflammatory response, with heterophils in the lumen of the tubules, degeneration of the tubule epithelium, and a moderate to severe heterophilic and early mononuclear interstitial nephritis (Fig. 5.9). Tubulointerstitial lesions are locally extensive and generally spare the glomeruli and the medulla in the affected lobules. With severe locally extensive lesions, it may be difficult to determine whether the infection began in the tubules and involved the interstitium or began in the interstitium and involved the tubules.

Bacteremia and septicemia commonly occur in a number of avian bacterial infections. Birds dying of overwhelming bacterial infections may have bacteria in both the renal veins and the arteries. For unexplained reasons, bacterial localization in the kidney may predominate in the cortical venous sinuses. Alternately, bacteria may be seen only in the glomeruli. Previous or ongoing bacteremias may result in subacute to chronic multifocal to locally extensive interstitial nephritis. These lesions are initially heterophilic but rapidly become granulomatous with necrosis and fibrosis.

A wide range of gram-positive and gram-negative bacteria are known to cause kidney disease, either as an

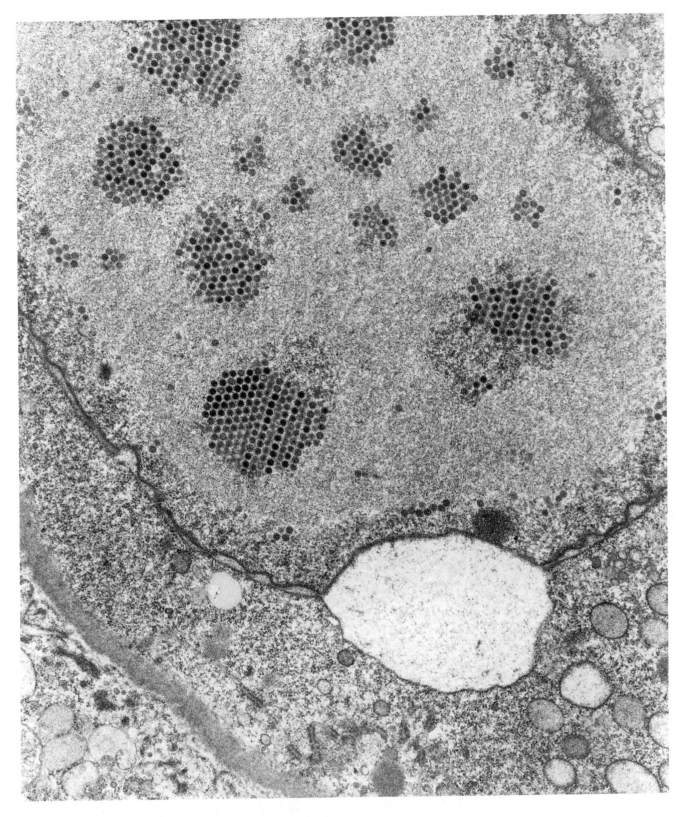

5.3. *Adenoviral particles in renal tubular epithelial cell nucleus.*

ascending infection or as part of a systemic disease. Staphylococci and streptococci are common pathogens in finches and canaries but are also reported to cause disease in psittacine birds. Other bacteria that can affect the kid-ney include members of Enterobacteriaceae, *Listeria* sp., *Erysipelothrix rhusiophathiae*, and *Pasteurella* sp.

Mycobacterial and *Chlamydophila psittaci* infections are generally systemic. They can cause lesions in the kidney

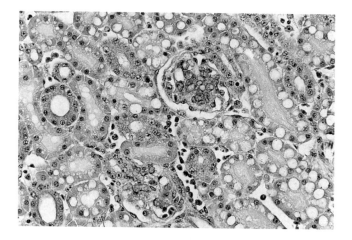

5.4. Polyomavirus infection. Glomerular mesangial cells have karyomegalic nuclei with pale intranuclear inclusion body formation and chromatin margination.

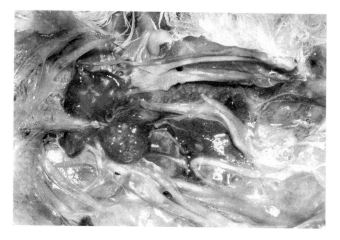

5.7. Severe nephritis due to bacterial infection. The enlarged kidneys have multiple yellow foci.

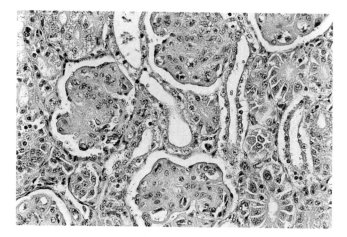

5.5. Membranous glomerulonephritis as a chronic change in polyomavirus infection. Glomerular capillary basement membranes are thickened.

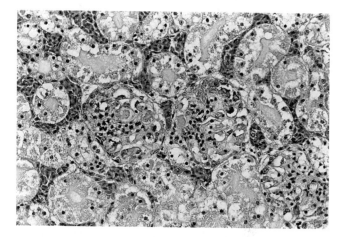

5.8. Glomerular hypercellularity and small fibrin thrombi associated with bacterial sepsis.

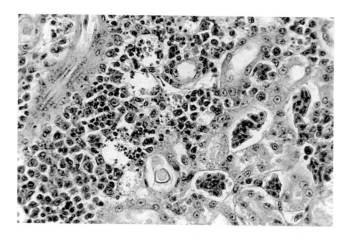

5.6. Nonsuppurative interstitial nephritis as a part of generalized West Nile virus infection.

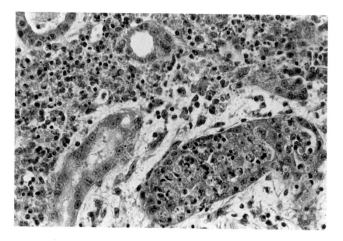

5.9. Bacterial nephritis with severe necrosis and inflammation involving tubules and interstitium.

99

but often do not. Mycobacterial lesions are similar to those found in other tissues; they include numerous macrophages and giant cells that contain acid-fast bacteria. Necrosis and abscess formation are not always present, particularly early in the disease. Lesions caused by *C. psittaci* are characterized by interstitial inflammation comprised primarily of histiocytes, plasma cells, and lymphocytes. Intracytoplasmic organisms are seen in histiocytes in some cases. Tubular involvement is variable.

Mycotic Disease. Fungal infection of the kidney occurs either as an extension of a fungal infection of abdominal air sacs or as a component of systemic infection where a fungus has invaded a vessel, resulting in fungal thrombosis of blood vessels. Fungal infections elicit a severe necrotizing inflammation with a pleocellular reaction involving blood vessels and renal parenchyma. Fungal hyphae in the lesion give it specificity.

Parasitic Disease. *Isospora* and *Eimeria* are found in the kidneys of nearly all species of wild ducks and geese. They are also commonly found in shorebirds and are less commonly seen in birds of prey. Organisms are predominantly found in the epithelium of perilobular collecting ducts and medullary collecting tract. Lesions in adult birds are minimal, with occasional obstruction of and dilation of the tubules and a mild lymphocytic and monocytic interstitial nephritis. *Eimeria truncata* can cause a more severe disease in juvenile waterfowl. Gross changes are often absent. Histologically there is variable tubular necrosis. Organisms are found in tubular epithelial cells or free in the lumen associated with inflammatory cells and necrotic debris (Fig. 5.10).

Cryptosporidial infection of the kidney of birds is rare. Grossly kidneys appear swollen and pale. There may be slight proliferation of tubular epithelial cells, and organisms are present on the surface of these cells. Necrotic cells are noted in the tubular lumens. An interstitial infiltrate of mononuclear cells and heterophils may be present.

Encephalitozoon hellem is a potential cause of nephritis (see chapter 4). Lesions are most commonly seen in lovebirds and budgerigars. Gross changes may be absent, or small pale foci may be present in the renal parenchyma. Histologically both cortical and medullary tubules are affected, but organisms predominate in the distal tubules. Necrosis and a mononuclear interstitial inflammatory response characterize the lesion (Fig. 5.11). Small protozoal organisms are present in cells and may be free in the necrotic foci and the lumen of the tubules. Infected cells are distended with the organisms. In chronic cases, there may be tubular hypertrophy. It is also fairly common to find the organisms in the kidney with little, if any, associated inflammation. These organisms are strongly gram positive.

Systemic sarcosporidial infection can lead to interstitial nephritis with an infiltrate that is primarily lymphoplasmacytic (Fig. 5.12). Organisms are usually not seen. Schizonts of *Leukocytozoon* can also be found in the kidney (Fig. 5.13).

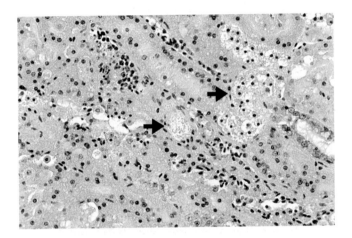

5.11.   Renal microsporidiosis. Minimal interstitial inflammation and aggregates of organisms are seen (arrows).

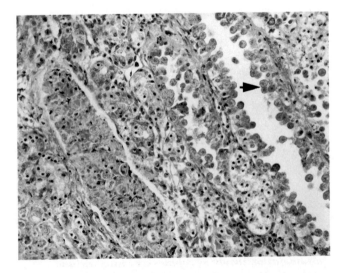

5.10.   Renal coccidiosis (Eimeria sp.). Variable tubular necrosis and numerous organisms are seen (arrowhead).

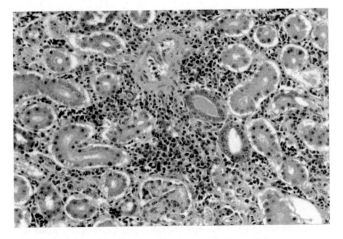

5.12.   Interstitial nephritis in a bird with systemic sarcosporidiosis. Organisms are rarely seen in the kidney in birds with this condition.

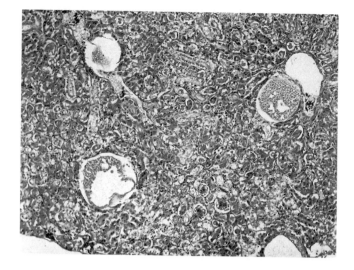

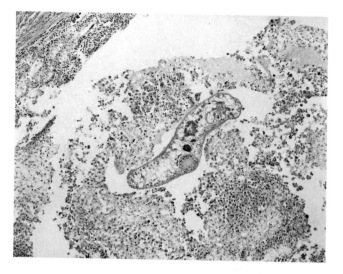

5.13.   Megaloschizonts of Leukocytozoon *in the renal parenchyma.*

5.15.   Necrosis and inflammation associated with renal trematodiasis.

Trematodes may be incidental findings or lead to clinical renal disease in some birds. These infections are most common in waterfowl. The flukes are found in collecting tubules in the medullary cone (Fig. 5.14). Affected tubules are dilated, and there is usually minimal or no inflammation. Severe infections result in obstruction of the tubules, variable inflammation, and necrosis and secondary dilatation proximal to the block (Fig. 5.15).

Schistosomiasis is common in waterfowl. These intravascular trematodes lay eggs that are trapped in small vessels, creating a foreign-body reaction and granuloma formation.

Inflammatory Disease of Undetermined Cause

Except as a sequela to polyomavirus infection (previously discussed), immune-complex glomerulonephritis is not well documented in birds. Based on cases examined by the authors (R.E.S. and D.R.R.), we believe it does occur.

In addition to the membranous glomerulonephritis described, we have seen examples of proliferative glomerulonephritis with hypercellularity of the glomerular tufts (Fig. 5.16), and membranoproliferative glomerulonephritis. In chronic cases, there may be proliferation of parietal epithelium and glomerular crescent formation (Fig. 5.17). Eventually there is glomerular shrinkage, fibrous connective tissue proliferation, and sclerosis (Fig. 5.18).

Noninfectious Disease

Dehydration. Dehydration results in reduced urine flow and sludging of the urate crystals within the tubules. If the dehydration is transient, this lesion is reversible. Persistent dehydration results in renal failure. Gross lesions are characterized by multifocal white to yellow-white foci or streaks that represent urate deposits (Fig. 5.19). The gross appearance is similar to that of mineralization and

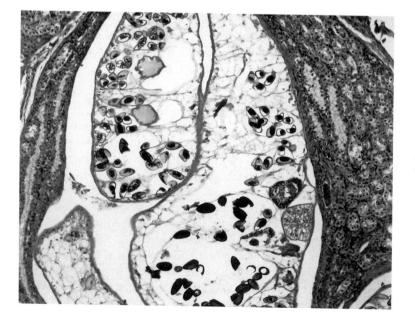

5.14.   Severe dilatation of a collecting tubule containing a trematode.

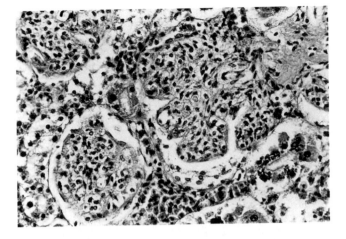

5.16. Hypercellularity of the glomerular tufts consistent with probable immune-mediated proliferative glomerulonephritis.

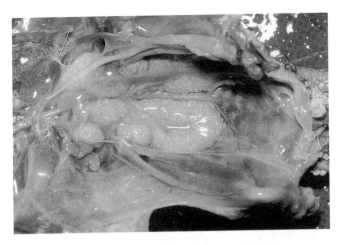

5.19. Swollen, pale kidneys with severe urate deposition.

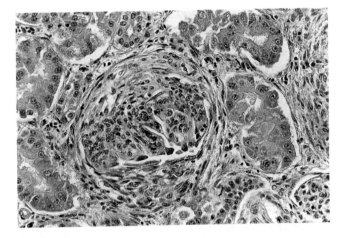

5.17. Severe chronic membranoproliferative glomerulonephritis with glomerular crescent formation.

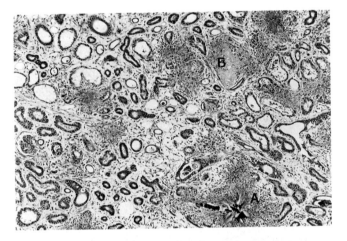

5.20. Severe renal urate deposition with both crystalline (A) and amorphous (B) urates noted.

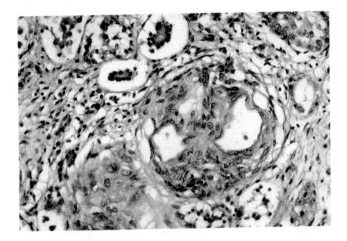

5.18. Severe chronic glomerulosclerosis.

severe nephritis; therefore histology is necessary for differentiation. Microscopically the urates will be dissolved during the fixation process but will leave behind the characteristic needle-shaped and amorphous spaces surrounded by an eosinophilic protein matrix where the

crystals had been. Secondary epithelial necrosis occurs, and the urate crystals induce inflammation that is primarily heterophilic (Fig. 5.20).

Disorders of protein metabolism may lead to elevation of uric acid. However, whether this in turn can result in urate deposition has not been proved.

Nutritional Disease. Metastatic mineralization of the kidney is a common lesion in nestling parrots and, to a lesser extent, in adult birds. It may vary from mild to severe, resulting in renal failure and systemic gout. This disease disproportionately affects nestling budgerigars, cockatiels, and blue and gold macaws. A nutritional imbalance is suspected. Experimentally diets containing 0.7% calcium or more cause metastatic mineralization of the kidney in nestling and adult budgerigars. Diets containing 0.3% calcium do not cause metastatic mineralization in this species of bird and are adequate for reproduction and growth. Vitamin D_3 concentrations ranging from 500 to 3300 IU/kg of diet did not result in metastatic mineralization in the low-calcium diet.

Mild cases of metastatic mineralization do not cause gross lesions. Advanced cases are grossly indistinguishable from severe nephritis or nephrosis associated with dehydration. Histologically mineralization occurs on the basement membranes of the tubules and within the tubules themselves. The mineral deposits are deeply basophilic and are round to crescent shaped. Necrosis of the tubular epithelium occurs when the mineralization is severe (Fig. 5.21). Inflammation may be absent, but, in some extensive lesions, mineralized tissue elicits a foreign-body reaction (Fig. 5.22). Renal failure follows, with urate precipitation in the kidneys, the development of a more extensive interstitial nephritis, and fibrosis.

Amyloidosis. Renal amyloidosis is most frequently observed in waterfowl and small passerine birds (chapter 4). Multiple organs, in addition to the kidney, are generally involved. Grossly there may be no discernible change, but, in severe cases, the kidneys are enlarged, pale, and

somewhat friable. Histologically amyloid is eosinophilic or amphophilic and may be deposited in glomerular or tubular basement membranes and the walls of renal arteries and arterioles (Fig. 5.23).

Vitamin Deficiency. Vitamin A deficiency leads to squamous metaplasia of the epithelium of the ureters and collecting ducts that in advanced cases results in the ureteral epithelium being transformed to a keratinized epithelium (Fig. 5.24). Partial or complete obstruction of the ureters follows. Tubule dilation and intratubular and interstitial urate crystal deposition occur. Secondary bacterial infections are also common.

Lipidosis. Renal lipidosis can be secondary to a high-fat diet or chronic hepatic disease. The latter is relatively common in Amazon parrots and cockatiels that have a high incidence of chronic-active hepatitis. Grossly the

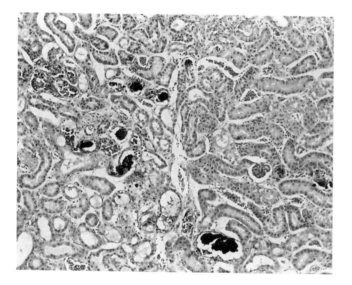

5.21. Multiple foci of renal mineralization involving tubules.

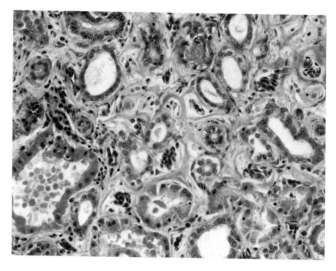

5.23. Amyloid deposition leading to thickened basement membranes and interstitium.

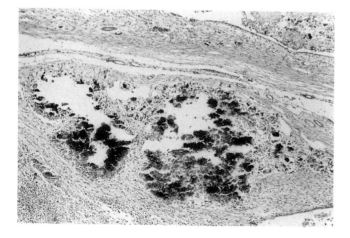

5.22. Severe mineralization and chronic inflammation and fibrosis involving the renal collecting duct.

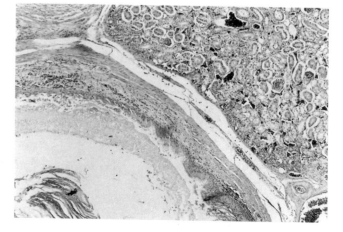

5.24. Squamous metaplasia and keratinization due to vitamin A deficiency. The affected collecting duct is markedly dilated.

kidneys are pale, and microscopically there is fat in tubular epithelial cells. Lipid-containing macrophages are usually present in glomerular capillaries.

Myoglobinuric nephrosis is possible as a sequela to exertional rhabdomyolysis or severe crushing injury to muscle, but this condition is rarely seen in common pet birds. The kidneys may be dark brown. Tubular degeneration and lumenal accumulation of amorphous eosinophilic material resembling myoglobin are seen microscopically in proximal convoluted tubules, and eosinophilic casts are noted in collecting tubules. Hemoglobinuric nephrosis is also possible but also infrequent due to the rarity of hemolytic disease in birds. Lesions would be similar.

Bile pigments are commonly found in the proximal tubules of birds with hepatitis. Polyuria is a common clinical feature of birds with biliverdinuria, but whether biliverdin has a physiologic affect on the kidney is not known.

Iron-storage disease (chapter 4) primarily affects the liver, but iron pigment is also seen in renal tubular cells in many affected birds. The iron does not cause an inflammatory or degenerative response (Fig. 5.25).

Toxic Nephropathies

Most renal toxins cause similar gross and histologic lesions, and therefore a definitive etiologic diagnosis is often not possible based on histopathologic changes alone. Grossly kidneys may be swollen and pale. They contain fine white to pale yellow linear striations that represent tubules dilated with urates. Numerous pinpoint, multifocal, white to pale yellow foci will also be present on the serosal and cut surfaces of the kidney.

Microscopically there is proximal tubule necrosis, proteinuria, tubule dilation, and urate tophi formation within the interstitium. If the insult was transient, the proximal tubules may regenerate. In acute cases, there will be little inflammation. If the bird survives for some time, the urate crystals may elicit an inflammatory response.

Interstitial fibrosis and glomerular sclerosis develop with chronicity.

Rodenticides. Vitamin D_3 and vitamin D_3-analog-based rodenticides are toxic to birds. These rodenticides cause increased intestinal absorption of calcium and a hypercalcemia. There may also be decreased urinary calcium excretion. Calcium is deposited in soft tissues, including the kidney. Affected kidneys are enlarged, firm, and contain numerous yellow-white foci (Fig. 5.26). There is variable renal tubular damage, with mineralization of tubular basement membranes. Necrotic epithelial cells and secondary urate deposition are seen.

Aminoglycosides. Gentamicin sulfate and amikacin are two aminoglycoside antibiotics that are commonly used in birds. Gentamicin sulfate is more nephrotoxic than is amikacin. Aminoglycoside toxicity results in kidney enlargement and changes resembling other causes of renal failure. Histologically there is tubular epithelial necrosis and secondary urate deposition and inflammation.

Heavy Metals. Lead and zinc toxicity both can cause acute tubular necrosis. Gross changes vary from none to swollen pale kidneys. Histologic lesions are similar to those previously described for other toxins. Occasionally, acid-fast intranuclear inclusion bodies are seen in some birds with lead toxicity. Cadmium, mercury, and arsenic also are nephrotoxic, but this type of poisoning would only be expected in wild birds.

Mycotoxins. Several mycotoxins, including oosporein, citrinin, and ochratoxin, have been shown to cause disease in poultry or domestic waterfowl. Gross lesions resemble those of other toxins, or there may be no gross lesion at all. Histologically there may be acute necrosis of tubular epithelial cells, followed by hypertrophy and hyperplasia of other cells. Aflatoxins cause degeneration of the proximal convoluted tubules and thickening of glomerular basement membranes.

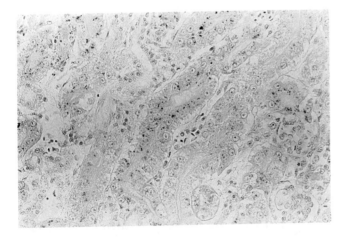

5.25. Deposition of iron in tubular epithelial cells of a toucan with an iron metabolic disorder. Prussian blue.

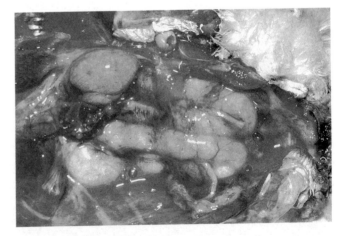

5.26. Renal swelling and discoloration secondary to vitamin D toxicity.

Salt. Excessive salt ingestion leads to renal problems that result in urate deposition and gross and histologic changes as previously described. It is documented in birds but rarely diagnosed in pet species.

Physical/Other Nephropathies

Acute Hypoxia/Ischemia. These changes are usually related to a localized or generalized vascular problem. The results are tubular necrosis, proteinuria, and urate deposition. Lesions are similar to the various problems discussed under metabolic disorders, and differential diagnoses include many of these conditions.

Hemorrhage. Renal hemorrhage may be secondary to trauma, ischemia, or a variety of primary disease conditions. The hemorrhage may be visible grossly and can affect both the interstitium and the tubules.

Renal Fibrosis. The end result of many of the aforementioned conditions can be chronic renal disease (end-stage kidney failure) with severe fibrosis (Fig. 5.27).

Neoplastic Disease

Renal tumors are reported in many species of birds but are particularly common in the budgerigar. Renal carcinoma is the most common tumor of the kidney, but adenoma, nephroblastoma, cystadenoma, fibrosarcoma, and lymphosarcoma are also reported to occur in the avian kidney.

The most common presenting sign of renal neoplasia is unilateral or bilateral lameness or paralysis. These signs result from compression of the roots of the ischiadic nerve as they pass through the kidney or from tumor growth into and adjacent to the synsacrum and ilium.

Renal adenomas are usually localized nodular swellings often in the cranial pole of the kidney. They are light tan to white and fluctuant. Histologically they are comprised of tubular structures lined by fairly well differ-

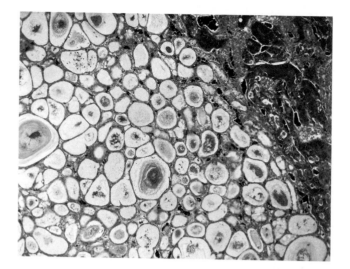

5.28. *Well-differentiated tubular structures in renal adenoma.*

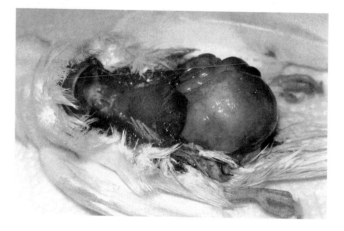

5.29. *Typical renal carcinoma that has become very large and displaced the abdominal viscera.*

entiated epithelial cells. There is usually slight to moderate stroma (Fig. 5.28). Renal carcinomas are large, somewhat friable, and vary from tan to red-brown (Fig. 5.29). Microscopically they are comprised of anaplastic epithelial cells forming tubules, nests, and sheets, usually with minimal stroma (Figs. 5.30 and 5.31). Extension into surrounding tissue is seen, and metastasis to the lung and liver is occasionally seen (chapters 3 and 4).

Embryonal nephromas (nephroblastomas) are most commonly reported in chickens but are also found in psittacine and small passerine birds. They are usually unilateral, but may be bilateral, and are grossly similar to carcinomas. Histologically there are tubules and glomerular-like structures as well as sheets of undifferentiated epithelial cells (Fig. 5.32). The latter may predominate in some cases. Some tumors have abundant amounts of stroma.

Lymphosarcoma may be isolated to the kidney but usually is a part of generalized neoplastic disease. Grossly

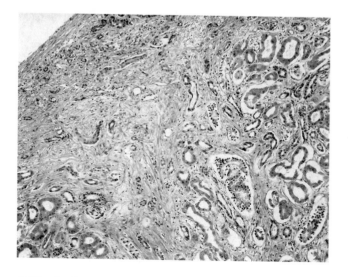

5.27. *End-stage renal disease with marked fibrosis. This can be the result of various insults.*

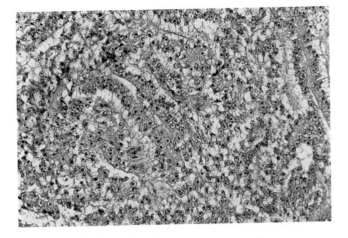

5.30. *One of the histologic presentations of renal carcinoma with poorly defined tubular structures and minimal stroma.*

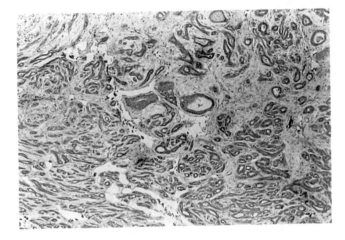

5.31. *Anaplastic renal carcinoma with marked scirrhous stroma.*

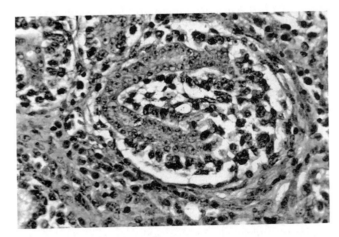

5.32. *Glomerular-like structures in nephroblastoma. Abundant stroma is present.*

the kidneys are pale and may appear mottled. They are moderately firm. The cell infiltration is either nodular or diffuse, with renal tissue effaced by immature lymphoid cells. Plasma cell tumors and myeloproliferative disease are also seen in the kidney, being grossly similar to lym-

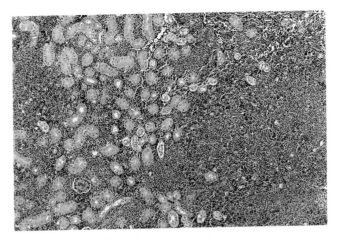

5.33. *Effacement of renal parenchyma by neoplastic myeloid cells. Lymphosarcoma has a similar appearance at low magnification.*

phosarcoma. Histologically there is parenchymal effacement, and diagnosis is based on the morphology of the infiltrating cells (Fig. 5.33).

Other primary sarcomas are possible but are rarely reported, and metastatic tumors are infrequent.

Metastatic tumors are not usually seen in the kidney, with the exception of malignant melanoma. Grossly there may be brown-black foci and masses. Microscopically, neoplastic cells are noted infiltrating the renal interstitium (Fig. 5.34).

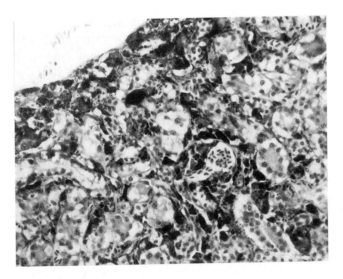

5.34. *Metastatic malignant melanoma. Neoplastic cells are infiltrating the interstitium.*

ADDITIONAL READING

Coleman CW, Oliver R. 1994. Lymphosarcoma in a juvenile blue and gold macaw (*Ara araruana*) and a mature canary (*Serinus canarius*). J Assoc Avian Vet 8:64–68.

Cross G. 1995. Paramyxovirus-1 infection (Newcastle disease) of pigeons. Semin Avian Exotic Pet Med 4:92–95.

Flammer K, Clark CH, Drewes LA, et al. 1990. Adverse effects of gentamicin in scarlet macaws and galahs. Am J Vet Res 51:404–407.

Gardiner CH, Imes GD. 1984 *Cryptosporidium* sp. in the kidneys of a black-throated finch. J Am Vet Med Assoc 185:1401–1402.

Glahn RP. 1993. Mycotoxins and the avian kidney: Assessment of physiological function. Worlds Poult Sci J 49:242–250.

Graham DL. 1993. A color atlas of avian chlamydiosis. Semin Avian Exotic Pet Med 2:184–189.

Holz P, Phelan J, Slocombe R, et al. 2000. Zinc toxicosis as a cause of sudden death in orange-bellied parrots (*Neophema chrysogaster*). J Avian Med Surg 14:37–41

Johnson OW. 1979. Urinary organs. In: King AS, McLelland J, eds. Form and function in birds, vol 1. New York: Academic Press, pp 183–235.

King AS, McLelland J. 1984. Urinary system. In: Birds: Their structure and function. London: Bailliere Tindall, pp 175–186.

LaBonde J. 1995. Toxicity in pet avian patients. Semin Avian Exotic Pet Med 4:23–31.

McLelland J. 1991. Urogenital system. In: A color atlas of avian anatomy. Philadelphia: WB Saunders, pp 66–84.

Mori F, Touchi A, Suwa T, et al. 1989. Inclusion bodies containing adenovirus-like particles in the kidneys of psittacine birds. Avian Pathol 18:197–202.

Page CD, Haddad K. 1995. Coccidial infections in birds. Semin Avian Exotic Pet Med 4:136–144.

Phalen DN, Wilson VG, Graham DL. 1996. Characterization of the avian polyomavirus-associated glomerulopathy of nestling parrots. Avian Dis 40:140–149.

Schmidt RE. 1992. Morphologic diagnosis of avian neoplasms. Semin Avian Exotic Pet Med 1:73–79.

Schmidt RE, Hubbard GB. 1987. Atlas of zoo animal pathology, vol 2. Boca Raton, FL: CRC, pp 83–96.

Schoemaker NJ, Lumeij JT, Beyen AC. 1997 Polyuria and polydipsia due to vitamin and mineral oversupplementation of the diet of a Salmon Crested Cockatoo (*Cacatua moluccensis*) and a Blue and Gold Macaw (*Ara ararauna*). Avian Pathol 26:201–209.

Sturkie PD. 1986. Kidneys, extrarenal salt excretion and urine. In: Sturkie PD, ed. Avian physiology. New York: Springer-Verlag, pp 359–382.

Styles DK, Phalen DN. 1998. Clinical avian urology. Semin Avian Exotic Pet Med 7:104–113.

Zwart P, Vroege C, Boostsma R, et al. 1974. Glomerular hypervascularity: A congenital defect in a canary (*Serinus canarius*). Avian Pathol 3:59–60.

6 Reproductive System

MALE REPRODUCTIVE SYSTEM

Normal Structure

The reproductive system of the male bird is composed of the testes, the efferent ducts, in passerines the seminal glomus, and, in several unrelated birds, a phallus. The paired testes are located on the cranioventral aspect of the cranial pole of each kidney just to the right and left of the midline. The cranial pole of the testes also partially covers the ventral surface of the adrenal gland. When a bird is in breeding season, the enlarged testes will completely cover the ventral surface of the adrenal gland.

Immature testes are smooth and somewhat flattened. However, they always have a smooth surface and rounded cranial and caudal poles. Usually, in immature birds, the left testicle is larger than the right. As male birds become sexually mature and come into breeding season, the testes enlarge from 10 to 500 times. The fully mature testes is yellow and rounded but is longer than it is wide and has prominent capsular blood vessels. White cockatoos, the golden conure, the blue and gold macaw, some species of passerine birds, and the keel-billed toucan have melanoblasts in the testicular interstitium, causing the testicles to be grossly black. During the nonbreeding season, the testicles will become small again but will never be as small as they were when the bird was a juvenile. Histologically the testis is similar to that in mammals. During the nonbreeding season, a single layer of cells lines each seminiferous tubule. Transition to breeding season is marked by the proliferation of spermatogonia and the development of spermatocytes, secondary spermatocytes, spermatids, and sperm. Following breeding season, spermatocytes and Sertoli cells die, and their debris occludes the lumens of the seminiferous tubules.

The efferent ducts include the rete testis, the epididymis, and the ductus deferens. The epididymis is under hormonal control and enlarges during the breeding season. Unlike in mammals, it is not divided into a head, body, and tail. The ductus deferens connects the epididymis to the urodeum and runs across the ventral surface of the kidney. In the nonbreeding season, it is narrow and straight. It becomes torturous and distended with semen during the breeding season. At the distal end of the ductus deferens in passerine birds is the seminal glomus. This structure enlarges many times in breeding birds and is believed to store sperm during its final stages of maturation.

A copulating organ is seen only in waterfowl, screamers, cracids, ratites, kiwi, and tinamous. In the ostrich, kiwi, and tinamous, there is no cavity. There are right and left erectile fibrolymphatic bodies within the organ. Dorsal sleeves are present in which the vas deferens ejects semen. A ventral elastic body with an inner layer of erectile tissue is seen. In the emu, cassowary, rhea, and in anseriforms, there is a cavity. It is a blind-ending tube in anseriforms. The superficial portion of the cavity is lined internally by keratinized stratified squamous epithelium. There is an opening at the tip into the deep blind end of the tube.

Diseases of the Testicle

Congenital Disease. Congenital abnormalities of the testes are uncommon to rare. They include abnormally shaped testicles, fusion of the cranial poles of the testes, hypoplasia, and agenesis.

Noninflammatory Disease. Noninflammatory testicular lesions include degeneration and atrophy. Due to the seasonal variation in the size of the avian testis and presence or absence of spermatogenesis, changes in size of the testes or an abscess of spermatogenesis must be carefully interpreted. Atrophy can be the end result of a degenerative process and has been associated with generalized malnutrition and can be caused by vitamin E deficiency.

Degenerative changes will usually affect mature spermatozoa first, with eventual involvement of immature germinal cells and the formation of spermatidic giant cells (Fig. 6.1). Eventually there may be nothing but irregular empty tubules. Hemorrhage is occasionally seen (Fig. 6.2).

A variety of toxins affects avian testicles. The changes are primarily degenerative without inflammation. In general, there will be reduced spermatogenesis regardless of the toxic agent. Cystic degeneration of seminiferous tubules has been reported with furazolidone toxicity.

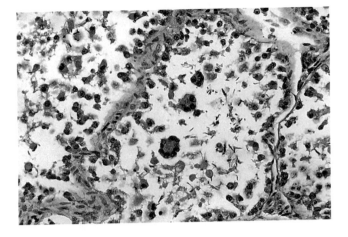

6.1. *Testicular degeneration with the formation of spermatidic giant cells. This is a nonspecific lesion whose cause is often not determined in individual cases.*

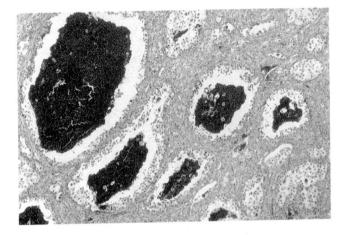

6.2. *Severe testicular degeneration with dilatation of tubules and hemorrhage.*

Copper fungicides can cause atrophy, and mercury has been reported to cause reproductive dysfunction.

Inflammatory Disease. Inflammatory disease of the testicle (orchitis) is not commonly reported but has been associated with a variety of causes. The characteristics of the lesion depend on the underlying cause. Bacterial and fungal infections may be due to extension from the peritoneal cavity or the air sacs, or these infections may be hematogenous. Mycobacterial and chlamydial infections are also seen as a part of a more generalized problem. Grossly the affected testicle is enlarged, reddened, and may contain yellow-white foci.

Histologically there is necrosis and a variable inflammatory cell infiltrate. In acute infections, heterophils predominate, with macrophages and giant cells seen in more chronic bacterial problems. Granulomatous lesions are predominantly associated with fungal or mycobacterial infections. Finding the specific organism within the lesion is necessary for an accurate etiologic diagnosis (Fig. 6.3).

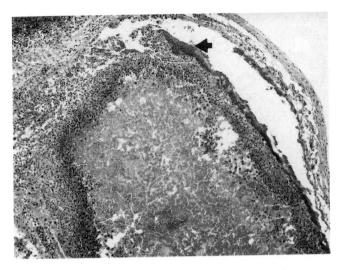

6.3. *Severe necrotizing orchitis. There is marked necrosis, inflammation, and bacterial colony formation (arrow).*

Neoplastic Disease. Tumors of the testicle cause obvious enlargement and usually abdominal distension. Reported tumors include seminoma, Sertoli cell tumor, interstitial cell tumor, lymphosarcoma, undifferentiated sarcoma, and teratoma. We have seen testicular tumors in several avian species, but, in our experience and that of others, the highest incidence of testicular neoplasia occurs in the budgerigar.

Seminomas are tumors of immature germ cells. Grossly they are yellow-red and cause enlargement of the testis (Fig. 6.4). On section, they are usually soft. Histologically the neoplastic cells are somewhat pleomorphic, with indistinct cytoplasmic boundaries and large vesicular nuclei (Fig. 6.5). There is minimal stroma, and there may be remnants of tubular architecture within the tumor.

Sertoli cell tumors are generally firm, gray-white neoplasms that may appear nodular on section. Cystic spaces

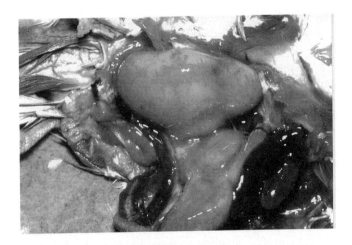

6.4. *Large seminoma that was displacing other abdominal organs. Note the smooth surface. Sertoli's cell tumors are usually firmer and more nodular grossly.*

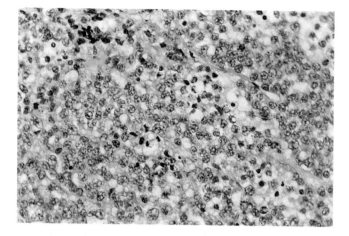

6.5. *Effacement of normal testicular architecture by neoplastic cells in seminoma.*

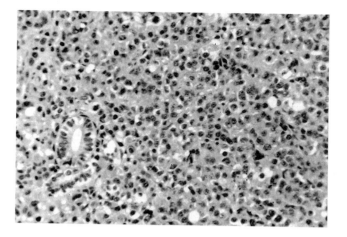

6.7. *Interstitial cell tumor. Tubules are effaced by a sheet of neoplastic cells with abundant cytoplasm.*

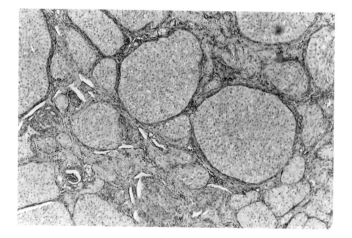

6.6. *Sertoli's cell tumor. Note the numerous tubular structures lined by neoplastic Sertoli's cells. There is abundant connective tissue stroma, which results in the gross firmness and nodularity.*

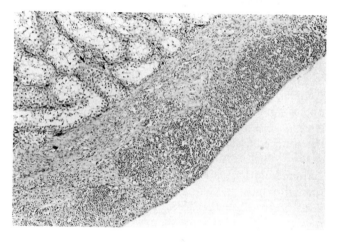

6.8. *Infiltration of the thickened testicular capsule by neoplastic lymphoid cells in lymphosarcoma.*

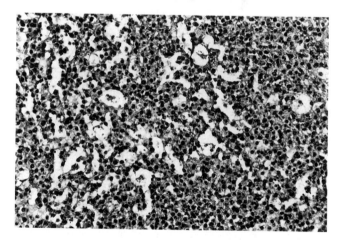

6.9. *Replacement of testicular parenchyma by neoplastic lymphoid cells. Note the similarity to seminoma.*

are sometimes present. Histologically there are numerous tubules containing pleomorphic immature Sertoli cells (Fig. 6.6). These tubules are separated by abundant stroma. Clinical signs of feminization, including a change in cere color from blue to brown in budgerigars, is reported in birds with Sertoli cell tumors.

Interstitial cell tumors may be cystic and are often orange-red due to steroid hormones and areas of hemorrhage. These tumors are comprised of large polyhedral cells with vacuolated cytoplasm. The neoplastic cells form trabeculae and sheets (Fig. 6.7). There can be variable hemorrhage and necrosis.

Lymphosarcoma can involve the testicle, and both grossly and histologically these tumors may be confused with seminomas (Figs. 6.8 and 6.9). However, testicular lymphosarcoma is usually just one manifestation of a multisystemic disease.

Undifferentiated testicular sarcomas may arise from connective tissue and are usually comprised of fusiform

cells forming interlacing bundles. Immunohistochemistry may be used to try to determine the exact cell type.

Teratomas do not have specific gross characteristics unless keratinaceous cysts or some other differentiated structure is seen. Histologically they contain a variety of structures comprising both epithelial and mesenchymal elements.

Diseases of the Epididymis

Inflammation and neoplasia are reported in the epididymis. Inflammation is generally due to the same causes as in orchitis. Both carcinomas and sarcomas can arise in the epididymis but are rare.

Diseases of the Phallus

Prolapse of the phallus is frequently reported. It can either lead to, or be caused by, trauma, inflammatory disease, or frostbite. It is usually diagnosed clinically.

FEMALE REPRODUCTIVE SYSTEM

Normal Structure

The ovary is located on the ventral surface of the cranial ventral surface aspect of the cranial division of the left kidney. In juvenile birds, the ovary is yellow, flattened, and somewhat triangular, with its apex pointing cranially. In contrast to the juvenile testis, the juvenile ovary has a granular surface. As a bird becomes sexually mature, secondary and tertiary follicles develop, forming grapelike clusters prior to ovulation. The ovary is tightly adhered to the surface of the kidney but becomes pendulous as the tertiary follicles fill with yolk. It is suspended by the mesovarium from the abdominal wall. Only the left ovary is present in most species of birds. Exceptions include many birds of prey and the brown kiwi. Pigmentation of the ovary also occurs in some species of birds, including the white cockatoos and the blue and gold macaw.

The ovary has a defined cortex and medulla in juvenile birds, but this distinction is lost in the mature ovary. The outer surface of the ovary is covered by a cuboidal flattened peritoneal mesothelium. The cortical region consists of numerous follicles in various stages of development. Unlike in mammals, an antrum does not develop in the avian follicle. The medulla contains blood vessels, nerves, smooth muscle, and interstitial cells.

A stalk of smooth muscle containing blood vessels and nerves suspends an enlarged tertiary follicle, which is comprised of a primary oocyte enclosed by a six-layered wall. From internal to external, these layers consist of radial processes of the oocyte cytolemma and the radial processes of granulosa cells. The layers include the stratum granulosum, the theca interna (comprised of fibroblasts and collagen), the theca externa, a connective tissue tunic, and the superficial "germinal" epithelium. The latter is essentially peritoneal mesothelium. Yolk, whose components originate in the liver, is supplied to the oocyte by the follicle. The follicle produces steroid hormones. Estrogen is produced within the thecal cells and progesterone within the granulosa cells. Thecal cells outside the follicle produce androgens.

Following ovulation, the follicle regresses and fills with granulosa cells that contain lipid. This is not a true corpus luteum as is seen in mammals, as there is no cellular multiplication. The thecal wall may rupture during this time, resulting in escape of yolk into the ovary or the peritoneal cavity.

Oviduct. The oviduct is divided into five functional zones: the infundibulum, magnum, isthmus, shell gland or uterus, and vagina. The most cranial region, adjacent to the ovary, is the infundibulum. The funnel portion of the infundibulum, which receives the ovum, has a folded nonglandular mucosa and is lined by nonsecretory pseudostratified ciliated cells. The tubular region has a thickened wall and secretory epithelial cells. The tubular glands are present at its junction with the magnum. The lamina propria of the infundibulum is loose collagenous tissue. Diffuse lymphocytic cell accumulations may be noted. The ovum is fertilized in this region, and the chalaziferous layer of the albumen is produced.

The magnum is the longest and thickest portion of the oviduct. The wall is thickened due to numerous tubular glands that are lined by cuboidal columnar epithelium. Nonciliated and ciliated epithelial cells are present on the mucosal surface. In the caudal few centimeters of the magnum is the mucous region. Glands in this region are reduced and contain abundant mucus. Most of the albumen and various minerals are deposited in the magnum.

The isthmus is shorter and has thinner walls and less prominent folds than in the magnum. Ciliated and nonciliated columnar epithelial cells line the isthmus. Branched tubular glands extend into the lamina propria. These glands contain sulfur-containing proteins. The outer and inner shell membranes are added in the isthmus.

The uterus or shell gland is a short region containing leaflike lamellae. The mucosal epithelium is pseudostratified and intermittently ciliated. Coiled tubular glands are noted within the uterus. The shell is formed in the uterus.

At the junction with the uterus is the vaginal sphincter. The vagina is S shaped due to its smooth muscle and connective tissue wall. It is thicker than any other part of the oviduct. Ciliated and nonciliated mucosal cells line the vagina. At the junction with the uterus are simple tubular glands lined by columnar epithelial cells containing lipid. These are so-called sperm-host glands that store and nourish spermatozoa.

Specific defects in abnormal eggs can sometimes be related to disease or dysfunction of a specific portion of the oviduct.

The length and diameter of the oviduct vary dramatically between the breeding season and nonbreeding season. During the nonbreeding season, the oviduct is slender, pink, linear, and of uniform diameter. The oviduct of juvenile birds is thin and nearly transparent, making it difficult to find at necropsy. The oviduct of female birds that are in the process of laying will be greatly elongated, festooned, and will have a thickened wall and a greatly widened lumen. The oviduct may fill much of the left caudal coelomic cavity, displacing the intestines to the right.

Diseases of the Ovary

A variety of congenital defects of the ovary are reported in birds. A retained right ovary is occasionally seen in birds that normally would have only a left ovary. Congenital ovarian cysts are most common in budgerigars and canaries. Grossly they are fluid filled and thin walled. Flattened cells line cysts caused by trapped surface mesothelium. Granulosa cells line follicular cysts. Follicular cysts may either be acquired or congenital.

Hermaphrodism has been seen in some hybrid ducks but is not commonly reported in pet birds.

Oophoritis can be secondary to infection of the peritoneal cavity or air sacs or can be associated with hematogenous infection. Viruses, bacteria, fungi, and mycobacteria are possible causes. Grossly the ovaries are enlarged, discolored, and possibly hemorrhagic.

The histologic appearance depends on the cause. Herpesvirus infection leads to acute necrosis and hemorrhage of ovarian stroma. Intranuclear inclusion bodies are noted in syncytial cells (Fig. 6.10). Acute necrosis and heterophil infiltration predominate in most bacterial infections (Fig. 6.11). Organisms may or may not be seen. Mycobacteria and fungi tend to produce granulomas containing large macrophages and giant cells (Figs. 6.12 and 6.13). Fungal organisms may be seen with routine stains, and acid-fast stains will confirm mycobacteria.

Noninfectious inflammation of the ovary is associated with rupture of follicles and extrusion of yolk material within the ovarian stroma. Grossly, affected ovaries may be slightly enlarged and contain variably sized yellow foci. Histologically the yolk material elicits a reaction initially comprised of macrophages and lymphocytes. The macrophages usually have abundant foamy cytoplasm. Eventually giant cells are seen (Fig. 6.14).

Toxic agents may cause noninflammatory ovarian disease. Aflatoxin leads to cessation of egg production and ovarian atresia.

Several types of ovarian neoplasms are seen in birds. Granulosa cell tumors, which are reported to be the most

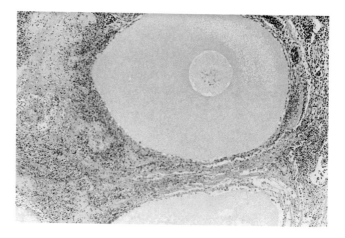

6.11.   Bacterial oophoritis characterized by necrosis, inflammatory cell infiltrate, and fibrin deposition in the ovarian stroma.

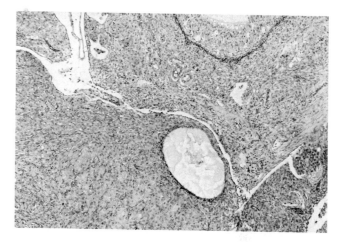

6.12.   Granulomatous oophoritis due to mycobacteria. Note the diffuse infiltration of large macrophages with abundant cytoplasm.

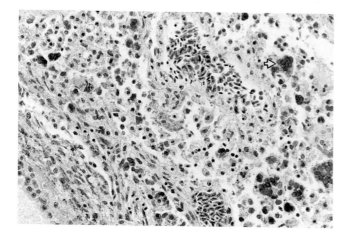

6.10.   Herpesvirus-induced oophoritis. Note the numerous cells, including syncytial cells, with intranuclear inclusion bodies (arrow).

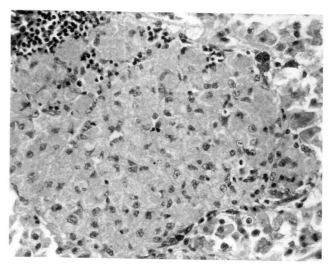

6.13.   Detail of inflammation in mycobacteriosis of the ovary. The granular cytoplasm of the macrophages contains numerous acid-fast bacteria.

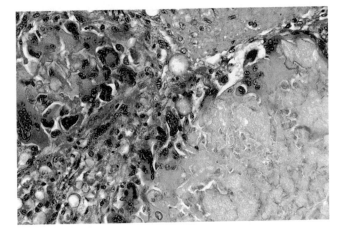

6.14. Yolk-induced oophoritis. A large mass of amorphous material is surrounded by macrophages and giant cells. Smaller granulomas are also seen.

common, are yellow lobulated irregular masses that are friable. They may become quite large and fill the abdominal cavity. Histologically the tumors are comprised of nests and trabeculae of slightly pleomorphic cells with eosinophilic cytoplasm and vesicular nuclei separated by variable amounts of stroma (Fig. 6.15).

Ovarian carcinomas are variably sized, firm, gray-white, and multilobular. They may also implant on the serosal surfaces of adjacent organs, the mesentery, and body wall. They may also metastasize. Histologically carcinomas are comprised of poorly differentiated epithelial cells forming cords, acini, and papillary structures (Figs. 6.16 and 6.17).

Dysgerminoma is the female analog of the seminoma and is infrequently seen. These tumors are comprised of sheets of pleomorphic round or ovoid cells with abundant cytoplasm and vesicular nuclei.

Arrhenoblastoma is histologically similar to the Sertoli cell tumor. In mammals, these tumors are usually called ovarian stromal tumor, Sertoli pattern. In chickens, they are associated with masculinization, but masculinization

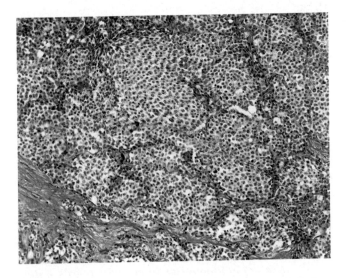

6.15. Granulosa cell tumor with predominant trabecular pattern.

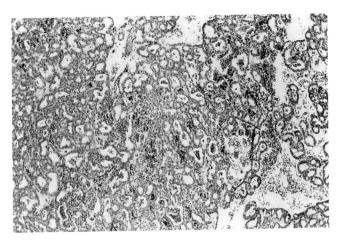

6.16. Ovarian carcinoma comprised of tubules and cords of neoplastic cells.

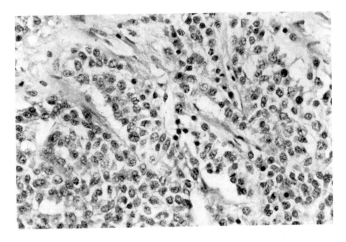

6.17. Cords and nests of anaplastic cells in ovarian carcinoma.

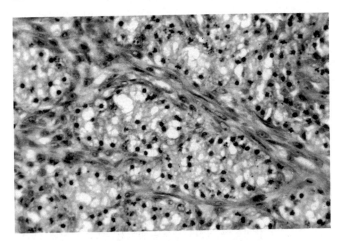

6.18. Ovarian stromal tumor, Sertoli's pattern (arrhenoblastoma). Nests and cords of neoplastic cells are separated by abundant stroma.

is not seen in pet birds in our experience. The tumors are gray-white lobulated masses comprised of structures resembling seminiferous tubules (Fig. 6.18).

Teratatomas can become quite large and histologically are comprised of tissues of various types, including both

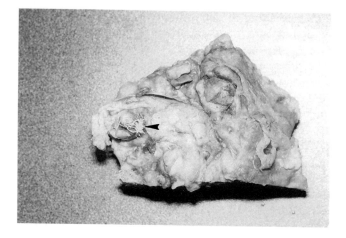

6.19. Ovarian teratoma. A large, irregular mass with an area of what appears to be attempted feather development (arrowhead).

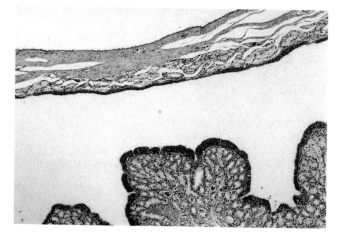

6.21. Area of oviductal cyst formation. The affected portion is lined by flattened epithelial cells.

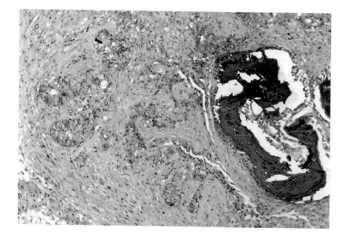

6.20. Irregular mixture of epithelial and mesenchymal elements in ovarian teratoma.

mesodermal and epithelial elements (Figs. 6.19 and 6.20).

Other tumors seen in the ovary include those of adipose tissue and connective tissue and hemangiomas, lymphosarcoma, and tumors of smooth muscle. The histology of these tumors is typical and is described in elsewhere in this book.

Diseases of the Oviduct/Uterus

Congenital malformations of the oviduct include atresia, segmental aplasia, and congenital cysts. These lesions may be associated with the developed left oviduct or a retained or incompletely regressed right oviduct. The cysts are usually fluid filled and lined by a flattened or low cuboidal epithelium (Fig. 6.21).

Inflammation of the oviduct can be caused by either infectious or noninfectious etiologies. Infectious etiologies include viruses, gram-negative and gram-positive bacteria, mycobacteria, fungi, and parasites. The source of infection can be the result of an organism ascending from the cloaca, hematogenous spread, or extension of disease from the peritoneal cavity.

The oviduct is usually enlarged, reddened, and friable, and a variable amount of exudate may be present. The appearance depends on the exact etiology and duration of the disease. Histologically necrosis, hemorrhage (Fig. 6.22), inflammation, and fibrosis are all potential changes. Bacterial salpingitis is characterized by an infiltrate of heterophils, lymphocytes, and macrophages (Fig. 6.23). Eventually there can be giant cell formation (Fig. 6.24).

Noninfectious causes of inflammation may be mechanical, secondary to improper egg maturation or formation. Inspissated yolk can elicit a chronic inflammatory response comprised of lymphocytes and macrophages. Often the macrophages contain phagocytosed yolk material. Free yolk, in the form of round, variably sized, basophilic globules, is seen in the lumen and sometimes in the tissue (Fig. 6.25).

Peritonitis (chapter 13) can be a secondary complication to either infectious or noninfectious salpingitis following penetration of the oviductal wall or rupture of the oviduct. Egg yolk peritonitis may result from internal ovulation or retrograde movement of the ovum back out through the infundibulum. Entire eggs may enter the

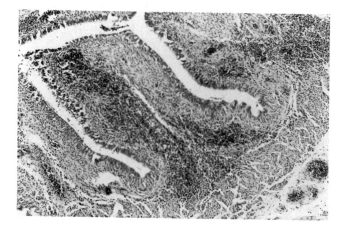

6.22. Hemorrhage due to herpesvirus infection within the oviduct wall.

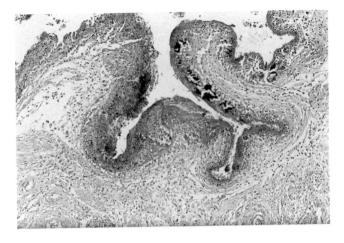

6.23.   Bacterial salpingitis. Note the mucosal necrosis and diffuse inflammatory cell infiltrate.

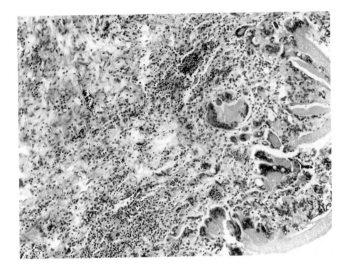

6.24.   Chronic bacterial salpingitis with giant cell formation.

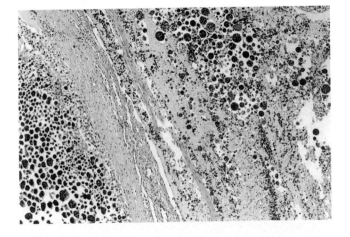

6.25.   Salpingitis secondary to rupture of the forming egg and infiltration of yolk protein into the wall of the oviduct.

abdomen either through a ruptured oviduct or by retrograde movement and expulsion through the infundibulum. If these eggs crack and leak their contents, they can also induce peritonitis.

Oviductal torsion occasionally occurs and, if not diagnosed, leads to the death of the bird. There is often vascular compromise, and the oviduct will be edematous, red-black, and friable.

Impaction of the oviduct is almost always a sequel to salpingitis or egg binding. In addition to finding an impacted egg (Fig. 6.26), there may be free yolk material, excess mucin, and purulent material in the lumen. The impacted egg can lead to pressure necrosis of the oviductal wall. Large neoplasms may also be associated with impaction.

Proliferative and neoplastic changes of the oviduct include cystic hyperplasia and neoplasia. In hyperplasia, numerous cystic structures are seen grossly. These cysts may contain clear or cloudy fluid and are lined by proliferative mucosa of the particular portion of the oviduct involved. The condition is probably of endocrine origin, but an exact cause/pathogenesis has not been established.

Neoplasms can be either adenomas or adenocarcinomas. These are firm, nodular, gray-white masses. Histologically cells of adenomas are arranged in acini, tubules, and sheets that resemble normal glands (Fig. 6.27). Carcinomas are comprised of less well differentiated cells forming acini and tubules that are infiltrative into the oviductal wall (Figs. 6.28 and 6.29).

In severe chronic cases, these tumors can also implant on peritoneal surfaces. Grossly it may be difficult to differentiate tumors of oviduct origin from those of ovarian origin, and histologically there are similarities between carcinomas from either site. Careful necropsy examination is necessary for differentiation in advanced cases.

Leiomyomas are a common tumor of the oviduct of chickens. Grossly these are red-brown masses comprised histologically of interlacing bundles of fusiform cells with oval or elongated nuclei.

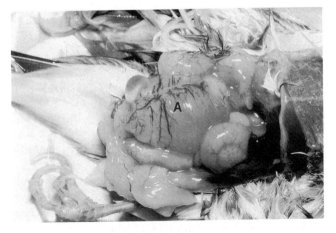

6.26.   Enlarged, impacted oviduct associated with egg binding (A).

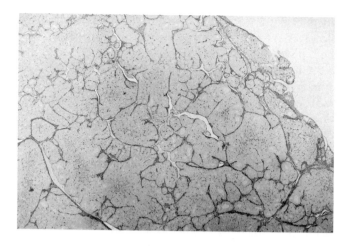

6.27. Oviductal adenoma. Numerous lobular structures are comprised of minimally undifferentiated mucosal epithelial cells.

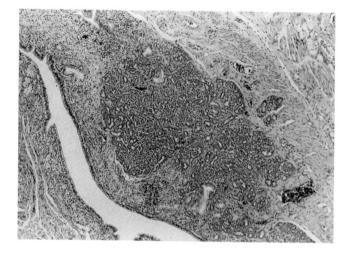

6.28. Focus of oviductal carcinoma formation. Note the infiltration of the oviduct wall by acini and tubular structures.

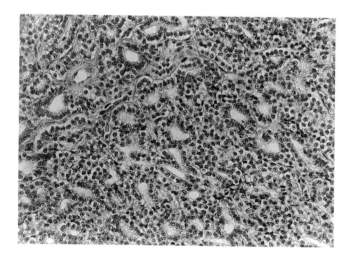

6.29. Nests and acini typical of oviductal carcinoma. Less well differentiated tumors can be difficult to distinguish from ovarian carcinomas, particularly if implanted on serosal surfaces.

Diseases of the Cloaca

The cloaca is affected by a variety of inflammatory and neoplastic diseases that can lead to problems with fertility and/or egg laying. These disease processes may lead to fibrosis and stricture or blockage due to mass lesions. They are discussed in chapter 3.

The Morphology of Egg Binding/Dystocia

Egg binding is the failure of eggs to pass through the oviduct at a normal rate. Dystocia is an egg obstructing the oviduct or causing oviduct prolapse. The most common cause of egg binding in companion birds is protracted egg laying. Birds naturally lay eggs and then brood the eggs and feed the young before beginning another cycle of egg laying, if they lay at all again that year. Finches, budgerigars, lovebirds, and cockatiels that are kept as pets often lay clutch after clutch of eggs. Many of these birds are not provided with sufficient dietary calcium and, as a result, cannot mineralize their eggs properly and may become hypocalcemic. It is assumed that hypocalcemia may result in weakness of the muscle of the oviduct and its inability to contract.

The retained egg then acts as a space-occupying mass placing pressure on the adjacent digestive organs and reducing the volume of the air sacs. The hypocalcemia, the mass effect, or both subsequently lead to the bird's death. Less commonly, adhesions form between the egg and the oviduct or rarely a portion of the oviduct is incorporated in the egg, preventing the egg from being passed. We have also seen egg binding in larger species of parrots that produce their first egg when they are older. The reason that these older birds become egg bound is not clear.

Other potential causes of egg binding are nutritional myopathies caused by a deficiency of either vitamin E or selenium, by obesity, and by a variety of environmental stressors.

Lesions associated with egg binding have been previously described. If there is dystocia, the oviduct may prolapse. If not corrected, the prolapsed oviduct may be found in the cloaca or extending from the vent at necropsy. Depending on the duration, affected tissue will be edematous, variably congested, and friable. Microscopically, necrosis, variable inflammation, congestion, and hemorrhage are seen.

Abnormal Eggs

Soft-shelled eggs are sometimes a manifestation of vitamin A or D deficiency or calcium deficiency. Infections with the avian bronchitis virus or an adenovirus also cause soft or thin-shelled eggs in poultry. Rough shells are sometimes a manifestation of salpingitis (Fig. 6.30). Organochlorine pesticides cause thin-shelled eggs. Other nutritional and toxic problems that can cause eggshell abnormalities include crude oil, nicotine, and furazolidone toxicity.

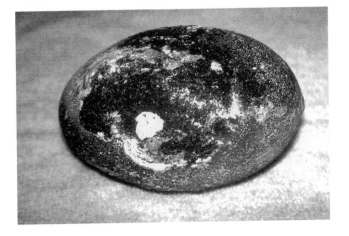

6.30.   *Roughening and discoloration of an eggshell secondary to bacterial salpingitis.*

Ectopic eggs are sometimes an incidental necropsy finding but can also be a cause of mortality, particularly if associated with peritonitis. Oviductal rupture or reverse oviductal peristalses are primary causes. At necropsy, the ectopic egg may have a complete normal shell, particularly if there is a rupture of the caudal oviduct. If the rupture is more cranial or if there was reverse peristalsis, the egg may be soft shelled or there may only be yolk and albumen present in the peritoneal cavity. There is usually some degree of peritonitis.

Infertility, Dead in Shell, and Fetal Necropsy

Investigation into hatching failure requires gross and histologic examination of the egg and its contents as well as the usual ancillary laboratory procedures. Egg necropsies are often disappointing. Aviculturists will often leave the egg in the incubator for an extended time after the embryo died because they are not aware of its death. As a result, many embryos are severely autolytic by the time they reach the pathologist. The pathologist must have some understanding of the environment of artificial incubation and what can go wrong that will eventually affect the developing embryo/fetus.

If there is failure to hatch, the first issue to be addressed is whether the egg is/was fertile. Fertilization of the ovum (yolk) initiates a series of cell divisions in the protoplasmic portion of the egg. This portion is seen grossly as a small white disc (blastodisc) present on the dorsal pole of the yolk. If there has been no fertilization, this small white area is all that is seen when the egg is examined.

Failure of fertilization is a potential reflection on a number of management issues. The most common cause of infertile eggs is pairing of two female birds. Other potential management problems include the use of inappropriate perches, inexperience of the male or the female parrot, immaturity of the male, improper nest boxes, and disturbances by other birds, wild or domestic animals, and caretakers. A properly formed egg usually implies that there is not a medical problem with the hen. The male, however, may not be producing sperm, or the sperm that he is producing may be abnormal.

A fertile egg will develop a blastoderm, which will appear as a small white area that enlarges and has a translucent center. Subsequently there is embryo formation and, by the end of the first third of incubation, organogenesis has usually taken place.

The first step of the egg necropsy is to evaluate the shell. If the shell is abnormal, then a problem with the hen should be suspected. Small or large cracks in the egg or small toenail punctures suggest rough handling by nervous or inexperienced parents. The egg should then be placed upright so that the its widest end is up. The top of the egg should be cleaned and disinfected. A circular incision is made around the top of the egg with a sterile instrument, and the top is removed. This will expose the air cell. The underlying shell membrane can be cut with a sterile instrument and a culture taken through this opening. If bacteria are growing in the egg, the contents of the egg are typically fetid, and if the infection occurred early in incubation, the contents may be curdlike and/or discolored.

Approximately 30% of embryonic deaths occur during the first third of incubation. Causes of deaths during this period include incubators that are too hot or have excessive vibration and rough handling of the egg. A study comparing the relatedness of macaw parents found that infertility and early embryonic death are more likely if macaws are closely related. Bacterial infections of the egg can also cause early embryonic mortality.

Mortality during the second third of incubation is less common. Bacterial infections and incubator problems are the most likely cause of fetal death during this period. The most common incubator problems that affect embryos at this stage are improper turning techniques that include rocking rather than turning (parrots) and excessive turning.

Another 30% of fetal deaths occur within 1 or 2 days of hatching. Mortality during the last third of incubation can still be of bacterial origin but is most often the result of an improper incubation technique. For an egg to hatch, it is critical that it loses a specific amount of moisture. The target for many parrot species is approximately 15% weight loss over the entire incubation period. Either excessive moisture loss or insufficient moisture loss will result in a weak chick that may not hatch. One of the main causes of late-term fetal death is failure to establish pulmonary respiration. If the incubator temperature is either too cold or too hot, weak and either dry or edematous chicks may be found. Weak chicks cannot penetrate the air cell with their beaks. Finally, airflow in the incubator is a critical factor. Insufficient airflow impacts chick development and moisture loss from the egg.

If the egg is near hatching, the position of the embryo should be examined carefully before it is removed from the egg. In the 2 or 3 days prior to hatching, the shell membrane contracts around the chick, making the air cell larger. At 1 to 2 days before hatching, the chick tears through the shell membrane, its head enters the air cell, and it begins to breathe air. Just prior to hatching, the chick should be positioned so that its tail is against the narrow end of the egg, the shoulders are against the air cell, and the head is tucked under the right wing. Seven abnormal positions are described. In position 1, the head is between the thighs. These chicks cannot hatch. In position 2, the head is at the small end of the egg. Some of these birds will pip, but others suffocate. In position 3, the head is to the left. This is a lethal position. In position 4, the body is rotated along the long axis of the egg, resulting in the beak not being near the air cell, and hatching is not possible. In position 5, the feet are over the head, and these birds usually fail to hatch. In position 6, the head is over the right wing. These chicks usually hatch. In position 7, the embryo is lying across the egg and cannot hatch. This position occurs if the egg is spherical and the embryo is small. With the exception of malformed eggs, an increase in the number of malpositioned chicks is often the result of improper turning techniques or possibly incubators with excess vibration.

Techniques of fetal necropsy vary. Small embryos and fetuses (finches) can be grossly examined, fixed, and processed for whole body sections. Larger chicks should be necropsied just as any posthatch bird. The yolk sac and other fetal and shell membranes should be examined histologically.

Gross and histologic lesions in chicks that are near hatching will be somewhat similar to those of posthatch chicks. Some things, however, are unique to developing chicks. Excessive humidity in the incubator can lead to a severely edematous fetus (Fig. 6.31). Inadequate humidity will have the opposite affect, and the fetus may be severely dehydrated (Fig. 6.32). Edema and dehydration are not, however, consistently this obvious.

Cockatiel and macaw late-term fetuses have a higher incidence of soft tissue, particularly renal, mineralization. This lesion may be the result of excessive vitamin D$_3$ in

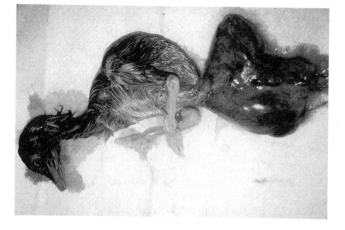

6.32. Fetal dehydration due to inadequate incubator humidity.

the diet of the hen, nutritional problems of the hen, or possibly improper incubation environments. The latter can lead to excessive loss of calcium from the shell and deposition of the calcium in the fetal soft tissues, particularly the kidney.

The yolk sac and chorioallantois mediate mobilization and transepithelial transport of mineral deposits from the egg. Mineral transport involves plasma proteins that bind mineral and are initially synthesized by the yolk sac and later by the liver. This change can be seen in developing fetuses and may appear grossly as white gritty foci in the kidneys. Typically there is variable tubular mineralization and no reaction histologically (Fig. 6.33). The underlying pathogenesis of the lesion cannot be determined based solely on its morphology.

Since fetal death is often associated with stress, examination of the bursa of Fabricius is very important in the fetal necropsy. Although not an etiology-specific lesion, the finding of severe bursal lymphoid depletion/necrosis or hypoplasia is indicative of stress to the developing chick.

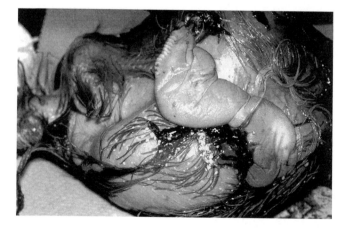

6.31. Severe fetal edema secondary to excessive humidity in the incubator.

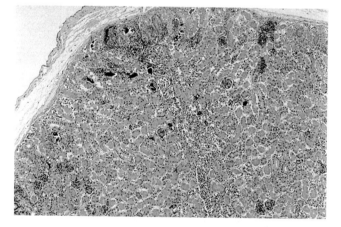

6.33. Fetal renal mineralization as one result of an improper incubation environment. If severe, this can lead to fetal death.

ADDITIONAL READING

Anderson Brown AF, Robbins GES. 1994. The new incubation book. Great Britain: BPC Wheatons, pp 69–102.

Beach JE. 1962. Diseases of budgerigars and other caged birds: A survey of post-mortem findings. Part I. Vet Rec 74:10–15; Part II. Vet Rec 74:63–68; Part III. Vet Rec 74:134–140.

Biswall G, Morrill CC. 1953. The pathology of the reproductive tract of laying pullets affected with Newcastle disease. Poult Sci 33:880–897.

Cooke AS. 1973. Shell thinning in avian eggs by environmental pollutants. Environ Pollut 4:85–152.

Degernes LA. 1994. Abdominal mass due to chronic salpingitis in an African grey parrot (*Psittacus erithacus*). Vet Radiol Ultrasound 35:24–28.

Gorham SL, Ottinger MA. 1986. Sertoli cell tumors in Japanese quail. Avian Dis 30:337–339.

Gupta BN, Langham RF. 1968. Arrhenoblastoma in an Indian Desi hen. Avian Dis 12:441–444.

Hasholt J. 1966. Diseases of the female reproductive organs of pet birds. J Small Anim Pract 7:313–320.

Helmbolt CF, Migaki G, Langheinrich KA, et al. 1974. Teratoma in a domestic fowl (*Gallus gallus*). Avian Dis 18:142–148.

Keymer IF. 1980. Disorders of the avian female reproductive system. Avian Pathol 9:405–419.

King AS, McLelland J. 1984. Female reproductive system. In: Birds: Their structure and function, 2nd edition. London: Bailliere Tindall, pp 145–165.

King AS, McLelland J. 1984. Male reproductive system. In: Birds: Their structure and function, 2nd edition. London: Bailliere Tindall, pp 166–174.

Lake PE. 1984. The male in reproduction. In: Freeman BM, ed. Physiological biochemistry of the domestic fowl. New York: Academic Press, pp 381–401.

Leach MW. 1992. A survey of neoplasia in pet birds. Semin Avian Exotic Pet Med 1:52–64.

Lofts B, Murton RK. 1973. Reproduction in birds. In: Farner DS, King JR, eds. Avian biology, vol 3. New York: Academic Press, pp 1–88.

Murton RK, Westwood NJ. 1977. Avian breeding cycles. In: Reproductive apparatus of the male. Oxford: Clarendon, pp 47–76.

Reece RL. 1987. Reproductive diseases. In: Burr E, ed. Companion bird medicine. Ames: Iowa State University Press, pp 89–100.

Reece RL. 1992. Observations on naturally occurring neoplasms in birds in the state of Victoria, Australia. Avian Pathol 21:3–32.

Rigdon RH. 1967. Gonads in hermaphroditic ducks: A pathologic study. Am J Vet Res 28:1125–1131.

Schmidt RE. 1992. Morphologic diagnosis of avian neoplasms. Semin Avian Exotic Pet Med 1:73–79.

Shivanandappa T, Krishnakumarii MK, Majunder SK. 1983. Testicular atrophy in *Gallus domesticus* fed acute doses of copper fungicides. Poult Sci 1983:405–408.

Sitler WG. 1956. A Sertoli cell tumor causing feminization in a brown leghorn capon. J Endocrinol 14:197–203.

Stoica G, Russo E, Hoffman JP. 1989. Abdominal tumor in a military macaw (Diagnosis: metastatic ovarian carcinoma). Lab Anim 18:17–20.

Thaxton JP, Parkhurst CR. 1973. Abnormal mating behavior and reproductive dysfunction caused by mercury in Japanese quail. Proc Soc Exp Biol Med 144:252–255.

Turk JP, Kim J, Gallera AM. 1981. Seminoma in a pigeon. Avian Dis 25:752–755.

Webb D, Van Vleet JF. 1990. Cystic testicular degeneration in furazolidone toxicosis of sexually immature ducks. Avian Dis 39:693–700.

7 Endocrine System

PITUITARY GLAND

Normal Structure

The pituitary gland is located in the sella turcica beneath the diencephalon and the optic chiasma. The pituitary is divided into the adenohypophysis and the neurohypophysis. The adenohypophysis consists of a pars tuberalis and a pars distalis; in contrast to mammals, birds do not have a pars intermedia. The pars tuberalis is further divided into cephalic and caudal zones. The acidophils of the cephalic zone stain lightly whereas the acidophils of the caudal zone are more intensely eosinophilic. The pars tuberalis contains secretory cells that are arranged in cords. Capillaries and vascular sinuses separate the cords. The neurohypophysis (pars nervosa) is a direct extension of the hypothalamus at the base of the brain. Subdivisions of the neurohypophysis are the median eminence, the infundibular stem, and neural lobe. Each has a three-layer structure of an ependymal layer that is in contact with the diverticulum of the third ventricle, a fiber layer, and a glandular layer.

Inflammatory Disease

Infections of the oral cavity can become severe and extend to involve the pituitary. Grossly these lesions are yellow-white and often have the appearance of an abscess. Histologically there is necrosis of the pituitary gland and the surrounding bone, with a pleocellular inflammatory infiltrate whose composition may be affected by the particular etiologic agent. Bacteria, fungi, and protozoa such as *Trichomonas* sp. have been implicated and may be seen in the lesion.

The neurohypophysis may be affected by encephalitis involving the hypothalamus. Bacterial and viral infections are possible, and their histologic appearance is similar to the lesion in nervous tissue.

Severe trauma can lead to hemorrhage and secondary inflammation of the pituitary. The gross and histologic appearance may be dominated by the hemorrhage, with necrosis and inflammation being more prominent if the bird survives the traumatic incident.

Neoplastic Disease

Adenomas and carcinomas have been reported, particularly in budgerigars. These tumors are usually red-brown and, if large, may extend outside of the sella turcica (Fig. 7.1). They may compress the optic chiasma, and the bird may have a history of blindness. There can be associated bone lysis. Adenomas grow by expansion, and there can be compression of adjacent brain. Adenomas are circumscribed whereas the margins of carcinomas are less well differentiated.

Histologically adenomas are comprised of large epithelial cells that are usually devoid of granules. These cells form nests and lobules with minimal stroma (Figs. 7.2 and 7.3). Cells making up carcinomas are more anaplastic and mitotic figures may be seen. Tumor lobules and cords are infiltrative into surrounding tissue. Metastasis is rarely reported.

THYROID GLANDS

Normal Structure

The thyroid glands are paired and round to slightly oblong. They are found immediately lateral to the carotid

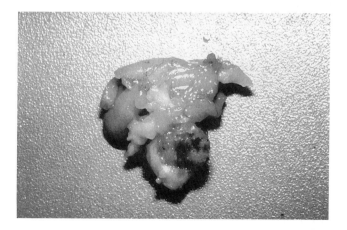

7.1. Pituitary adenoma that was compressing the adjacent brain.

121

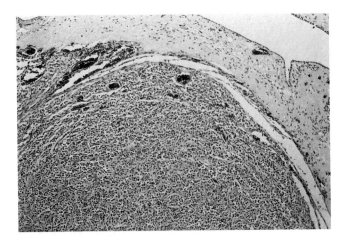

7.2. Pituitary adenoma growing by expansion and compressing the brain.

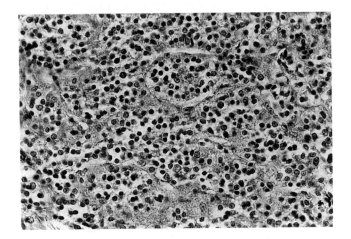

7.3. Pituitary adenoma. Note the nests of neoplastic cells separated by fine stroma.

arteries within the thoracic inlet. They are red-brown, similar to the syringeal muscle, and the latter is sometimes thought to be thyroid gland by prosectors with minimal avian experience. Anatomically they are very similar to the thyroids of other animals, being composed of closely packed spherical follicles. A flattened single layer of epithelial cells lines the follicles in adult birds. In young growing birds, the epithelial cells are cuboidal, and the follicles contain less colloid. Calcitonin-secreting cells are not present in avian thyroids except in doves and pigeons, where they are within the follicular epithelium. In other birds, they are in the ultimobranchial glands.

Congenital Lesions

Partial persistence of the caudal portion of the thyroglossal duct can lead to cyst formation within or adjacent to the thyroid gland. These cysts are lined by epithelium similar to that of thyroid follicles.

Inflammatory Disease

Lymphocytic thyroiditis similar to autoimmune disease in humans and dogs has been seen in certain strains of

chickens, and a morphologically similar lesion is seen sporadically in young African grey parrots. Affected glands are small, pale, and may be slightly irregular. Histologically there is variable follicle degeneration and connective tissue proliferation associated with lymphoid cell infiltration and lymphoid follicle formation (Figs. 7.4 and 7.5).

Disseminated mycobacteriosis may involve the thyroid. Grossly the glands are enlarged, yellow-white, and irregular. Histologically there is necrosis associated with an infiltrate of large histiocytes with blue-gray cytoplasm that contain acid-fast bacteria.

Inflammation of the soft tissue of the neck secondary to trauma or infection that has spread may involve the thyroid glands. The specific changes depend on the underlying cause.

Noninflammatory Disease

Apparent degenerative lesions are sporadically seen, particularly in budgerigars and cockatiels. Some older litera-

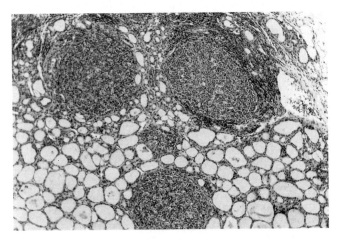

7.4. Multiple lymphoid follicles in the thyroid gland of an African gray parrot with thyroiditis histologically similar to autoimmune thyroid disease seen in other species.

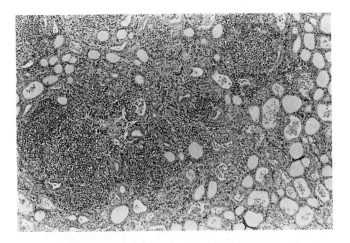

7.5. Severe lymphocytic thyroiditis and effacement of normal thyroid parenchyma.

ture refers to the condition as dystrophy. Affected glands may be both slightly enlarged, pale and irregular, or occasionally slightly small. Foci of red-brown mottling may be seen.

Histologically, variable follicular collapse and colloid loss characterize these glands. A few follicles may be cystic. Remaining colloid is usually granular and often discolored. Hemorrhage may be seen in follicles and interstitium (Fig. 7.6).

Experimentally, organotin compounds cause atrophy of the thyroid gland of chickens. Organotin compounds can be found in disinfectants, pesticides, and antihelmintics. Whether pet birds are exposed to these compounds is not known, and whether they cause some of the degenerative thyroid lesions described remains speculative.

Amyloid deposition is occasionally seen in the interstitium of the thyroid and is just one manifestation of generalized amyloidosis.

Proliferative Disease

Thyroid hyperplasia (goiter) has been most commonly reported in budgerigars but occurs in a wide variety of pet and nonpet birds. Goiter in the budgerigar is common in parts of the world where the grain they are fed is grown on iodine-deficient soils. The soils of the midwestern United States are iodine deficient, and budgerigars in the eastern and midwestern United States are at high risk for goiter. Goiters in budgerigars are readily preventable by supplying trace amounts of iodine in the diet or drinking water.

The highest incidence in pet birds seen in our practice is in blue and gold macaws. The underlying cause of the condition has not been conclusively determined. Iodine deficiency or excess or ingestion of plant material containing goitrogenic substances are possible causes. Experimentally in Japanese quail it has been shown that hens deposit thyroid hormones into eggs in proportion to their own thyroid status, and, if deficient, the chicks may also be deficient.

Congenital hyperplasia with a possible genetic link may also be possible. This genetic defect could result in loss of enzymes responsible for biosynthesis of thyroid hormone and resulting decrease in T_4 and T_3, which stimulates production of thyrotrophic hormone (TTH) and hyperplasia of follicular epithelial cells.

Thyroid hyperplasia is bilateral, resulting in enlarged, red-brown or purple glands that put pressure on the trachea, esophagus, and other soft tissues of the neck and collapse the interclavicular air sac. Hyperplastic glands have a smooth surface (Fig. 7.7). Histologically, affected glands are comprised of numerous follicles lined by enlarged epithelial cells. There is no colloid and often no apparent follicular lumen (Figs. 7.8 and 7.9).

Colloid goiter is considered the involutionary phase of thyroid hyperplasia. Colloid is produced, but endocytosis is decreased after T_4 and T_3 return to normal and TTH concentration is reduced. Affected glands are enlarged and red-brown and have a translucent or glassy appearance on section. Histologically the gland is comprised of large follicles containing colloid and lined by epithelial cells that

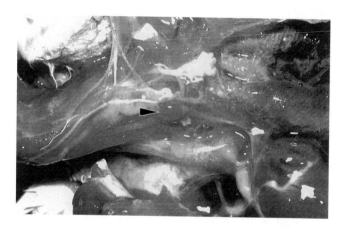

7.7. Enlarged thyroid gland typical of hyperplastic goiter (arrowhead). The enlargement is bilateral, but the second gland is not seen due to the orientation of the photo.

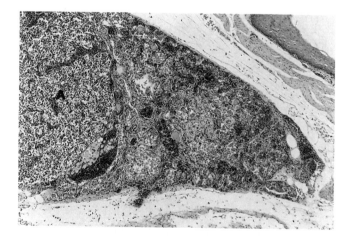

7.6. Thyroid degeneration, hemorrhage, and atrophy. Note the adjacent, histologically normal parathyroid gland (A).

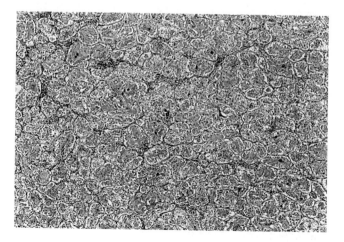

7.8. Thyroid hyperplasia. Follicles contain enlarged epithelial cells and minimal amounts of residual colloid.

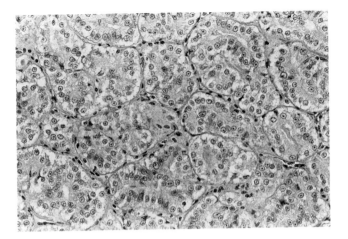

7.9.   Detail of hyperplastic thyroid follicles.

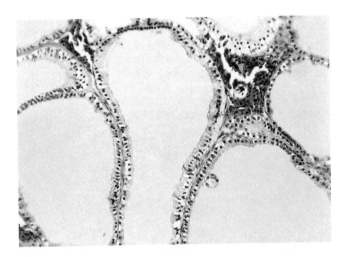

7.10.   Early colloid goiter. Cuboidal or columnar cells line enlarged follicles.

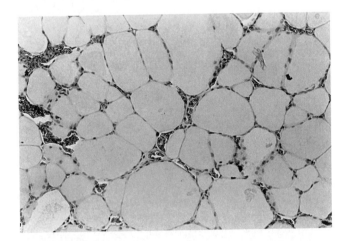

7.11.   Diffuse colloid goiter with follicles lined by flattened atrophic epithelial cells.

may be cuboidal or columnar initially but eventually become flattened atrophic cells having a smooth interface with the colloid (Figs. 7.10 and 7.11).

Thyroid gland neoplasia presents as a unilateral swelling of the affected gland. The highest incidence of

thyroid neoplasia occurs in budgerigars and cockatiels. Thyroid adenomas are most common. Thyroid adenomas are usually smooth, red-purple, and may displace associated soft tissue. Histologically several forms are noted. Follicles may be variably enlarged and lined by cuboidal or low columnar cells. Colloid is usually minimal or absent. In some cases, cystic follicles are seen (Figs. 7.12 and 7.13). Some adenomas are primarily papillary with numerous papillae seen in dilated follicular structures (Fig. 7.14). Carcinomas lead to distortion and enlargement of the thyroid gland. The mass may be firm and gray-white with indeterminate boundaries. Histologically carcinomas are comprised of poorly differentiated cells that form nests and trabeculae and infiltrate the capsule and surrounding tissue. Papillary and cystic structures may be present in some tumors.

PARATHYROID GLANDS

Normal Structure
The avian parathyroid glands are paired structures that lie immediately caudal to the thyroid gland and immediately

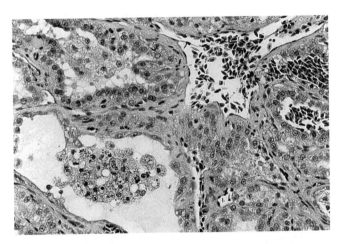

7.12.   Thyroid adenoma with proliferative epithelium and irregular follicle formation.

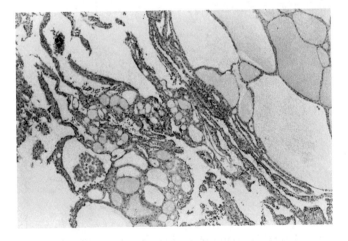

7.13.   Cystic follicles adjacent to an area of cystadenoma formation in thyroid gland.

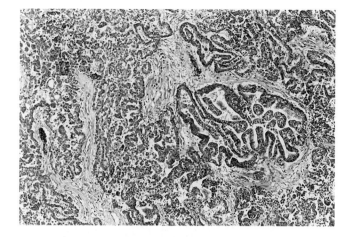

7.14.   Papillary adenoma of the thyroid gland. Moderate amounts of stroma are also seen.

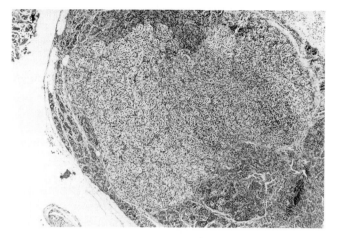

7.16.   Parathyroid hypertrophy/hyperplasia. Affected cells have large amounts of clear cytoplasm.

lateral to the carotid artery. They are ivory colored, round, and smooth. The parathyroids are often so small that they cannot be seen grossly if the bird is eating a diet with sufficient calcium. The parathyroids of birds that are in a negative calcium diet may reach 2 to 3 mm in diameter. Histologically, chief cells are in cords that in cross section appear as clusters of cells, each surrounded by a thin layer of connective tissue. The chief cells in birds that are eating a diet that is sufficient in calcium are small round cells that are closely packed together. They have scant cytoplasm and a dense nucleus.

Proliferative Disease

Hypertrophy and hyperplasia of the parathyroid may be obvious grossly (Fig. 7.15) but can be difficult to detect if minimal. The enlarged parathyroid is gray-white to yellow, and the condition is bilateral. Affected birds may also have grossly observable bone problems (chapter 9). Histologically, chief cells are variably enlarged with granular cytoplasm that will become foamy to clear in severe cases. The chromatin of the chief cells becomes less condensed,

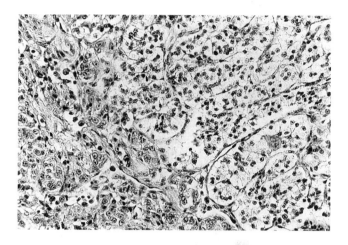

7.17.   Detail of hypertrophied parathyroid gland cells.

and the nucleus enlarges. The cells form trabecular structures, and the entire gland is involved (Figs. 7.16 and 7.17).

Parathyroid adenomas can be unilateral or occasionally bilateral. Grossly they cannot be differentiated from severe hyperplasia in most birds. The histologic appearance of adenoma is similar to severe hyperplasia, but there will be compression of adjacent normal tissue and some indication of capsule formation.

We have not seen any example of parathyroid carcinoma.

ADRENAL GLANDS

Normal Structure

The avian adrenal glands are paired in most species, but in a few birds they may be fused. Jackdaws have several small accessory glands embedded in the epididymis. They are pink to orange, flattened, and lie at the medial and cranial aspect of the ventral surface of the cranial division of the each kidney. Birds, unlike mammals, do not have a defined cortex and medulla to their adrenal glands.

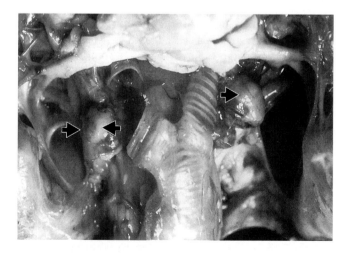

7.15.   Marked bilateral enlargement of severely hypertrophied parathyroid glands (arrows).

Instead, cords or islands of mesodermal-derived (interrenal or cortical) cells and neuroectodermal-derived (chromaffin or medullary) cells are intermixed within the adrenal gland.

Interrenal cells are rounded to polygonal and have substantial eosinophilic cytoplasm and a small, dense, centrally located nucleus. These cells contain carotenoids, which impart the yellow color seen grossly. Chromaffin cells are of similar size and shape but have a densely basophilic and nearly granular cytoplasm.

Noninflammatory and Inflammatory Diseases

Generalized disease processes may involve any portion of the gland. Scattered foci of mineralization, which are usually only seen histologically, are sometimes found in the adrenal (Fig. 7.18). Amyloidosis occurs sporadically, and, when severe, the affected gland may be enlarged and have a uniform pale appearance. Histologically amyloid is deposited primarily in sinusoidal walls, which are thickened by a diffuse amphophilic or slightly eosinophilic material. There is variable loss of both interrenal and chromaffin cells (Fig. 7.19).

Generalized inflammatory disease is usually the result of hematogenous extensions of systemic bacterial infections or extension from bacterial or fungal peritoneal or air-sac infections. The exact character of the lesion depends on the etiologic agent. Grossly, in bacterial and fungal disease of the adrenal, there may be hemorrhage and mottling, with necrotic foci and exudate seen in severe cases.

Histologically there is necrosis and an infiltrate of heterophils, macrophages, and variable numbers of lymphocytes and plasma cells. Finding the organism is often the only way to differentiate the type of infectious process. In chronic infections, there can be giant cells.

Systemic mycobacteriosis may involve the adrenal glands. Grossly there is often no obvious change, and the histologic lesion is comprised of infiltrating large macrophages with abundant lightly basophilic cytoplasm.

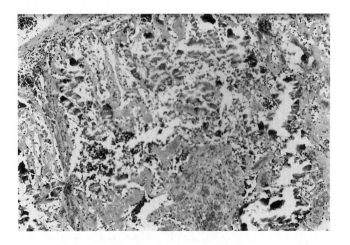

7.18. *Severe mineralization and degeneration of the adrenal gland.*

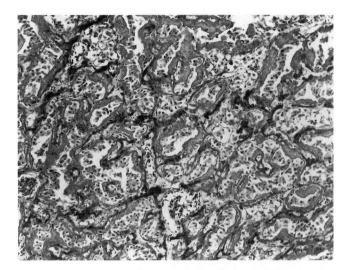

7.19. *Generalized amyloidosis of the adrenal gland. Affected basement membranes are thickened by amorphous, darkly eosinophilic amyloid.*

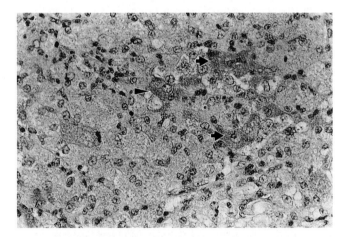

7.20. *Mycobacterial infection of the adrenal gland. Numerous macrophages containing granular material are seen. This material represents acid-fast bacteria. The infiltrating macrophages are morphologically similar to the interrenal cells (arrows) they are displacing.*

These cells can be mistaken for normal chromaffin cells if not carefully evaluated (Fig. 7.20).

A few lesions specific to the interrenal cells can be seen. Vacuolation of interrenal cells associated with no other lesion is seen in birds that die suddenly, particularly African grey parrots. The cause of the condition is not known. This lesion can be severe and may indicate that the bird was in adrenal failure, but, as of yet, antemortem tests that might confirm the possibility have not been done. Grossly the gland may be yellow-brown and slightly mottled (Fig. 7.21). Histologically there is diffuse swelling and vacuolation of the interrenal cells (Fig. 7.22).

Several viral diseases affect the chromaffin cells. Polyomavirus inclusions may be seen in karyomegalic nuclei. Paramyxovirus inclusions have been noted in chromaffin

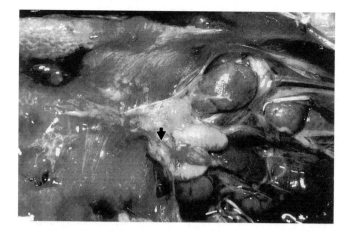

7.21.   Degeneration of the adrenal glands. The glands are small, dark, and nodular (arrow).

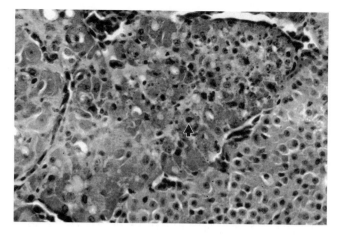

7.23.   Necrosis of chromaffin cells and intracytoplasmic inclusion bodies (arrow) in the adrenal gland of a bird with paramyxovirus infection.

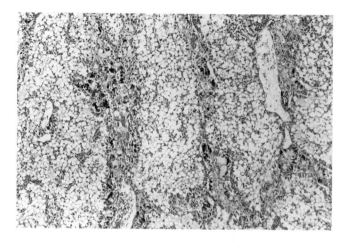

7.22.   Severe swelling and vacuolation of interrenal cells that is typical of idiopathic adrenal degeneration.

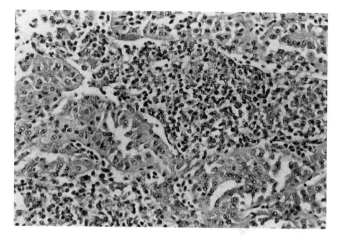

7.24.   Proventricular dilatation disease. Diffuse infiltration of chromaffin portion of the adrenal gland by lymphocytes and plasma cells.

cell cytoplasm (Fig. 7.23). Birds with proventricular dilatation disease may have adrenal gland involvement. Affected glands are slightly enlarged and may have mild red-gray mottling. Microscopically there is a variable infiltrate of lymphocytes and plasma cells within the chromaffin portions of the gland (Fig. 7.24).

Proliferative Disease

Hyperplasia as seen in the cortex of mammalian adrenal glands is not documented in birds. Hypertrophy of interrenal cells does occur, associated with vacuolar changes consistent with degeneration, and may indicate chronic stress and eventual adrenal exhaustion. In a few severe cases, necrosis of interrenal cells is seen.

Adenomas and carcinomas of interrenal cell origin are reported and occur sporadically. Grossly these tumors are lobulated and gray-yellow. Histologically adenomas are comprised of irregular cords of enlarged pale cells with amphophilic or eosinophilic cytoplasm (Fig. 7.25). Carcinomas contain pleomorphic anaplastic cells with vesicular nuclei and variable amounts of cytoplasm. These cells form

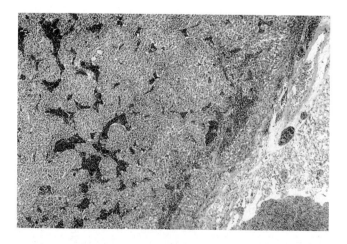

7.25.   Adrenal gland adenoma comprised of proliferative interrenal cells forming cords and nests and growing by expansion.

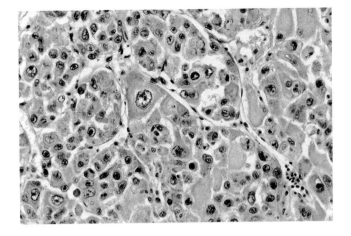

7.26.   *Anaplastic, pleomorphic interrenal cells typical of adrenal carcinoma.*

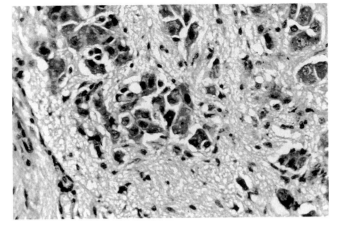

7.28.   *Portion of ganglioneuroma with neuropil-like substance and neoplastic cells.*

poorly defined trabeculae separated by minimal stroma. There is moderate mitotic activity (Fig. 7.26). Occasional metastasis is seen, primarily involving liver or lung.

Pheochromocytomas are not well documented. We have seen one case in a budgerigar in which the tumor was comprised of small cells with minimal cytoplasm. Tumor cells formed nests and trabecular structures (Fig. 7.27).

Ganglioneuromas of the adrenal gland of birds are not distinctive grossly, presenting as a nonspecific enlargement adjacent to the gland or of the gland itself. Histologically they are comprised of large cells with basophilic cytoplasm resembling neurons. These cells form clumps and sheets, which are embedded in a stroma or ground substance that is lightly eosinophilic or amphophilic and resembles normal neuropil (Fig. 7.28).

PANCREATIC ISLETS

Normal Structure

Avian pancreatic islets are of three types: light, comprised of A and D cells; dark, comprised of B and D cells; and mixed, which contain A, B, and D cells. A cells produce glucagon, B cells produce insulin, and D cells produce somatostatin. Histologically light islets blend with surrounding exocrine pancreas whereas dark islets are separated by collagen. Islet distribution is not uniform in all species of birds, so multiple sections of the pancreas should be evaluated.

Inflammatory Disease

Paramyxovirus infections can cause pancreatitis in several pet avian species (see chapter 3). The inflammation can be severe enough to involve the pancreatic islets in some cases.

Degenerative Disease

Degenerative changes in the pancreatic islets usually lead to diabetes mellitus. This condition is seen in a variety of pet species, supposedly being somewhat more prevalent in toucans, although in our experience most cases are in psittacine birds. No gross lesion is seen, and histologically there may be hypoplasia, atrophy, and/or vacuolation of islet cells (Fig. 7.29). Inflammation is rarely reported.

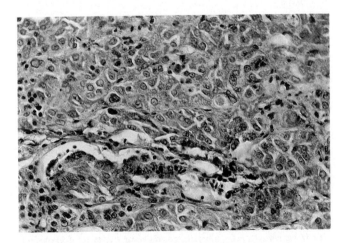

7.27.   *Sheet of neoplastic chromaffin cells in pheochromocytoma. Poorly defined trabeculae are seen.*

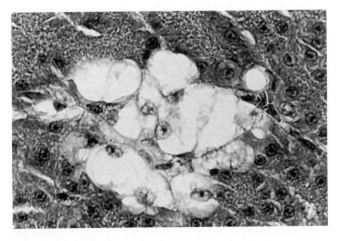

7.29.   *Typical swelling and vacuolation of islets of Langerhans seen in birds with diabetes mellitus.*

Proliferative Disease

Islet cell hyperplasia and hypertrophy are occasionally seen. In most of our cases, they are due to proliferation and enlargement of A cells associated with vague clinical signs and death. There is no grossly observable change. Histologically the enlarged islets are comprised of large cells forming trabeculae (Fig. 7.30).

Islet cell tumors are rare in birds. Reported cases are described as nodular masses that are comprised of poorly differentiated epithelial cells with hyperchromatic nuclei. The cells form trabeculae that extend into surrounding pancreatic parenchyma (Fig. 7.31).

ULTIMOBRANCHIAL BODY

Normal Structure

Avian ultimobranchial bodies are paired structures posterior to the parathyroid glands and immediately lateral to the carotid arteries. The ultimobranchial body in companion birds is typically 1.0 to 3.0 mm in diameter. The left body may attach to the parathyroid. They are difficult to locate in birds that have a moderate or excessive amount of fat. The avian ultimobranchial body contains cords or islands of C cells, small vesicles, and parathyroid nodules in a loose connective tissue stroma. The C cells produce calcitonin.

Lesions

If there is long-term hypercalcemia, there may be hypertrophy of the ultimobranchial bodies, and they can be greater than 3.0 mm and will be obvious grossly. Histologically the C cells are enlarged and have abundant cytoplasm. Cysts may develop in the ultimobranchial bodies. These cysts may be lined by C cells or by squamous epithelium in some cases.

CAROTID BODIES, PINEAL GLAND, AND GASTROINTESTINAL ENDOCRINE SYSTEM

Normal Structure

The carotid bodies are paired at each side of the thoracic inlet in contact with the medial surface of the parathyroid glands. In some birds, they may be embedded in the parathyroid gland. Accessory carotid bodies may occur in other sites, including the adventitia of arteries. The cells of the carotid body are epithelioid with a round nucleus and a finely granular cytoplasm. A thick capsule surrounds the carotid bodies.

The pineal gland, which is located between the cerebral hemispheres and the cerebellum, is a dorsally divided projection of the diencephalon.

Cells of the gastrointestinal endocrine system are found in the mucosa of the gastrointestinal tract, with the greatest concentration in the proventriculus.

Lesions

A chemodectoma has been reported in a budgerigar, but no detailed description was given. Pinealomas are rarely seen and are present as lobulated nodular growths of the gland. Histologically the cells have vesicular nuclei and form rosettes.

Lesions of the gastrointestinal endocrine system have not been reported.

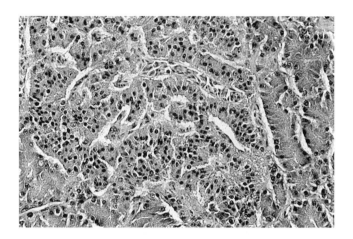

7.30. *Marked hyperplasia of islets of Langerhans. Based on histochemistry, the granular material is glucagon.*

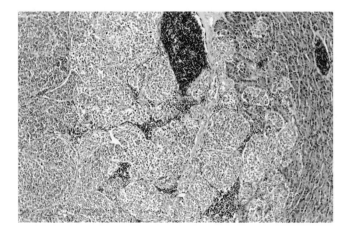

7.31. *Infiltrative growth of low-grade islet cell carcinoma.*

ADDITIONAL READING

Blackmore DK. 1966. The clinical approach to tumors in cage birds: I. The pathology and incidence of neoplasia in cage birds. J Small Anim Pract 6:217–223.

Dillberger JE, Citino SB, Altman NH. 1987. Four cases of neoplasia in captive wild birds. Avian Dis 31:206–213.

Harms CA, Hoskinson JJ, Bruyette DS, et al. 1994. Development of an experimental model of hypothyroidism in cockatiels (*Nymphicus hollandicus*). Am J Vet Res 55:399–404.

Ito M, Kameda Y, Tagawa T. 1986. An ultrastructural study of the cysts in chicken ultimobranchial glands, with special reference to C-cells. Cell Tissue Res 246:39–44.

King AS, McLelland J. 1984. Birds: Endocrine system. In: Birds: Their structure and function. London: Bailliere Tindall, pp 200–213.

Lumeij JT. 1994. Endocrinology. In: Ritchie BW, Harrison GJ, Harrison LR, eds. Avian medicine: Principles and application. Lake Worth, FL: Wingers, pp 582–606.

Oglesbee BL. 1992. Hypothyroidism in a scarlet macaw. J Am Vet Med Assoc 201:1599–1601.

Olson JM, McNabb A, Jablonski MS, Ferris DV. 1999. Thyroid development in relation to the development of endothermy in the red-winged blackbird (*Agelaius phoeniceus*). Gen Comp Endocrinol 116:204–212.

Rae M. 1995. Endocrine disease in pet birds. Semin Avian Exotic Pet Med 4:32–38.

Randall CJ, Reece RL. 1996. Color atlas of avian histopathology. London: Mosby-Wolfe, pp 223–228.

Reece RL. 1992. Observations on naturally occurring neoplasms in birds in the state of Victoria, Australia. Avian Pathol 21:3–32.

Sasipreeyajan J. 1988. Goiter in a cockatiel (*Nymphicus hollandicus*). Avian Dis 32:169–172.

Schmidt RE. 1992. Morphologic diagnosis of avian neoplasms. Semin Avian Exotic Pet Med 1:73–79.

Socaciu C, Baba AI, Rotaru O. 1994. Histopathologic investigations of acute and subchronic toxicities of some organotin compounds in chickens. Vet Hum Toxicol 36:535–539.

Swaryo K, Tewari Srivastav AK. 1986–87. Ultimobranchial body and parathyroid gland of the parrot *Psittacula psittacula* in response to experimental hypercalcemia. Arch Anat Microsc Morphol Exp 75:271–277.

Treihou-Lahille F, Lasmoles F, Taboulet J, et al. 1984. Ultimobranchial gland of the domestic fowl: Two types of secretory cells involved in calcitonin metabolism. Cell Tissue Res 235:439–448.

Wadsworth PF, Jones DM. 1979. Some abnormalities of the thyroid gland in non-domesticated birds. Avian Pathol 8:279–284.

8 Lymphatic and Hematopoietic System

Immunity is defined as a state or power of resisting the development of a (given) disease (*Webster's Dictionary*). In birds, there are many redundant and integrated mechanisms to accomplish this. The innate immune system includes the epidermis, secretions into the gastrointestinal, urogenital, and respiratory tracts, inflammation, and cell phagocytosis. These systems function at birth and do not require antigenic stimulation. Adaptive resistance responds to antigens and combats pathogens that can evolve much faster than in any vertebrate immune system. This system can improve resistance upon repeated challenge.

NORMAL STRUCTURE

The immune system is composed of two types of lymphoid tissue: primary and secondary. The thymus and the bursa of Fabricius are primary lymphoid tissues. The thymus, which is derived from the third and fourth pharyngeal pouches, is comprised of three to eight pale pink, flattened, irregularly shaped masses that extend along the length of both sides of the neck close to the jugular vein. The thymus has both epithelial and lymphoid components. The epithelial tissue is present as both the onionskin layers of keratinized epithelioid cells called Hassall's corpuscles and the loose network supporting the lymphoid cells. In domestic fowl, the thymus will involute at around 4 months of age, at the onset of sexual maturity. The thymus can enlarge and regain function in adult chickens if they are exposed to thyroxine. The thymus of cage birds involutes at approximately the same time that the birds are weaned. Histologically the thymus is made up of lobes, each having a cortex and medulla. The junction between the cortex and medulla is less well defined in birds as compared with mammals. The thymus contains T-lymphocytes (T cells) that are derived from stem cells produced in the para-aortic region that then migrate to the yolk sac before they enter the thymus. T cells mature and differentiate in the thymus. The thymus also contains a small number of B-lymphocytes (B cells) that migrate to the thymus after hatching. Unlike in mammals, the thymus can function as a secondary lymphoid organ.

In most birds, the bursa of Fabricius is a dorsal median diverticulum of proctodeum that contains the bursal lymphoid follicles. It appears grossly as a light cream–colored saccular organ with inner folds. Ratites are unusual in that the bursa of Fabricius is diffuse and contained submucosally in the dorsal wall of the cloaca and has a reversed cortex and medulla. The bursa of Fabricius reaches its maximum size before a bird is sexually mature and then undergoes involution. Each bursal follicle has a cortex of lymphocytes, macrophages, and plasma cells, and a medulla of lymphocytes, lymphoblasts, and plasma cells. In a normal bursa, the follicle-associated epithelium should be difficult to see (Fig. 8.1). Aggregates of granulocytic extramedullary hematopoiesis may be present between the follicles in young birds. Antigens from the cloaca move into the bursa of Fabricius by retrograde movement up the infundibulum and are presented to the developing B cells in the follicles. The bursa of Fabricius also functions as a secondary lymphoid organ for intestinal antigens.

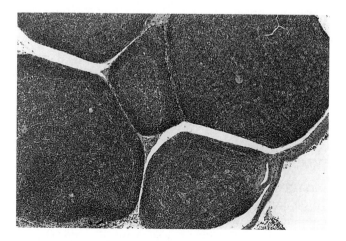

8.1. Normal psittacine bursa. The follicle-associated epithelium is barely visible.

The secondary lymphoid tissues include the spleen, harderian gland, pineal gland, bone marrow, and a diffuse system of perivascular lymphoid aggregates. Solitary and aggregated lymphoid nodules are more numerous in the digestive tract, with scattered nodules in the oropharynx around the choanal opening and the pharyngeal opening of the auditory tubes. These nodules are nonencapsulated aggregates of lymphocytes and small numbers of plasma cells and macrophages. Ducks have an esophageal tonsil that is located at the terminal part of the thoracic esophagus and is an aggregate of lymphoid nodules. In some birds, prominent lymphoid nodules called cecal tonsils are found in the wall of cecum, near the junction of rectum. In nestling budgerigars, and possibly other nestling psittacine birds, there are extensive areas of lymphocytes and plasma cells in the lamina propria of the isthmus of the stomach. These likely represent normal gut-associated lymphoid tissue.

The spleen, which is located at the right side of the junction of proventriculus and ventriculus, is round to oval in most psittacines, elongated with a slight curve in passerines, triangular in ducks and geese, and spherical in many poultry species. The spleen has a thinner capsule compared with the spleen in mammals and does not have a distinct red-and-white pulp. Birds have distinct sheathed arterioles, which are surrounded by the histiocytic reticular cells. These are very prominent structures in the spleen of owls. In birds, the spleen is not a significant reservoir of blood. The splenic circulation is open, with no direct vascular connection between arteries and veins. Within the spleen, worn-out erythrocytes are phagocytosed, and lymphopoiesis and antibody production occur.

The harderian gland, which is located ventrally and posteromedially to the globe of the eye, is infiltrated with plasma cells and is a site of immunoglobulin A (IgA) production. The pineal gland, which contains B-lymphocytes and T-lymphocytes and has germinal centers, contributes to the granulocytic extramedullary hematopoiesis of hatched chickens.

The bone marrow is the main source of granulocyte production in late embryonic life and after hatching. Histologically erythropoiesis and possibly thrombopoiesis occur within the vascular sinuses (intravascular) whereas granulopoiesis is outside the vascular sinuses (extravascular). Some long-lived IgM-secreting lymphocytes are found in bone marrow. The precise role of the bone marrow in avian immunology is unclear, although it is not a primary organ as in mammals.

IMMUNITY

Innate Immunity

This is a static immunity, where the organism responds to immunologic stimulation the same way each time. The components of the innate system include complement proteins, acute-phase proteins, iron-binding proteins, natural killer cells, and phagocytes. The avian phagocytic cells are the macrophages/monocytes, heterophils, and thrombocytes. An example of an innate system is the chicken respiratory system resident macrophages. In chickens, there are low numbers of these macrophages present in the respiratory system. However, when stimulated by a pathogen, there is a *preventive activation* of the respiratory phagocytes, resulting in an induced influx of phagocytes to the area and enhanced phagocytosis.

Adaptive or Acquired Immunity

The adaptive immune system of all vertebrates (including birds) can be divided into two arms: humoral immunity and cellular immunity. Humoral immunity develops in the bursa of Fabricius and is characterized by antibodies secreted by B cells. The bursa of Fabricius is a primary lymphoid organ unique to birds and not found in mammals. The cellular immune system develops in the thymus. The thymus is essential for the maturation of T-lymphocytes, the principal cells of cellular immunity.

Humoral Immunity

Adaptive or acquired immunity has a memory with a primary and a secondary response. In the primary response, there is a lag time of approximately 10 to 15 days before there is measurable serum antibody. The predominant antibody generated is IgM. With sustained antigenic stimulation, there is a transition to IgG secretion, and high antibody titers will develop. The secondary response occurs if a bird is subsequently exposed to the same antigen. In this case, antibody production occurs more quickly because of the presence of a population of memory cells. IgG is the primary antibody. In the secondary response, the B-lymphocyte receptors also have a higher affinity for antigen, and the T-lymphocytes adhere more strongly to other cells to transduce extracellular signals more efficiently.

The avian antibody is structurally similar to mammalian immunoglobulins. There are five classes in mammals, but only three classes have been completely described in birds: IgG (this may be listed as IgY in some literature), IgM, and IgA.

IgM, a pentameric molecule, is the predominant immunoglobulin until 20 days of development in the chicken. It is confined to the vasculature and is an efficient agglutinin (the clumping of bacteria or other immunologically reactive material) and cytolytic antibody.

IgG, which is the major serum immunoglobulin, forms the largest class. It functions to enhance phagocytosis, neutralize toxins, and inactivate some viruses. In ducks and chickens, there is passive transfer of IgG through the egg yolk. The intestinal lamina propria lymphocytes are rich in cells secreting IgG.

IgA, generally a trimer molecule, is the most common immunoglobulin found in external secretions. Both the intestinal lamina propria and the lungs are relatively enriched in cells actively secreting IgA. As in mammals, a secretory polypeptide that is synthesized by epithelial cells attaches to the IgA before secretion. In the chicken embryo, IgA and IgM are found in low concentrations in egg white and are believed to be derived from oviduct secretions. IgM and IgA that are swallowed by embryos via amniotic fluid during development are believed to provide some protective immunity to newly hatched chicks.

The immunoglobulins in nonpoultry species have only recently been examined. In ostriches, both IgG and IgM classes have been identified. They are distinct from chicken classes by both molecular weight and structure. Pigeons have all three groups: IgG, IgM, and IgA. IgA is transferred to squabs via crop milk. It appears that in the crop milk it exists in a dimeric state and probably does not have a secretory component.

Maternal IgG is present in the egg yolk and reaches the embryo via the circulation of the yolk sac as in chickens. The maximum values of IgG resorption are reached on the second day of life. In psittacine birds, monoclonal antibodies made to the IgG heavy chain of IgG from the blue and gold macaw cross-reacted with the sera of other macaws, conures, and a few other New World psittacines, but did not cross-react with IgG from African and Australian psittacines. There is some evidence, from studies showing protection from circovirus in hatchlings and low levels of hemagglutination inhibition activity in psittacine chicks, that maternally derived antibody is passed to psittacine chicks in budgerigars. Although maternal IgG is present in the yolk sacs, the antibody does not reach the nestling circulation in measurable amounts.

Cell-Mediated Immunity

Cell-mediated immunity, which is mediated by T cells, includes the cytotoxic, helper, and suppressor responses. The T-lymphocytes are different from B-lymphocytes in that they have a lower affinity to antigen, interact with other cells, do not produce antibody, and recognize digested foreign peptides on cell surfaces. These actions help them to protect the host primarily from viruses by mediating the destruction of virus-infected cells. They also have actions against intracellular bacteria, parasites, fungi, and some tumor cells.

Antigen receptors on chicken T cells are described as CD3/TCR complexes. T-cell receptors (TCRs) define the lymphocytes as T cells and function to recognize foreign antigen when displayed on the surface of a target cell. TCR1 and TCR2 correspond to the mammalian counterparts, and TCR3 is unique to birds. The T cells have coreceptors that do not bind antigen and are invariant and nonpolymorphic. The receptors in poultry are designated CT1, that is, different molecularly from the mammalian CD1, but appears to have the same functions. CD4 receptors bind to MHC2 (major histocompatibility complex 2) and are expressed in helper T cells. CD8 receptors bind to MHC1 and are expressed in cytotoxic T cells.

Chickens have a unique T cell. CD3/TCRs are not expressed on its surface, but it does have CD3 in the cytoplasm. It is designated as TCR0 and can be found in spleen, bursa, thymic medulla, and intestine. These may be natural killer cells. The TCR genes are rearranged and gain diversity in the hematopoietic precursor cells in the thymic microenvironment along with T-cell differentiation and proliferation in chickens.

Immune Suppression

Direct immune suppression can occur with drug toxicity, aflatoxicosis, and lead poisoning. Aflatoxin depresses complement activity, decreases phagocytic activity, and impairs cell-mediated immunity through inhibition of thymic-associated lymphocytes in chickens. All fungal toxins interfere with protein synthesis, which affects both T-cell and B-cell immunity. In poultry, tetracycline, tylosin, and gentamicin are immunosuppressive and decrease antibody production. Lead poisoning may have immunosuppressive effects in birds. Poisoned mallards have decreased hemagglutinating antibody as compared with normal controls.

Stress-induced immunosuppression is mediated by the adrenal gland. Corticosteroids are reported to inhibit antibody-forming cells and inhibit the production and action of immunoregulatory cytokine interleukin 1 in mammals. Acute feed restriction or fasting elevates plasma corticosterone dramatically in chickens. Injectable dexamethasone reduces serum IgG in ducks and suppresses the humoral response in other species of birds. In pigeons, a single oral dose or ocular dose of glucocorticoids has caused suppression of the pituitary-adrenocortical system.

Nutrition plays a critical role in maintaining the immune system. In people, chronic malnutrition, particularly protein malnutrition, suppresses the immune system, preventing a response to immunogens. A calorie-deficient diet suppresses antibody responses in chickens. The weight of the bursa of Fabricius is reduced in vitamin A-deficient chickens.

DISEASE

Bursa of Fabricius

Atrophy. The bursa of Fabricius normally involutes as the bird matures leaving only a small number of follicular remnants (Fig. 8.2). During this process the lymphocytes

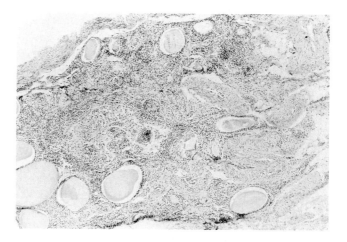

8.2. Severe atrophy and involution of psittacine bursa. It may take over a year for this to occur.

of both the medulla and cortex undergo apoptosis. Medullary cysts may form, and these may contain mineralized material. The follicular associated epithelium becomes more prominent and is transformed into a pseudostratified layer separating the cortex from the medulla. There will be variation in the size and shape of the follicles with increased interfollicular connective tissue separating the follicles. Nonspecific stresses, such as malnutrition, poor management, or infection, can result in premature atrophy of the bursa and potential immunosuppression (Fig. 8.3).

Viral Disease

Psittacine Circovirus Disease. The psittacine beak and feather disease virus (PBFDV) is a 14- to 16-nm nonenveloped virion belonging to the family Circoviridae. All psittacine species are considered susceptible to infection by this virus, but disease is predominantly confined to parrots of African and Australasian distribution and is most common in birds less than 3 years of age. Unique circoviruses infect doves, racing pigeons, canaries, finches, geese, and the Southern black-backed gull.

Three main clinical presentations exist. A common presentation occurs in wild and recently imported wild-caught cockatoos, several other species of Australasian parrots and, rarely, New World parrots. This chronic form of the disease is insidious in its development and progression. Typically, dystrophic feathers gradually replace normal ones as they are molted. Affected birds are usually 8 months to 3 years of age. An acute form of the disease also occurs in nestling cockatoos, lorikeets and, less commonly, other parrot species. In these birds, all growing feathers are affected simultaneously; the birds show generalized signs of disease and die within a few days to weeks. Nestling budgerigars also show generalized feather dystrophy, but it may not be fatal. Another acute form of PBFDV infection may not result in feather lesions, or the feather lesions may be localized and minimal. These birds generally die from secondary infections due to virally induced immunosuppression.

Primary PBFDV replication occurs at the portals of entry in the bursa of Fabricius and/or gastrointestinal tract lymphoid tissue. Secondary virus replication occurs in the liver, thymus, and probably other tissues. A common target organ is the epidermis, where the virus attacks cells in developing feathers.

Atrophy of the primary lymphoid organs is the typical finding on gross examination. The thymus and bursa of Fabricius may be difficult to find. The bone marrow can appear pale and yellowish.

Histologically, if the PBFDV attacks B cells prior to bursal regression, there will be extensive necrosis of the lymphoid follicles, with lymphocytolysis. Proteinaceous fluid and cell debris may accumulate within medullary cysts, and the follicular-associated epithelium will be prominent. Bursal hemorrhage may also be prominent. Inclusion bodies both intranuclear and intracytoplasmic can be found in macrophages and lymphocytes (Fig. 8.4). The intracytoplasmic inclusions that are more common in macrophages form clumps of globular basophilic to magenta pigments (Fig. 8.5). Eosinophilic intranuclear inclusions are characteristic of epithelial cells. In chronic cases, the bursa of Fabricius is greatly distorted by loss of lymphoid follicles and severe lymphocytic depletion (Fig. 8.6).

Young African grey parrots have a specific presentation of peracute PBFDV infection characterized by severe leukopenia, anemia, or pancytopenia and liver necrosis in the absence of feather and beak abnormalities. The liver will be enlarged and pale orange, with necrotic foci. Splenomegaly and mycotic pneumonia are also common. The definitive viral inclusions are generally restricted to the bursa of Fabricius.

Avian Polyomavirus. Avian polyomavirus disease (APV) is described extensively in chapter 4. Nestlings dying of APV

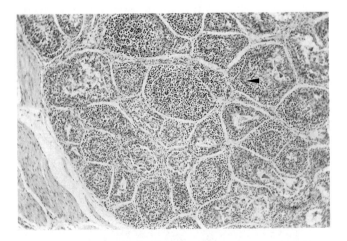

8.3.   Nonspecific bursal atrophy. Follicles are irregular, there is loss of lymphoid cells, and the follicle-associated epithelium is easily seen (arrowhead).

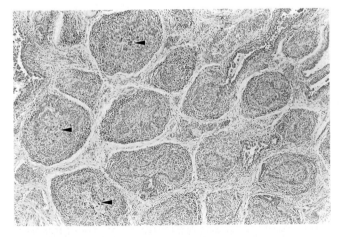

8.4.   Severe bursal lymphoid depletion due to circovirus infection. Inclusion bodies can be seen in some follicles (arrowheads).

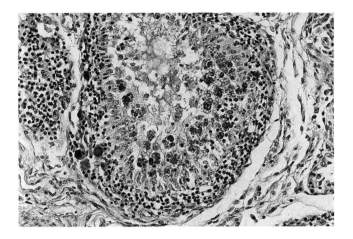

8.5. *Detail of circovirus inclusions in the cytoplasm of bursal reticular cells.*

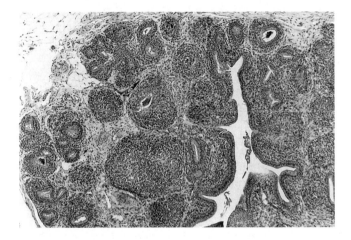

8.6. *Severe bursal depletion and loss of follicles in chronic circovirus infection.*

disease will have swelling and often hemorrhage of the bursa of Fabricius. Depletion and necrosis of lymphocytes in medulla of bursa of Fabricius are seen histologically. Karyomegaly with typical clear to lightly basophilic intranuclear inclusion bodies is occasionally seen in lymphocytes within the bursa of Fabricius.

Other Viruses. Many of the common pet bird viral infections will result in damage to the lymphoid follicles of the bursa of Fabricius. These include Pacheco's disease, parvovirus of ducks and geese, avian influenza, and adenovirus in poultry and psittacine birds. Intranuclear inclusion bodies may be found in bursal reticular cells in Pacheco's disease. Infectious bursal disease virus of chickens has a direct cytopathic effect on immature B cells. There will be extensive necrosis characterized by lymphocytolysis. Chickens infected with this virus are often subsequently immunocompromised. We have recognized a similar virus by electron microscopy in the bursa of Fabricius of ostriches.

Bacteria. Bacterial infections of the bursa of Fabricius are uncommon. They may represent localization of a systemic disease or an extension from a cloacal infection. The bursa of Fabricius may be enlarged and irregular and have caseous foci. Usually the follicles are diffusely and severely depleted of lymphocytes. Multiple foci of necrosis and microabscesses with intralesional bacteria are seen. The abscesses may be surrounded by macrophages and giant cells, some containing intracytoplasmic bacteria.

Yeast. Yeast infections of the bursa of Fabricius are very uncommon. They are most likely a localization of a systemic disease and are more commonly recognized in young cockatiels. The bursa of Fabricius may be difficult to identify grossly. Usually the follicles are diffusely and severely depleted of lymphocytes. Multiple foci of necrosis with intralesional yeast and pseudohyphae are seen. Mixed inflammation of heterophils, lymphocytes, plasma cells, macrophages, and giant cells may be present.

Protozoal Disease. Cryptosporidia are 2- to 5-μm intracytoplasmic, apicomplexid coccidian parasites that parasitize the apical portions of the occulorespiratory, gastrointestinal, and genitourinary epithelia. Infections are rare in pet birds. The majority of cases described have been confined to the gastrointestinal tract. The intestines will have excessive intraluminal fluid and gas. The proventriculus will also have intraluminal fluid and a thickened mucosa. The bursa of Fabricius may appear edematous. The spherical to ovoid cryptosporidia proliferate within the epithelium of the bursa of Fabricius and mucosa epithelium of the proventricular glands and intestinal mucosa. These gram-negative organisms have a foamy, pale eosinophilic cytoplasm with a distinct basophilic nuclei and occasional periodic acid-Schiff-positive internal structures. Many crytosporidial infections occur in birds that are concurrently infected with PBFDV.

Toxins. A number of toxins have resulted in severe lymphocytic depletion and lymphocytolysis of the bursa of Fabricius in wild birds and poultry. These have included crude oil, excessive vitamin D, selenium, mycotoxins, and organotin compounds used as pesticides, stabilizers, disinfectants, molluscicides, antihelminthics, and antitumor agents.

Nutrition. Calorie-deficient diets and hypovitaminosis A will result in atrophy of the bursa of Fabricius of young birds.

Neoplastic Disease. Tumors of the bursa of Fabricius are rare in psittacine birds. There is a single report of a spindle cell sarcoma arising within the bursa of a budgerigar. Lymphosarcoma, the classic poultry tumor of the bursa of Fabricius, is induced by a chicken retrovirus.

Thymus

Cysts. Thymic cysts are rarely found as incidental lesions in birds. The etiology of the cystic development in birds is unknown; however, thymic cysts may be dilations of persistent thymopharyngeal ducts. Another possibility is that they develop during thymic involution from clefts forming in the condensed thymic epithelium. The cysts may be lined by a columnar or stratified squamous epithelium of variable thickness and filled with a colloidlike material (Fig. 8.7).

Atrophy. Premature thymic atrophy is characterized by loss of the lymphocyte population and a loss of cortex and medulla differentiation. In both psittacine birds, the viral diseases commonly associated with the atrophy or widespread lymphocytolysis of the thymus include circoviruses and Pacheco's disease virus. Avian influenza, Marek's disease virus, and some strains of infectious bursal disease virus cause similar lesions in poultry. Nutritional stress and exposure to corticosterone hormone can also induce thymic atrophy.

Neoplastic Disease: Thymoma. Neoplasms of the thymus may arise from the epithelial cells or lymphocytes. The epithelial tumors are classified as thymomas, and the lymphoid tumors are thymic lymphosarcomas. The tumor masses may form anywhere in the subcutis of the neck from the mandible to the thoracic inlet. These masses may be cystic and hemorrhagic (Fig. 8.8).

Thymomas are comprised of a pleomorphic population of small to moderately sized lymphocytes, lymphoblasts, and large reticular cells. The reticular cells are arranged in sheets with large, round to oval vesicular nuclei and a strongly eosinophilic cytoplasm. Mitotic figures are common. These cells may be positive for cytokeratin and proliferating cell nuclear antigen. Thymic lymphosarcomas are typical lymphosarcomas and are composed of sheets of neoplastic lymphocytes effacing the normal architecture of the thymus (Fig. 8.9). Thymic lymphosarcomas often metastasize by the time the primary mass is recognized.

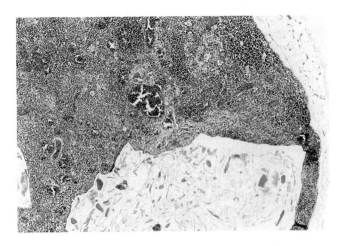

8.7.   Thymic cyst containing amorphous debris.

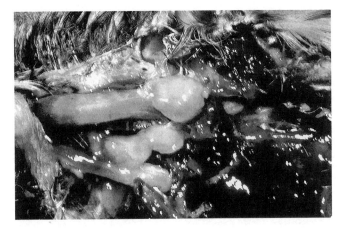

8.8.   Lymphosarcoma involving several lobes of the thymus.

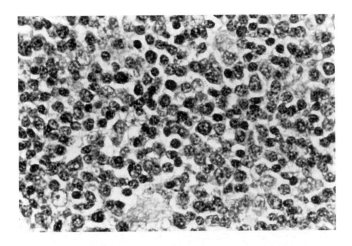

8.9.   Sheet of monomorphic neoplastic lymphoid cells effacing the thymus.

Spleen
Viral Disease

Avian Polyomavirus. Birds with APV disease typically have an enlarged and often hemorrhagic spleen. Histologically there is multifocal splenic necrosis (Fig. 8.10). Karyomegaly with typical lightly basophilic to clear intranuclear inclusions are usually prominent and may be massive (Fig. 8.11), particularly in macrophages of the splenic periarteriolar sheaths (Fig. 8.12). Karyomegaly can be prominent in splenic reticular cells. A nonspecific lymphocytic depletion may also occur. Rarely a bird will survive APV disease. These birds may have little functional tissue remaining in their spleen.

Herpesvirus (Pacheco's Disease). The Pacheco's herpesvirus disease viruses commonly cause lesions of the spleen. Often there is splenomegaly, although this may be absent in birds with peracute disease (Fig. 8.13). Necrosis of the cells in the periarterial lymphatic sheaths and of the mononuclear cells and lymphocytes is common. Pale

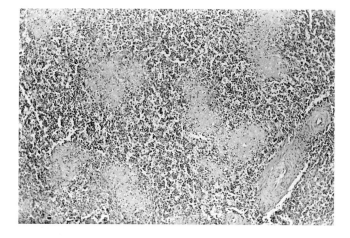

8.10. *Multifocal splenic necrosis in a bird with poly-omavirus infection.*

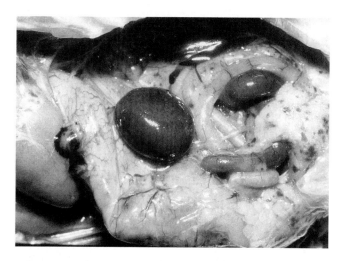

8.13. *Enlarged, mottled spleen in a psittacine bird with Pacheco's disease.*

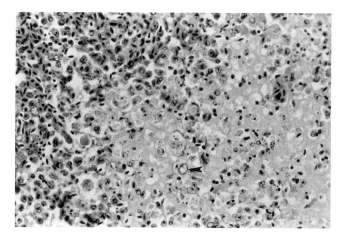

8.11. *Detail of splenic necrosis and minimal inclusion body (arrowhead) formation seen in many large psittacine birds.*

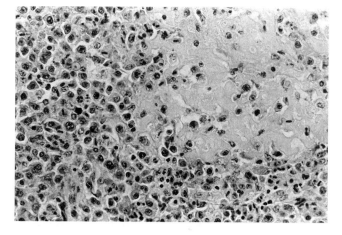

8.14. *Splenic necrosis and mononuclear cell infiltrate in Pacheco's disease.*

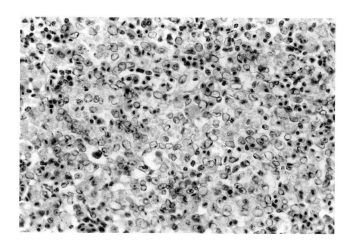

8.12. *Numerous intranuclear inclusion bodies in reticular cells of spleen typical of the presentation in budgerigars and some eclectus parrots.*

to deeply staining eosinophilic intranuclear viral inclusions are generally common. Syncytial cell formation is rare (Fig. 8.14). Pacheco's disease is described in more detail in chapter 4.

Avipoxvirus. Avipoxvirus infection can result in a systemic disease, as well as the classic cutaneous infection. The systemic disease, which is more common in house sparrows, canaries, and other finches, is characterized by a proliferative rhinitis, bronchopneumonia, air sacculitis, and necrosis of the liver and heart. Splenomegaly has been described, although commonly there will be marked lymphocytic depletion. An unusual lesion of marked splenic lymphoid proliferation has been associated with systemic canary pox infections (Fig. 8.15).

Bacterial Disease

Salmonella. This gram-negative bacterium is a member of the large family Enterobacteriaceae and is cosmopolitan

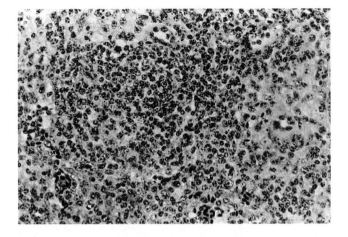

8.15.   Marked lymphoid proliferation typical of systemic canary pox infection. The proliferation can have a "pseudolymphomatous" appearance.

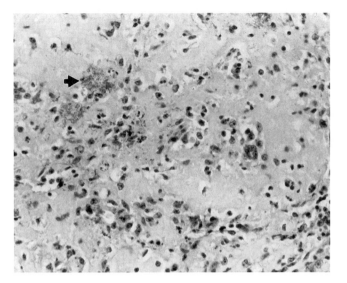

8.17.   Detail of necrotic area from Fig. 8.16. Note the clumps of bacteria (arrow).

in distribution. Salmonella is considered a primary pathogen, with some serotypes able to penetrate the mucosal barrier. Noninvasive serotypes may result in the carrier state. Domestic poultry are the single largest reservoir for *Salmonella*. *Salmonella typhimurium* is the most common psittacine and free-living avian isolate.

The disease progression in birds depends on the number of organisms present, the serotype, and the age, species, and condition of the host. It ranges from peracute, to acute, to chronic, to a subclinical infection.

The classic lesions are hepatomegaly, splenomegaly, pneumonia, and a catarrhal to hemorrhagic enteritis. Salmonellosis may also result in meningitis and osteoarthritis. In most cases, there is a multifocal to coalescing necrotizing splenitis with nodular aggregates of lymphocytes, macrophages, and heterophils (Fig. 8.16). Bacteria may be present within these foci (Fig. 8.17).

Yersinia. *Yersinia pseudotuberculosis*, which is a gram-negative, non-spore-forming, rod bacterium with a zoonotic

potential, is indigenous to Europe and the Soviet Far East but has a worldwide distribution. The organisms can be found in water and on vegetables and fish. Free-living birds and rodents that have access to aviaries are considered to be significant reservoirs of *Y. pseudotuberculosis*. Toucans are reported to be very susceptible. It has been incriminated in major epornitics in canaries, lorikeets, and mynahs. The disease in birds is an acute septicemia, followed by a chronic focal infection, with caseous swellings and nodules resembling avian tuberculosis.

Postmortem lesions include focal necrosis and miliary abscesses of the liver and spleen, as well as a severe catarrhal or hemorrhagic pneumonia. In canaries and related passerine species, there is an impressive swelling of the spleen. Histologically the spleen has irregular multifocal to coalescing areas of necrosis characterized by central cores supporting large numbers of bacteria in a granular eosinophilic matrix and surrounded by a band of degenerate macrophages and cell debris (Fig. 8.18).

Other Bacterial Splenitis. Both systemic and localized bacterial disease may affect the spleen. With bacteremias, the spleen will enlarge and appear deep red with vascular congestion. The bacteremia usually results in peracute to acute lesions with the bacterial organisms confined to the vascular spaces. Peracute lesions may result in perivascular edema and fibrin deposition, and an associated vasculitis characterized by numerous heterophils transmigrating across necrotic vessel walls. The acute lesions will include random foci of acute necrosis characterized by cell debris supported in lacy to homogeneous eosinophilic matrix that may be infiltrated with small numbers of heterophils. Erythrophagocytosis and histiocytic hemosiderin may be present.

Lymphocytic depletion or lymphoid hyperplasia with a plasmacytosis may occur. Heterophils may be a promi-

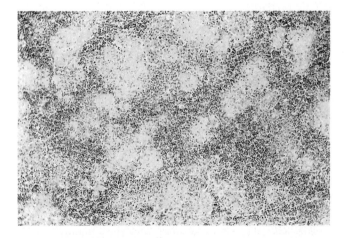

8.16.   Multifocal to confluent splenic necrosis in a bird with salmonellosis.

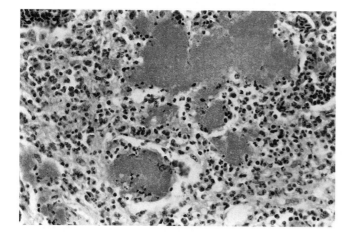

8.18. Splenic necrosis and numerous large bacterial colonies typical of Yersinia infection.

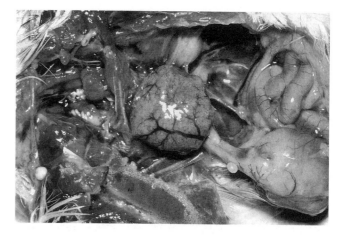

8.20. Markedly enlarged, pale spleen from a bird with avian mycobacteriosis.

nent cell type in spleens from birds with the systemic bacterial disease. Bacteria may be present within multifocal areas of acute necrosis comprised of pools of homogeneous eosinophilic material that represent hemorrhage, fibrin, edema, and cell debris.

Some bacterial organisms will produce more chronic lesions of granulomas. These will have a central core of bright granular material that is proteinaceous fluid or fibrin supporting cell debris and surrounded by variable numbers of macrophages, degenerate heterophils, and occasional multinucleated giant cells (Fig. 8.19).

Mycobacteria. Mycobacteria are acid-fast and weakly gram-positive rods. The typical gross lesions are of organ enlargement, especially the liver and spleen (Fig. 8.20), and a regional thickening of the intestines. Multiple focal to large coalescing firm, white masses may develop through the coelomic body cavity. In pet birds, the nodular masses (tubercles) do not calcify. The granulomas and

granulomatous inflammation are commonly found in the liver, intestine, spleen, lung, air sacs and, uncommonly, bone marrow and kidney.

The splenic parenchyma will be effaced by proliferation of macrophages, lymphocytes, and plasma cells, with granulocytic extramedullary hematopoiesis (Fig. 8.21). Mott cells with numerous intracytoplasmic globular pale eosinophilic pigments are not uncommon within the cell population. Multifocal granulomas and/or foci of necrosis within the splenic parenchyma are characterized by central cores of granular eosinophilic background matrix supporting cell debris and surrounded by vacuolated macrophages as well as infiltrates of mixed inflammatory cells. Multinucleate giant cells may surround a number of these granulomas (Fig. 8.22). Outlines of rod-shaped bacteria may be recognized within the cytoplasm of macrophages as well as

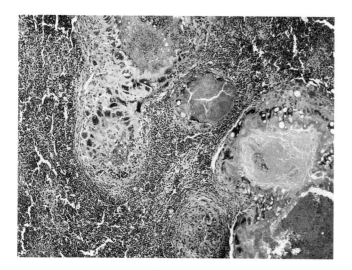

8.19. Chronic bacterial splenitis with granuloma formation.

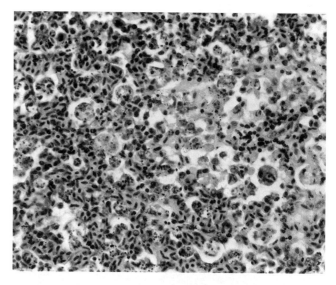

8.21. Early mycobacterial infection with lymphoid depletion and macrophage infiltration. Organisms may not be found on special stains in early inflammatory lesions.

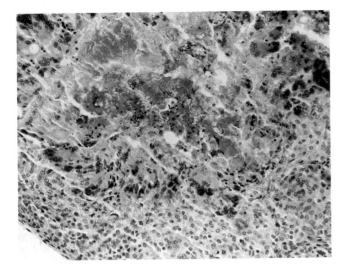

8.22. Chronic avian mycobacteriosis with granuloma formation. Organisms will be seen on special stains at this stage of the infection.

identified within the core of the granulomas on hematoxylin-eosin preparations.

Chlamydophila psittaci. *Chlamydophila* infections in birds commonly cause splenomegaly. The spleen may range from dark red to purple, a change characteristic of a congested spleen. Alternatively the spleen may be pale as the result of increased numbers of histiocytes and plasma cells (Fig. 8.23). On histologic examination, the single most consistent lesion is histiocytosis. There will be hyperplasia of histiocytes of the perivascular sheaths and a diffuse proliferation of plasma cells. Occasionally *Chlamydophila* organisms can be recognized as punctate basophilic structures within the cytoplasm of macrophages. Special stains are often necessary to demonstrate these bacteria. Fluorescent antibody and Gimenez staining of impression smears of the spleen are sensitive and rapid means of identifying this infection. Polymerase chain reaction assays of splenic swabs are also valuable diagnostic tools. The differential

diagnosis for the lesions can include chronic bacterial infections and *Sarcocystis*.

Protozoal Disease

Atoxoplasmosis. *Atoxoplasma* is an apicomplexa coccidian with a prolonged life cycle involving the reticuloendothelial system and intestinal epithelium. It is more commonly recognized as a pathogen of passerines. Asexual reproduction (merogony) occurs in intestinal and blood cells and in the lymphocytic/histiocytic system. Sexual (gametogony) reproduction occurs in enterocytes. The primary gross lesion is the great enlargement of the spleen and occasionally the liver. The small intestines may be edematous and congested. The spleen will have a profound lymphohistiocytic inflammatory response. Mononuclear infiltrates will be present in the liver and lamina propria of the intestines. Oocysts may be recognized in epithelial cells of the intestinal mucosa. Macrophages within the spleen that have an intracytoplasmic, 3- to 5-μm diameter, poorly stained organism indenting the host nucleus can occasionally be found by careful examination (Fig. 8.24). *Atoxoplasma* organisms are readily identified on exfoliative cytology imprints of the spleen and lung. A polymerase chain reaction assay for this organism is commercially available.

Malaria (*Plasmodium*). *Plasmodium* is one of three avian blood parasites that have life cycles with a schizogenous tissue phase and gametogenous sexual phase in host erythrocytes. It has an additional asexual replication phase in erythrocytes, where invading merozoites develop into trophozoites and then undergo schizogony and produce hemozoin. Briefly the life cycle includes a female mosquito that bites a bird and releases sporozoites, which form cryptozoites at point of entry. The first-stage exoerythrocytic schizogony (asexual reproduction) occurs in tissue macrophages adjacent to the mosquito bite. From here, the merozoites develop into metacryptozoites and

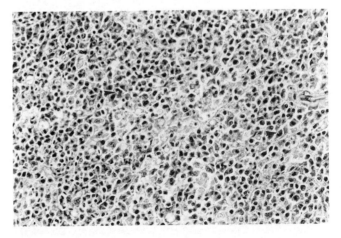

8.24. Atoxoplasma infection with splenic lymphoid depletion and histiocyte infiltration. Organisms are usually difficult to see, but a few indented nuclei are noted (arrowheads).

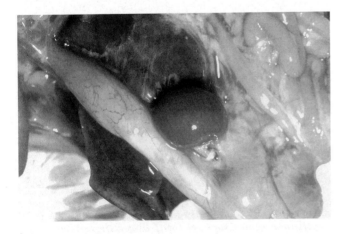

8.23. Splenic enlargement and minimal necrosis (small white foci) as a part of systemic Chlamydophila infection.

can infect erythrocytes and other cells such as endothelial cells (*P. relictum*) and hematopoietic cells (*P. elongatum*). In erythrocytes, the merozoites round up, form trophozoites, and undergo schizogony, during which they incompletely catabolize hemoglobin, leaving a brown pigment, hemozoin, within food vacuoles. Trophozoites can produce more merozoites as well as differentiate into gametocytes. Merozoites will continue on to infect other cells. With infections of nonadapted hosts, the exoerythrocytic schizogony is more prominent, and merozoites from erythrocytic schizonts are able to infect cells of the reticuloendothelial system.

Although there are 25 *Plasmodium* species of birds, these parasites rarely cause disease in psittacines. Some *Plasmodium* can be associated with significant disease in gyrfalcons, peregrines, penguins, and canaries. The liver and spleen can be black in some infected birds, particularly raptors. Hepatosplenomegaly and pulmonary edema are common gross lesions. The most striking histologic lesion is exoerythrocytic schizogony in the lungs, spleen, liver, and other organs. The parasitic hemozoin pigment, which is dark brown and coarsely granular, can be identified in Kupffer's cells and histiocytes of the spleen along with intracellular schizonts (Fig. 8.25). The pigment is birefringent and iron negative. A marked histiocytic and plasmacytic splenitis develops.

Sarcocystis. *Sarcocystosis* is predominantly a disease involving the skeletal muscle and lung. An extensive description of this disease is provided in chapter 2. Birds surviving the acute pulmonary disease develop a histiocytic, plasmacytic splenitis (Fig. 8.26).

Degenerative Disease

Amyloid. This is an insoluble pathologic proteinaceous substance deposited between cells in various tissues and organs of the body. In birds, the amyloid is usually considered to be secondary. This amorphous, eosinophilic, hyaline, extracellular substance encroaches on, and

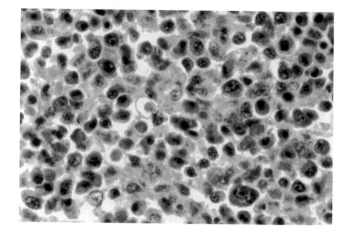

8.26. Mixed mononuclear infiltrate in the spleen of a bird with systemic sarcosporidiosis. The infiltrate is similar to that seen in Chlamydophila infection, and organisms are usually not seen.

results in, pressure atrophy of adjacent cells. Systemic amyloidosis has been reported in finches, in captive domestic and wild Anseriformes especially of the Anatidae family (swans, geese, and ducks), and in gallinaceous birds (domestic fowl and turkeys). The incidence in Pekin ducks ranges from 5% to 40%. Amyloidosis is less common in psittacine birds but, when it does occur, generally involves both the spleen and the kidney. In finches, amyloid deposition is more common in the liver and spleen. The presence of amyloid can be confirmed with special stains (e.g., Congo red) and by examination under polarized light.

Grossly the spleen will appear pale and will be firm when sectioned. Amyloid is a homogeneous, pale, eosinophilic to amphophilic material. It may be found randomly within the splenic parenchyma expanding and filling spaces. Deposits may thicken the basement membranes of blood vessels (Fig. 8.27) or accumulate around

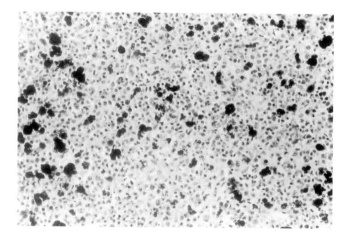

8.25. Macrophages containing malaria pigment in the spleen. The pigment is seen primarily in raptors but not in small passerines with the infection.

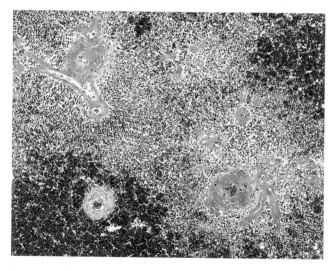

8.27. Mild splenic amyloidosis primarily involving the walls of blood vessels.

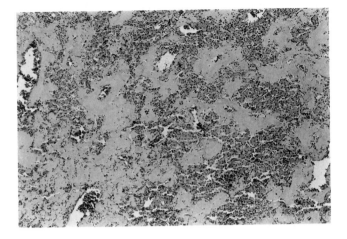

8.28. *Severe splenic amyloidosis with marked tissue effacement.*

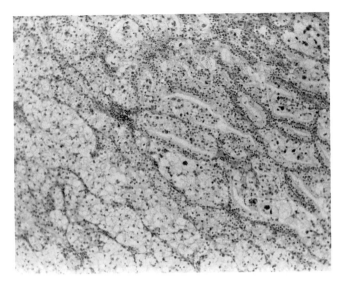

8.29. *Severe infiltration of spleen by macrophages containing lipid in their cytoplasm.*

the periarterial sheaths and extend into the surrounding parenchyma (Fig. 8.28).

Hemosiderin. The accumulation of this iron-containing pigment is typically due to previous hemorrhage (including hemolytic anemia) or severe tissue congestion resulting in breakdown and phagocytosis of the red blood cell debris. Impaired use of iron, such as from systemic bacterial infections or from anemia of chronic disease, also leads to the increased presence of hemosiderin. This is a common mechanism in pet birds. In the spleen, hemosiderin accumulates within sinusoidal macrophages. It is a golden brown granular cytoplasmic pigment that stains positive with Prussian blue.

Histiocytic Lipid Accumulation. The presence of histiocytes with a vacuolated cytoplasm in the spleen of pet birds seems to be associated with chronic liver disease or reproductive disease in female birds. The majority of histiocytes throughout the splenic parenchyma and periarterial sheaths are expanded with a finely vacuolated cytoplasm to coalescing vacuoles (Fig. 8.29). Commonly, in the liver, both hepatocytes and Kupffer's cells will also be enlarged, with cytoplasmic vacuolization. The lesion suggests altered fat metabolism.

Neoplastic Disease

Lymphosarcoma. Multicentric lymphosarcoma is the most common lymphoid neoplasia in psittacine and passerine birds. Diffuse or nodular involvement is characteristic of pet-bird lymphosarcoma. Organs typically infiltrated include liver, spleen, kidneys, skin, bone marrow, gastrointestinal tract, thyroid gland, oviduct, lungs, sinus, thymus, testes, brain, mesentery, trachea, fat, periorbital muscles, and pancreas. The liver is most frequently involved, followed by the spleen and kidneys. These organs generally are enlarged and pale. Other diseases that grossly resemble visceral lymphosarcoma include amyloidosis, fatty liver syndrome, atoxoplasmosis (in

mynahs and canaries), hepatitis, systemic mycobacteriosis, and other neoplasms.

Histologically a solid sheet of a uniform population of lymphoblasts and mature lymphocytes effaces the splenic architecture. The lymphoblastic cells have a large, round to indented vesicular nuclei, one or more prominent nucleoli, and a basophilic cytoplasm (Fig. 8.30). Mitotic figures are common.

Although lymphosarcoma in chickens commonly is associated with retrovirus (avian leukosis virus) or herpesvirus (Marek's) infection, there is no evidence to date of a viral link to the tumor formation in pet birds. Recent molecular investigations suggested a retroviral cause for multicentric lymphosarcoma in a starling. Retrovirus-induced lymphosarcoma has been suspected in other passerine birds, but this remains to be proven.

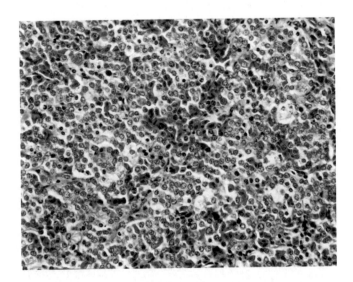

8.30. *Effacement of splenic parenchyma by neoplastic lymphoid cells.*

Myeloproliferative Disorders. Myeloproliferative disorders are neoplastic proliferations of nonlymphoid hematopoietic cells. These neoplastic cells generally infiltrate the spleen, liver, and bone marrow. The infiltration can result in massive enlargement of both the liver and the spleen (Fig. 8.31). In the spleen, the neoplastic proliferation can be difficult to differentiate from excessive granulocytic extramedullary hematopoiesis. The blast forms of the various cell lines are difficult to distinguish on hematoxylineosin stains, making it difficult to determine the neoplastic cell line. In poultry, this type of neoplasm is associated with infections by retroviruses of the leukosis/sarcoma group. A viral etiology has not been proven in psittacines.

Hemangioma and Hemangiosarcoma. Hemangiomas are benign tumors of vascular endothelium. The malignant version is hemangiosarcoma, also known as malignant hemangioendothelioma or angiosarcoma. Hemangiomas are more commonly reported in budgerigars (*Melopsittacus undulatus*) than in other birds and usually occur in the skin or spleen. They are uncommonly described in larger psittacines. Hemangiosarcomas occur in the skin, liver, myocardium, and metacarpus. With the exception of the budgerigar, they are rarely described in the spleen. They are locally invasive, metastatic, and multicentric. Both tumors are characterized by the formation of vascular channels. The endothelial cells of hemangiosarcomas are less well differentiated than those lining the vascular spaces of hemangiomas (Fig. 8.32).

In chickens, hemangiomas and hemangiosarcomas are induced by a recently described strain of avian retrovirus, avian hemangioma virus (AHV). The typical type C retrovirus particle was demonstrated in the tumor by electron microscopy. Retroviruses or viral particles have not been found by electron microscopy in budgerigar hemangiomas.

Myelolipoma. This uncommon tumor has been reported in the subcutis, spleen and, multifocally, in the liver.

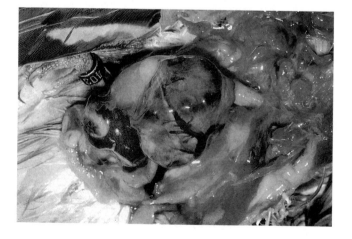

8.31. Markedly enlarged spleen in a bird with myeloproliferative disease.

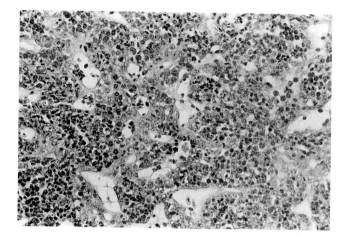

8.32. Low-grade splenic hemangiosarcoma. Irregular vascular channels are separated by proliferating, moderately undifferentiated endothelial cells.

Myelopomas behave like lipomas, with slow progressive growth. They are considered choristomatous (histologically normal tissue in an abnormal location) hematopoietic stem cell elements. Grossly they appear as masses of fat with hemorrhage and can resemble lipomas, xanthomas, and fibrosarcomas. They may contain focal areas of mineralization or bone formation.

Myelolipomas histologically are well-delineated, expansile, benign, extramedullary neoplasms composed of varying proportions of fat and hematopoietic cells. The differential diagnoses based on histologic examination of the tumor in the spleen include hemangiolipoma, osseous metaplasia, hematopoietic neoplasms, and extramedullary hematopoiesis. Hemangiolipomas are fatty neoplasms with endothelium-lined vascular channels. They occur as solitary tumors of the skin and ovary in fowl and as a solitary subcutaneous tumor in budgerigars. Osseous metaplasia, the formation of bone from soft tissue, is comprised of osteoid and spicules of mineralized bone associated with the hematopoietic cells.

Hematopoietic neoplasms (e.g., myelocytoma and myeloblastoma) result from proliferation of a single cell line, with a shift to immaturity. These tumors are relatively common in domestic fowl but rare in exotic birds.

Extramedullary hematopoiesis is a nonencapsulated, dense aggregate of hematopoietic cells that lacks a fatty component. Extramedullary hematopoiesis is seen most frequently in the liver, spleen, kidney, yolk sac remnant, and bursa of Fabricius. It is common in birds with chronic bleeding disorders.

Fibrosarcoma. This tumor originates from fibrous connective tissue and is a common neoplasm in birds. Based on literature reports, fibrosarcomas (malignant) appear to be more common than fibromas (benign). The common sites of occurrence include the limbs, face, beak, syrinx, liver, small intestine, cloaca, spleen, air sacs, and lungs. Fibrosarcomas are white-to-gray, raised or rounded, firm masses that have indistinct borders within the spleen. The spindle-shaped tumor cells are arranged in bundles forming interwoven fascicles. The cells are numerous and closely placed with indistinct cytoplasmic borders (Fig. 8.33). Fibrosarcomas are locally invasive and have a low to moderate metastatic potential.

Metastatic Carcinomas. Metastatic carcinomas to the spleen are rare, with only metastatic gastric carcinoma reported. Gastric carcinomas may reach the spleen from local implants or through the vascular system. In the spleen, gastric carcinomas form irregular tubular structures as well as individualized neoplastic cells. The cells are pleomorphic, with variably distinct cytoplasmic borders and variable amounts of either lacy basophilic pale cytoplasm or deeply granular basophilic cytoplasm. The cell nuclei are variably sized and hyperchromic, with indistinct nucleoli (Fig. 8.34).

Bone Marrow

Lesions of the bone marrow are either hypocellular or hypercellular. Interpretation of erythrocytic-versus-granulocytic responses typically requires comparison with the peripheral blood counts and cytologic examination of the bone marrow cells.

Infectious Disease. Inflammatory diseases caused by bacteria, *Chlamydophila*, and fungi can result in granulocytic hyperplasia (Fig. 8.35). Anemia induced by many disease processes will produce a similar appearance due to erythroid hypoplasia.

Mycobacterial infections can result in severe myeloid hyperplasia and bone marrow infiltrations of macrophages (Fig. 8.36). Granulomas similar to those seen in other organs may also be found in the bone marrow (Fig. 8.37). The macrophages generally have intracytoplasmic acid-fast-positive bacteria (Fig. 8.38).

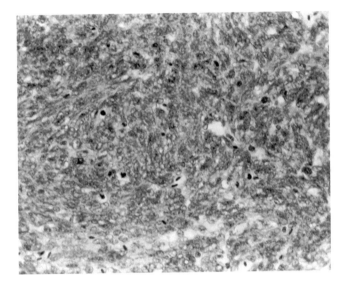

8.33. *Primary splenic fibrosarcoma. Neoplastic cells are poorly differentiated and have indistinct cytoplasmic boundaries.*

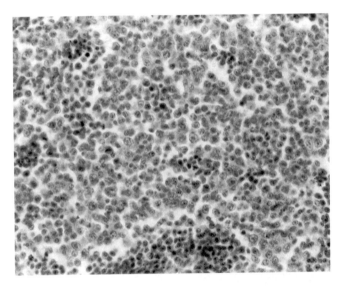

8.35. *Diffuse nonspecific myeloid hyperplasia of the bone marrow.*

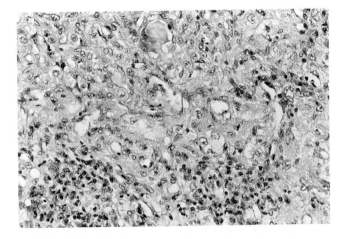

8.34. *Proventricular carcinoma metastatic to the spleen. Tumor cells are individualized, and a few contain mucin in their cytoplasm.*

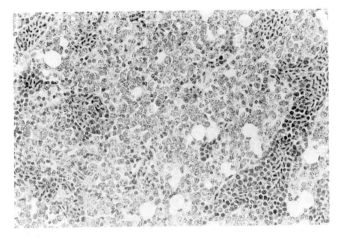

8.36. *Severe myeloid hyperplasia and early macrophage infiltration of the marrow in a bird with avian mycobacteriosis.*

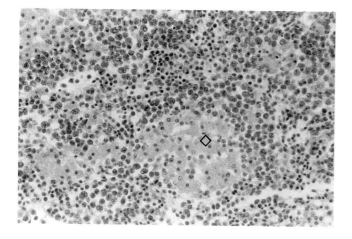

8.37.   Avian mycobacteriosis with focal granuloma formation in the marrow (diamond).

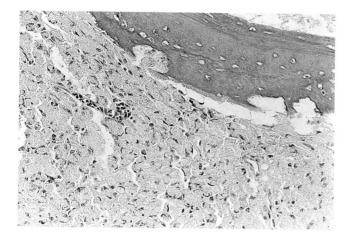

8.38.   Severe avian mycobacteriosis. Diffuse replacement of bone marrow by large macrophages containing acidfast bacteria.

Bone marrow hypoplasia is described with several viral infections. Severe leukopenia and anemia from bone marrow hypoplasia is common in young African grey parrots and pigeons infected with circovirus. Occasionally the typical cytoplasmic basophilic to amphophilic globular inclusions can be found in histiocytic-type cells. Other viruses have been isolated from bone marrow; however, specific lesions are not described. These viruses include herpesvirus, poxvirus, reovirus, and avian polyomavirus.

Toxins. A number of toxins can result in bone marrow hypocellularity. Ochratoxin A produced by *Aspergillus ochraceous* results in bone marrow depression, as does sulfaquinoxaline and cisplatin [*cis*-dichlorodiammineplatinum (II)] toxicity. The myelosuppression of cisplatin is suspected to be due to binding and cross-linking of DNA, with interference of DNA replication. At published dosages for birds, several benzimidazoles, such as fenbendazole, result in a marked heteropenia followed by a progressive anemia and bone marrow suppression. The inhibition of microtubule polymerization is suspected of interfering with mitosis in rapidly dividing cells of the bone marrow and the mucosa of the gastrointestinal tract.

Lead poisoning interferes with several stages of heme synthesis. It acts to inhibit delta-aminolevulinic acid dehydratase, heme synthetase, and the delivery of iron to the site of ferrochelatase action. The bone marrow will be hypocellular, with a marked decrease in mature erythrocytes and an increase in early and late polychromatic erythroblasts. Mitotic figures will be common. In birds, the nuclei of the erythrocytes may serve as lead-storage sites. Grossly the bone marrow can appear fatty or edematous. Other lesions of lead toxicity include hepatocyte necrosis and Kupffer cell hemosiderosis, nephrosis and sloughing of renal tubular epithelium with variable acid-fast intranuclear inclusion bodies in the cells of the proximal convoluted tubules, degeneration of the heart, pectoral skeletal muscles and muscular tunics of the ventriculus, neuronal degeneration of the brain and meningeal edema, and degenerative changes in peripheral nerves (vacuolated myelin sheath with rare swollen axonal segments).

Proliferative Disease

Xanthoma. Xanthomas are not neoplasms but are locally invasive and appear as masses commonly in the skin. They rarely occur in internal organs and even more rarely have been identified within the bone marrow. The masses are of foamy macrophages, multinucleated giant cells, and cholesterol clefts (Fig. 8.39). Xanthomas have been reported most frequently in psittacine and gallinaceous birds. They are considered common in cockatiels and female budgerigars.

Neoplastic Disease

Myeloproliferative Disorders. Myeloproliferative disorders are neoplastic proliferations of nonlymphoid hematopoietic cells that originate in the bone marrow. These neoplastic cells generally infiltrate the spleen, liver, and bone marrow. Hematopoiesis is suppressed by marked

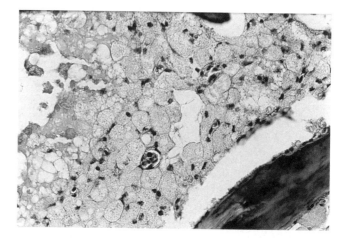

8.39.   Xanthoma of the bone marrow. On routine sections, this must be differentiated from mycobacterial infection (Figure 8.38).

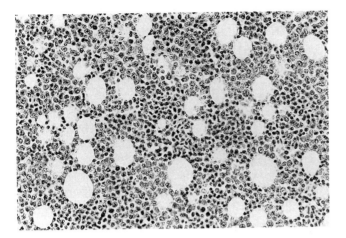

8.40.   Myeloproliferative disease. Monomorphic imma-ture myeloid cells replacing normal marrow elements.

proliferation of tumor cells in the bone marrow (Fig. 8.40). Since blast forms of the various cell lines are difficult to distinguish on hematoxylin-eosin stains, other cytochemical stains are required to identify the neoplastic cell line. Although in poultry this neoplasm is associated with retrovirus infections, a viral etiology has not been proven in psittacine birds.

Hemangiosarcoma. Hemangiosarcomas, also known as malignant hemangioendotheliomas or angiosarcomas, are malignant tumors of vascular endothelium. In birds, they are locally invasive, metastatic, and multicentric. In the diaphysis of long bones, they have an aggressive osteolytic radiographic appearance. Histologically they are typical of hemangiosarcoma in any location (Fig. 8.41).

Metastatic Tumors. Only one metastatic neoplasm to the bone marrow has been reported in pet birds. A leiomyosarcoma, which presented as a nodular growth attached to a rib cage, developed metastases to the bone marrow. This tumor also had metastases in the liver, spleen, and kidneys. The primary site was not determined.

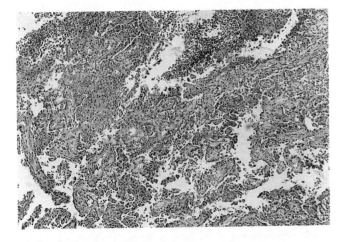

8.41.   Hemangiosarcoma of the marrow. Primary bone involvement may be seen in some cases.

ADDITIONAL READING

Atoji Y, Yamamoto Y, Suzuki Y. 1999. Thymic epithelial cysts in the pigeon. Anat Anz 181:365–370.

Bauck L. 1986. Lymphosarcoma/avian leukosis in pet birds: Case reports. In: Proceedings of the Association of Avian Veterinarians, Miami, FL, pp 241–245.

Balaguer L, Romano J, Mora A. 1995. A poorly-differentiated squamous cell thymoma in a chicken with lymphoma. Avian Pathol 24:737–741.

Cacho ED, Gallego M, Bascuas JA. 1991. Granulopoiesis in the pineal gland of chickens. Am J Vet Res 52:449–452.

Cadman HF, Kelly PJ, Dikanifura M, et al. 1994. Isolation and characterization of serum immunoglobulin classes of the ostrich. Avian Dis 38:616–620.

Carlson HC, Allen JR. 1969. The acute inflammatory reaction in chicken skin: Blood cellular response. Avian Dis 13:817–831.

Chan AS. 1986. Ultrastructure of epithelial thymic cysts of the chick. Poult Sci 65:177–182.

Chand N. 1979. Pharmacological basis of immediate hypersensitivity in the domestic fowl. J Vet Pharmacol Ther 2:151–171.

Coleman CW, Oliver R. 1994. Lymphosarcoma in a juvenile blue and gold macaw (*Ara araruana*) and a mature canary (*Serinus canarius*). J Assoc Avian Vet 8:64–68.

Coleman CW. 1995. Lymphoid neoplasia in pet birds: A review. J Avian Med Surg 9:3–7.

Cook ME. 1991. Nutrition and the immune response of the domestic fowl. Crit Rev Poult Biol 3:167–189.

Daoust PY. 1978. Osteomyelitis and arthritis caused by *Salmonella typhimurium* in a crow. J Wildl Dis 14:483–485.

Fitzgerald SD, Reed WM, Fulton RM. 1995. Development and application of an immunohistochemical staining technique to detect avian polyomaviral antigen in tissue sections. J Vet Diagn Invest 7:444–450.

Fox JH, Greiner EC, Bain P, Jones R. 1996. Malaria in a captive emu (*Dromaius novaehollandiae*) from Florida. Avian Dis 40:477–479.

García A, Latimer KS, Steffens WL, Ritchie BW. 1998. Granulocytic sarcoma in a budgerigar (*Melopsittacus undulatus*). In: Annual international virtual conference in veterinary medicine (IVCVM), University of Georgia College of Veterinary Medicine.

Gardner MB, Rongey RW, Sarma P, Arnstein P. 1981. Electron microscopic search for retrovirus in spontaneous tumors of the parakeet. Vet Pathol 18:700–703.

Glick B. 1986. Immunophysiology. In: Sturkie PD, ed. Avian physiology. New York: Springer-Verlag, pp 87–100.

Goodwin MA. 1989. Cryptosporidiosis in birds: A review. Avian Pathol 18:365–384.

Graczyk TK, Cranfield MR, Shaw ML, Craig LE. 1994. Maternal antibodies against *Plasmodium* sp. in African black-footed penguin chicks. J Wild Dis 30:365–371.

Graham DL. 1993. Special presentation a color atlas of avian chlamydiosis. Semin Avian Exotic Pet Med 2:184–189.

Grimes JE, Arizmendi F. 1992. Survey of clinical psittacine bird sera for *Salmonella typhimurium* agglutinins. Avian Dis 36:813–815.

Hacking MA, Sileo L. 1974. *Yersinia enterocolitica* and *Yersinia pseudotuberculosis* from wildlife in Ontario. J Wildl Dis 10:452–457.

Harrington R, Blackburn BO, Cassidy DR. 1975. Salmonellosis in canaries. Avian Dis 19:827–829.

Hill JE, Burke DL, Rowland GN. 1986. Hepatopathy and lymphosarcoma in a mynah bird with excessive iron storage. Avian Dis 30:634–636.

Johnson-Delaney CA. 1989. The avian immune system and role in disease. In: Proceedings of the Association of Avian Veterinarians, Miami, FL, pp 20–28.

Jones MP. 1994. Avian immunology: A review. In: Proceedings of the Association of Avian Veterinarians, Miami, FL, pp 333–336.

Ketz CJ, Carpenter JW, Bacmeister C. 1999. What is your diagnosis? J Avian Med Surg 13:218–222.

Latshaw JD. 1991. Nutrition: Mechanisms of immunosuppression. Vet Immunol Immunopathol 30:111–120.

Latimer KS, Rakich PM, Kircher IM, et al. 1990. Extracutaneous viral inclusions in psittacine beak and feather disease. J Vet Diagn Invest 2:204–207.

Latimer KS. 1994. Oncology. In: Ritchie BW, Harrison GJ, Harrison LR, eds. Avian medicine: Principles and applications. Lake Worth, FL: Wingers, pp 667–669.

Latimer KS, Ritchie BW, Campagnoli RP, Harris DJ. 2000. Cutaneous T-cell-rich B-cell lymphoma and leukemic blood profile in an umbrella cockatoo (*Cacatua alba*). In: Annual international virtual conference in veterinary medicine (IVCVM), University of Georgia College of Veterinary Medicine.

Leach MW. 1992. A survey of neoplasia in pet birds. Semin Avian Exotic Pet Med 1:52–64.

Lung NP, Thompson JP, Kollias GV, Klein PA. 1996. Development of monoclonal antibodies for measurement of immunoglobulin G. Am J Vet Res 57:1157–1161.

Lung NP, Thompson JP, Kollias GV, et al. 1996. Maternal immunoglobulin G antibody transfer and development of immunoglobulin G. Am J Vet Res 57:1162–1167.

Maeda H, Ozaki K, Fukui S, Narama I. 1994. Thymoma in a Java sparrow (*Padda oryzivora*). Avian Pathol 23:353–357.

Marsh AE, Barr BC, Tell L, et al. 1997. In vitro cultivation and experimental inoculation of *Sarcocystis falcatula* and *Sarcocystis neurona* merozoites into budgerigars (*Melopsittacus undulatus*). J Parasitol 83:1189–1192.

Moore FM, Petrak ML. 1985. Chlamydia immunoreactivity in birds with psittacosis: Localization of chlamydiae by the peroxidase-antiperoxidase method. Avian Dis 29:1036–1042.

Nakamura K, Ogiso M, Tsukamoto K, et al. 2000. Lesions of bone and bone marrow in myeloid leukosis occurring naturally in adult broiler breeders. Avian Dis 44:215–221.

O'Toole D, Haven T, Driscoll M, Nunamaker C. 1992. An outbreak of Pacheco's disease in an aviary of psittacines. J Vet Diagn Invest 4:203–205.

Page CD, Schmidt RE, English JH, et al. 1992. Antemortem diagnosis and treatment of sarcocystosis in two species of psittacine. J Zoo Wildl Med 23:77–85.

Panigrahy B, Grimes JE, Rideout MI, et al. 1979. Zoonotic diseases in psittacine birds: Apparent increased occurrence of chlamydia. J Am Vet Med Assoc 175:359–361.

Phalen DN, Wilson VG, Graham DL. 1995. Failure of maternally derived yolk IgG to reach detectable concentrations in the sera of nestling budgerigars (*Melopsittacus undulatus*). Avian Dis 39:700–708.

Phalen DN, Wilson VG, Graham, DL. 1996. Characterization of the avian polyomavirus-associated glomerulopathy of nestling parrots. Avian Dis 40:140–149.

Quiroga MI, Aleman N, Vazquez, S, Nieto JM. 2000. Diagnosis of atoxoplasmosis in a canary (*Serinus canarius*) by histopathologic and ultrastructural examination. Avian Dis 44:465–469.

Rae MA, Shafer D. 1996. Thymoma in caged birds. In: Proceedings of the Association of Avian Veterinarians, Tampa, FL, pp 101–108.

Ramos-Vara JA, Smith EJ, Watson GL. 1997. Lymphosarcoma with plasmacytoid differentiation in a scarlet macaw (*Ara macao*). Avian Dis 41:499–504.

Redig PT. 1993. Avian malaria. In: Proceedings of the Association of Avian Veterinarians, Miami, FL, pp 173–181.

Ritchie BW, Niagro FD, Latimer KS, et al. 1992. Antibody response to and maternal immunity from an experimental psittacine beak and feather disease vaccine. Am J Vet Res 53:1512–1518.

Schmidt RE. 1997. Neoplastic diseases. In: Altman RB, Clubb SL, Dorrestein GM, Quesenberry K, eds. Avian medicine and surgery. Philadelphia: WB Saunders, pp 590–600.

Schmidt RE. 1997. Immune system. In: Altman RB, Clubb SL, Dorrestein GM, Quesenberry K, eds. Avian medicine and Surgery. Philadelphia: WB Saunders, pp 645–652.

Schoemaker NJ, Dorrestein GM, Latimer KS, et al. 2000. Severe leukopenia and liver necrosis in young African grey parrots (*Psittacus erithacus erithacus*) infected with psittacine circovirus. Avian Dis 44:470–478.

Sela-Donenfeld D, Korner M, Pick M, et al. 1996. Programmed endothelial cell death induced by an avian hemangioma retrovirus is density dependent. Virology 223:233–237.

Sharma JM. 1991. Overview of the avian immune system. Vet Immunol Immunopathol 30:13–17.

Socaciu C, Baba AI, Rotaru O. 1994. Histopathologic investigations of acute and subchronic toxicities of some organotin compounds in chickens. Vet Hum Toxicol 36:535–539.

Toth TE, Veit H, Gross WB, Siegel BP. 1988. Cellular defense of the avian respiratory system: Protection against *E. coli*. Avian Dis 32:681–687.

Trust KA, Miller M, Ringelman JK, Orme IM. 1990. Effects of ingested lead on antibody production in mallards (*Anas platyrhynchos*). J Wild Dis 26:316–322.

Vainio O, Imhof BA. 1995. The immunology and developmental biology of the chicken. Immunol Today 16:365–370.

Wade LL, Polack EW, O'Connell PH, et al. 1999 Multicentric lymphoma in a European starling (*Sturnus vulgaris*). J Avian Med Surg 13:108–115.

Westerhof I, Pellicaan CHP. 1995. Effects of different application routes of glucocorticoids on the adrenocortical axis in pigeons. J Av Med Surg 9:175–181.

9 Musculoskeletal System

SKELETAL MUSCLE

Normal Structure

Birds have both red and white muscle fibers, both of which are found in most muscles. Red and white fibers are differentiated by their myoglobin content. In the pectoral muscles of birds like the hummingbird, there may be only red fibers, which fatigue slowly. Two-joint muscles, which span two articulations between their origin and insertion, comprise most of the important strong muscles of birds. Histologically, avian skeletal muscle resembles mammalian skeletal muscle.

Disease

Congenital Disease. Muscular dystrophy is reported in chickens and turkeys but not in pet birds. The lesion is characterized by irregular atrophy, with myofibers lost and replaced by fat. The number of nuclei is increased, and fiber size is reduced.

Arthrogryposis is a term for congenital flexure or contracture of joints secondary to failure of proper skeletal muscle development (Fig. 9.1). There is atrophy of mus-

cles that is secondary to congenital neurologic problems. Affected myofibers are lost and replaced by fibrous tissue. The condition can also be secondary to congenital toxicity due to alkaloids from plants such as tree tobacco (*Nicotiana glauca*), lupines (*Lupinus* sp.), and poison hemlock (*Conium maculatum*).

Noninflammatory Disease

Atrophy. Muscle atrophy is a common reaction to many problems, including disuse, denervation, generalized chronic disease, local compression, and aging. Grossly there is a diminution of muscle size (Fig. 9.2). In birds, particularly budgerigars, disuse atrophy may occur secondary to nerve damage caused by renal tumors.

Histologically a decrease in fiber size and cross-sectional area alterations of contractile elements is seen. There may be shrinkage of the plasma membrane, which pulls away from the external lamina, which in turn may become convoluted. The sarcoplasmic reticulum becomes more prominent, as do other organelles.

Hypertrophy. This is usually a compensatory change that results in an enlarged muscle mass. There may be

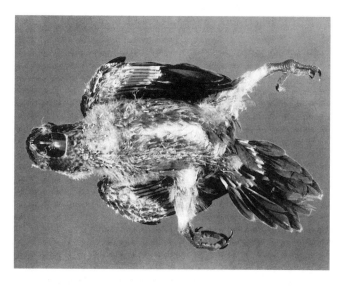

9.1. *Multiple congenital joint flexures secondary to improper skeletal muscle development.*

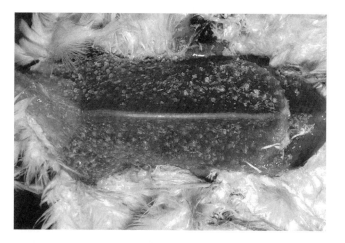

9.2. *Severe pectoral muscle atrophy secondary to chronic disease and malnutrition.*

increased numbers of fibrils, but histologic changes are often difficult to detect.

Steatosis. This is seen sporadically in birds, particularly obese Amazon parrots and other obese psittacine birds. An extensive increase in intramuscular fat, with replacement of myofibers, is noted. The cause is usually malnutrition, but metabolic disorders should be considered.

Trauma. Trauma results in hemorrhage, edema, and gross disruption of muscles. The affected area may become yellow-brown with chronicity (Fig. 9.3). The extent of the muscle reaction will depend on whether the injured area develops a secondary infection. Intramuscular injections usually lead to some necrosis and mononuclear inflammatory infiltration, with macrophages, lymphocytes, plasma cells, and giant cells present in severe reactions. Free and phagocytosed amorphous material with variable tinctorial properties may be seen. The extent of the muscle necrosis varies with the nature and volume of the drug. Massive muscle necrosis is associated with some forms of compounded long-acting doxycycline formulations.

Nutritional Disease. Pectoral muscle mass is an important indicator of how long a bird had been in a catabolic state prior to death. Birds that die acutely will have substantial body fat, adequate heart fat, and a robust pectoral muscle mass. Subacute disease with decreased food consumption will result in a loss of heart fat, followed by muscle wasting. Birds with chronic disease often have severe loss of pectoral muscle mass. The rate of loss of pectoral muscle mass is at least, in part, proportional to the size of the bird. Smaller birds with higher metabolic rates lose fat and muscle mass faster than larger species. Typically, however, a robust, medium-sized parrot that is not eating or eating very little will lose most of its pectoral muscle in 5 to 7 days.

Vitamin E or selenium deficiencies are implicated in muscle disease in picivorous birds that are fed a diet of improperly frozen and thawed fish. Any diet containing rancid polyunsaturated fat may cause similar lesions. A similar disease is seen in other species of birds, including companion birds.

Gross lesions of vitamin E and selenium deficiency are white streaks and patches in striated muscle (Fig. 9.4). Histologic changes include muscle fiber degeneration without inflammation. Individual fibers may be enlarged and hypercontracted, with loss of striations and with hypereosinophilia (Fig. 9.5). Fibers eventually become shrunken and fragmented, and there may be an infiltration of macrophages that phagocytose necrotic debris. Fibrosis and mineralization can be seen in chronic lesions (Figs. 9.6–9.8). Myocardial, hepatic, and central nervous system lesions may also accompany the muscle lesions (chapters 4 and 10).

The great-billed parrot is an uncommon avicultural species that has experienced a high mortality rate in captivity. A review of necropsies of these birds (D. Phalen 2001, unpublished data) shows that most have some degree of skeletal and cardiac muscle degeneration that

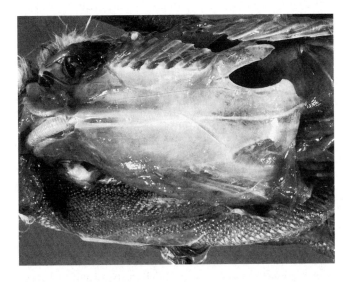

9.4.   Large area of pale pectoral muscle fibers in a bird with vitamin E deficiency.

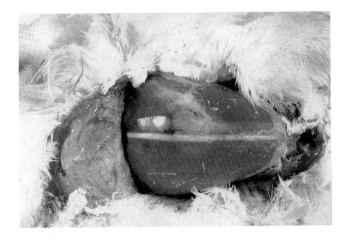

9.3.   Focal area of traumatic hemorrhage and necrosis in the pectoral muscle.

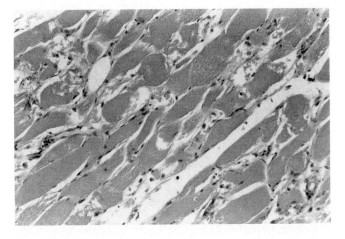

9.5.   Early noninflammatory skeletal muscle degeneration in vitamin E deficiency. Fibers are swollen and fragmented.

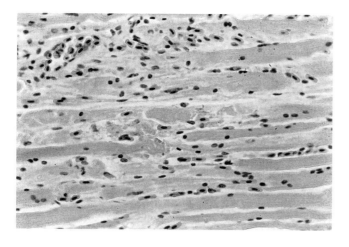

9.6. *Shrinkage and fragmentation of myofibers in subacute to chronic vitamin E deficiency. There is some sarcolemmal nuclear proliferation and macrophage infiltration.*

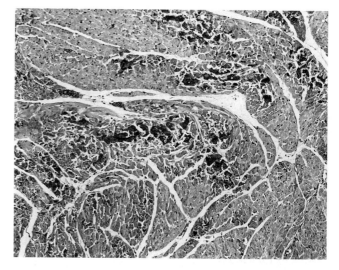

9.8. *Severe mineralization in chronic nutritional myodegeneration.*

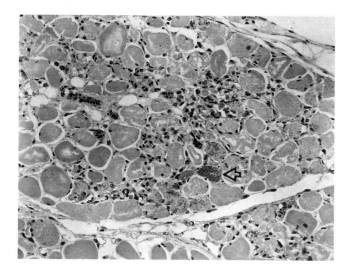

9.7. *Chronic nutritional myodegeneration. In addition to degeneration and cell infiltration, there is early mineralization of myofibers (arrow).*

resembles that seen in other species with vitamin E or selenium deficiency. An additional lesion that is also consistent with this etiology is a spongiform encephalopathy. Although the pathogenesis of this lesion is not proven, it is thought that a diet low in fat (the major source of vitamin E) may be the cause.

Exertional/Capture Myopathy. Stress-related or exertional rhabdomyolysis results in muscle necrosis with grossly noted yellow foci and hemorrhage in acute cases. With chronicity, firm white streaks are noted. At times, entire muscles or muscle groups will be affected and will be uniformly pale. Histologically necrosis and hemorrhage with variable fragmentation of myofibers are seen in acute cases. As the lesion ages, there is macrophage infiltration, fibroplasia, and mineralization.

Endocrinopathies. Hyperthyroidism and hyperadrenocorticism can lead to myofiber degeneration or atrophy. The morphologic changes are as described previously.

Toxic Myopathy. Toxins such as ionophores used as coccidiostats and growth promoters, gossypol, and plants such as *Cassia* sp. have caused skeletal muscle lesions in birds, including ostriches, quail, and other African wild birds. Gross changes may not be noted, and histologic lesions can be minimal. Loss of striations, fragmentation, macrophage infiltration, and mineralization are reported. Although not specifically reported in common pet birds, the potential for exposure exists.

Other Disease. Myasthenia gravis is an autoimmune disease of people and is seen in dogs and cats. Affected animals have clinical muscle weakness. The condition may be associated with thymic hyperplasia. Occasionally adult birds that die acutely are found to have thymic hyperplasia as an isolated lesion. Whether these birds have myasthenia gravis remains unproven. Consistent morphologic changes in skeletal muscle of these birds have not been demonstrated. Immune-mediated myositis has not been documented in birds.

Inflammatory Disease: Infectious Disease. Although not common, a variety of infectious agents can cause myositis. The infections can be associated with trauma, extension from adjacent tissue, or hematogenous dissemination.

Viral myositis is uncommon. A proliferative, but nonneoplastic, fibromatosis of skeletal muscle has been produced experimentally by cloned recombinant avian leukosis virus. Polyomavirus infection in large psittacine birds may cause skeletal muscle lesions. Gross pallor and occasional hemorrhage are seen (Fig. 9.9). Myofiber necrosis, sarcolemmal karyomegaly, and inclusion body formation may be noted histologically.

Bacterial infections can be aerobic or anaerobic. They rarely are limited to skeletal muscle, usually also involving

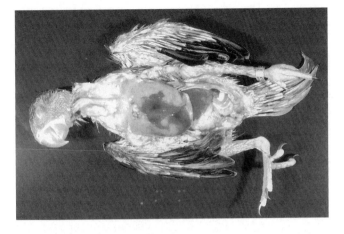

9.9. *Marked skeletal muscle hemorrhage due to polyomavirus infection.*

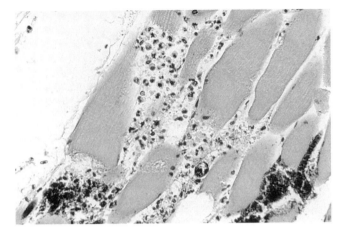

9.11. *Bacterial myositis. Note the inflammation and large bacterial colonies.*

subcutis, fascia, or bone. Necrosis and accumulation of yellow caseous material is seen in severe lesions. Heterophils predominate in early lesions, with increasing numbers of macrophages and plasma cells with chronicity. Eventually granulation tissue may form. Organisms may or may not be seen (Figs. 9.10 and 9.11).

Mycotic infections are often due to local extension from air sacs or due to systemic disease. They are most common in immunosuppressed birds, although overwhelming infections are seen in otherwise normal birds. Grossly nonspecific areas of necrosis and, in some cases, abscess formation are present. Histologically the lesion is similar to that of bacterial infection, with specificity due to finding fungal organisms (Fig. 9.12). Infarction of an entire pectoral muscle was seen in a starling that had fungal-induced thromboembolism of the pectoral artery.

Parasitic infections of skeletal muscle associated with visceral larva migrans (*Baylisascaris procyonis*) are possible as incidental findings, with the parasite causing clinical signs when it invades the central nervous system (chapter

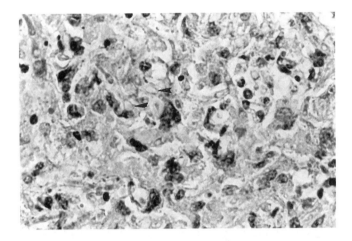

9.12. *Mycotic myositis. Severe necrosis and an infiltrate of macrophages are seen. Fragments of fungal hyphae are difficult to see in many cases (arrowheads).*

10). Mites (*Laminosioptes cysticola*) can invade skeletal muscle in some cases. These mites have been found in a variety of birds. Gross changes vary from small white foci that may be mineralized to abscess formation and tracts that may lead to the skin. Finding the parasite or fragments is necessary for a definitive diagnosis.

Sarcocystosis is a disease of many species of birds. Most *Sarcocystis* sp. are generally adapted to their host and cause little disease. Ducks are commonly affected with *S. riyeli*. The definitive host for this parasite is the skunk. Large protozoal cysts (rice grains) are found in the pectoral muscles of these birds. Sarcocystosis is generally an incidental finding in most species of New World parrots. Mature sarcocysts filled with bradyzoites are seen within the muscle but do not elicit inflammation or muscle degeneration (Fig. 9.13). By contrast, sarcocystosis can cause severe myositis in Old World species of parrots, particularly the eclectus parrots. Gross changes may not be seen, but, if the infection is severe, small white foci or steaks may be present. Histologically necrosis, mononuclear inflammatory infiltrates, and myodegeneration can

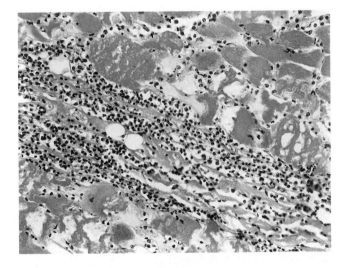

9.10. *Myodegeneration and heterophil infiltration in acute bacterial myositis.*

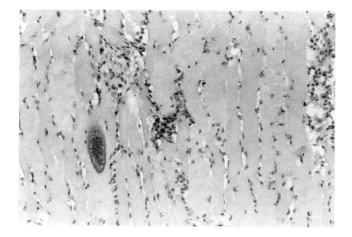

9.13. *Cyst of* **Sarcocystis** *found incidentally in skeletal muscle of a New World psittacine bird.*

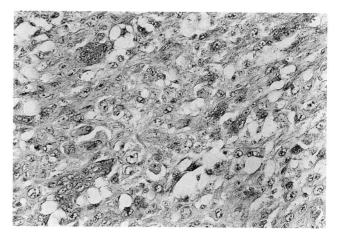

9.15. *Rhabdomyosarcoma. Note the large, multinucleated cells and strap cells.*

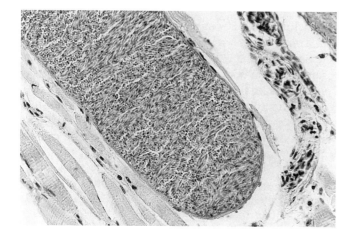

9.14. *Multifocal myositis and cyst of* **Sarcocystis falcatula** *in skeletal muscle.*

be found, with or without organisms (Fig. 9.14). The primary host for *Sarcocystis falcatula*, the species believed to infect parrots in the New World, is the opossum. Birds become infected when they ingest an insect that has fed on opossum feces, or the insect itself acts to move the sporocysts onto the bird's food. Experimentally infection of budgerigars indicated that cysts are found in skeletal muscle by 8 days after inoculation. In breast muscle most cysts degenerated, but in other locations they matured in 44 to 77 days.

Neoplastic Disease

Rhabdomyoma and Rhabdomyosarcoma. Primary tumors of skeletal muscle are infrequently reported in pet birds. A site predilection for these tumors is not observed. Grossly, benign tumors are tan-red and resemble normal skeletal muscle. They are comprised of striated myofibers, and cross striations are usually visible. Rhabdomyosarcomas have irregular borders and may be tan to gray. Histologically, strap cells and large multinucleated cells are present (Fig. 9.15).

As in mammals, lymphosarcoma is one of the few tumors that will commonly invade skeletal muscle. Grossly there are gray-white masses, which are comprised of diffuse sheets of immature lymphoid cells. Marek's disease and fibromatosis (described previously) are caused by viruses and have not been documented in pet birds. Malignant melanoma can invade skeletal muscle and is usually associated with skin and subcutaneous lesions. Tumor cells are usually pigmented but amelanotic types are seen.

Metastatic tumors are rare in skeletal muscle.

TENDONS AND LIGAMENTS

Specific conditions of either tendons or ligaments are infrequently diagnosed. Possible problems include physical damage following trauma, inflammation of tendon sheaths, and neoplasia. Cranial luxation of the tibiotarsus is an uncommon but regular lesion seen in nestling parrots. Ligaments supporting the knee in these birds are completely disrupted. The ligament of the extensor propatagialis muscle is often injured when wings are immobilized as part of the treatment for fracture of the bones of the wings. Bandages cause pressure necrosis of the overlying skin and the ligament. Resulting inflammation causes contracture and scarring of the ligament. Birds with this lesion are unable to extend their wing fully and fly. In systemic gout, urate tophi commonly form on the sheaths of the flexor tendons of the antebrachium and on the tendons of the feet.

Infectious agents that affect the tendons of poultry include *Mycoplasma synoviae*, other bacteria, and a reovirus. These diseases first start as an arthritis and spread locally to involve the tendons. A pleocellular inflammatory infiltrate is seen with all infections, and fibrin may be present. Organisms may or may not be seen. Although studies have found a few conures with antibodies to *M. synoviae*, and budgerigars have been experimentally infected with this organism, its role in clinical disease in pet birds has not been documented.

Noninfectious inflammation associated with trauma or immune-mediated disease is usually mononuclear. Although lesions suggestive of immune-mediated disease are seen occasionally, the exact underlying cause is usually not determined.

Tendon sheath sarcomas are possible but rarely seen.

BONE AND CARTILAGE

Normal Structure

There are several unique aspects to the avian skeleton. Birds have only a single ear ossicle (columella/stapes). They have an additional bone in the shoulder, the coracoid, which is not present in other animals. The coracoid articulates with the clavicle, humerus, and sternum. Birds also have articulated ribs, and their ribs have a prominent uncinate processes, a feature shared with reptiles. The bird's sternum is a broad bone that covers most of the ventrum of the coelomic cavity. A prominent keel or carina that projects from the sternum acts as an attachment for the pectoral muscles. The keel is absent in ratites (ostrich, rheas, emus, and kiwis). There are eight thoracic vertebrae. Thoracic vertebrae 1 through 6 are fused to form the notarium. Thoracic vertebrae 7 and 8 are fused together with the combined lumbar vertebrae, ilium, pubis, and ischium to form the synsacrum.

The bird's wing also has a reduced number of bones. In the manus, they have a large major digit and a small, nearly vestigial minor digit. The three metacarpal bones are fused. A third short digit, the alula, articulates with the leading edge of the fused metacarpal bones just distal to the articulation with the carpal bones. There are only two carpal bones: the radial and the ulnar. In contrast to mammals, the ulna is a larger bone than the radius.

The hind limb also has several fused bones. The tibia is fused with the proximal tarsal bones and is referred to as the tibiotarsus. The distal tarsal bones fuse with a single tarsal bone to become the tarsometatarsus. The number of toes present and their orientation will vary with the species. Most birds have four toes, but several species only have three, and the ostrich only has two.

Air sacs extend into many bones, replacing the marrow. The degree of pneumatization is somewhat species specific. In most birds, the femur, humerus, sternum, skull, and at least some of the vertebrae are pneumatized.

Avian bone matrix varies with the skeletal site, reflecting the differing functions of bone. The avian physis has four zones from epiphysis to medulla: the zones of proliferation, prehypertrophy, hypertrophy, and ossification.

Relationship of Bone to Eggshell Formation

Female birds, in order to lay an egg, must transport a considerable amount of calcium to the shell gland and subsequently the eggshell itself within a short period. There is insufficient calcium in the average bird's diet to support this demand; therefore birds have evolved a type of bone —medullary bone—that can serve as a storage site for readily mobilized calcium. Medullary bone develops in long bones that are not pneumatized. As a hen prepares to lay, spicules and then trabeculae develop from the endosteum of the surrounding compact bone. If breeding behavior persists, but the hen does not lay, the medullary bone will completely fill the medullary cavity. The medullary bone is strongly basophilic and clearly distinguishable from the cortical bone. During the cycle of ovulation/ovipositioning, periods of medullary bone formation alternate with periods of depletion. If dietary calcium is insufficient to replace the calcium lost to egg laying, the medullary bone is lost completely and the cortical bone is reabsorbed.

Disease/Lesions of Bone

General Reactions to Injury. Direct physical injury leads to osteoblastic proliferation (from the osteogenic layer of the periosteum) and new bone formation. Bone necrosis is seen secondary to neoplasia, vascular lesions, or osteomyelitis.

Fracture repair is similar to that in mammals. There is initial hematoma formation followed by mesenchymal cell proliferation, which matures into osteoblasts that form the woven bone of the callus. Eventually, the woven bone is replaced by lamellar bone. Birds are unique in that if the fracture site is stabilized, they will form an endosteal callus instead of a periosteal callus. However, if movement continues to occur at the fracture site, a periosteal callous will also form.

If a limb is not used, bone resorption will increase and bone formation will diminish.

Abnormalities of Development. Developmental anomalies can be genetic, adaptational, or due to teratogens. Congenital long-bone deformities are the most commonly recognized bone malformations. Other miscellaneous anomalies include brachygnatha, polydactylia, syndactyly, and spina bifida (Figs. 9.16 and 9.17). These conditions are primary structural defects associated with localized problems during embryogenesis and occur sporadically in pet birds. Other congenital anomalies result-

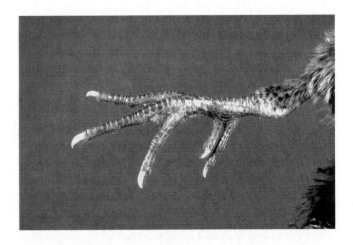

9.16. *Congenital polydactylia. These lesions are sporadic and have not been related to any specific cause.*

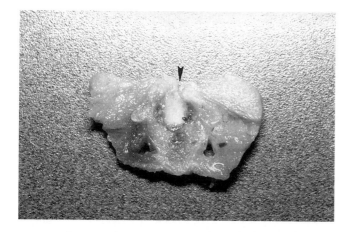

9.17.   Cross section of the vertebral column through an area of spina bifida. The dorsal portions of the vertebra were missing, and there was a space that communicated with the surface (arrowhead).

ing in deformities may arise late in fetal life and are alterations in a previously normal structure. Their cause is often not apparent but may include the position of the embryo in the egg and the turning frequency of the egg.

Chondrodystrophies. Tibial dyschondroplasia is seen in turkeys, chickens, and ducks but is not reported in pet birds. Copper deficiency, specific toxins, excessive dietary cysteine, and acidosis are all implicated in its pathogenesis. Grossly an unmineralized core of cartilage extends from the articular cartilage of the tibia distally into the diaphysis. Histologically the cartilage core is comprised of hypertrophic chondrocytes. This lesion is believed to be the result of a defect in vascularization of the cartilage, resulting in an insufficient supply of mineral ions and nutrients to cartilage. As a result, matrix vesicle formation and subsequent mineralization are not properly supported, and some chondrocytes in the growth plate do not reach normal size and thus undergo premature necrosis.

Nutritional/Metabolic Disease
Nutritional Chondrodystrophy. Deficiencies of manganese, choline, biotin, nicotinic acid, zinc, or pyridoxine cause a generalized disorder of growth of long bones in poultry, and similar lesions are seen in companion birds. Linear growth is primarily impaired, but mineralization and appositional growth are not affected. Bones become short, and joints enlarge. Varus or valgus leg deformities with gastrocnemius tendon displacement are other manifestations of this disorder. Histologically the zone of proliferation is hypoplastic and disorganized.

Osteoporosis (Osteopenia). Osteopenia is characterized by a reduction in bone mass, with the remaining bone normally mineralized. It is a failure of bone matrix formation. It is not a simple loss of apatite and collagen; there are changes in the collagen molecule biochemistry and therefore the physical properties of the collagen fiber. Increased lysine hydroxylation and change in the inter-

molecular cross-link profile lead to increased turnover of collagen and increased bone fragility. Causes of osteopenia/osteoporosis include starvation; calcium, copper, phosphorus, or vitamin D_3 deficiencies; and reduced physical activity. Grossly the cortical bone has reduced thickness and is more porous. The bone is easily fractured and may bend when pressure is applied (Fig. 9.18). The trabecular bone becomes thinner and is eventually lost (Figs. 9.19 and 9.20).

Rickets and Osteomalacia. The name applied to this condition depends on the age of the bird. Rickets is seen in birds in which the skeleton is still growing. Osteomalacia occurs in birds that are fully grown. These problems are due to a failure of mineralization of matrix leading to bone deformities and fractures.

Rickets is the result of the failure of mineralization of newly deposited osteoid. Insufficient dietary calcium, vitamin D_3, or phosphorus and excess phosphorus or calcium will all cause rickets. Grossly the joints of birds with rickets are swollen. Bones are soft and the metaphyses

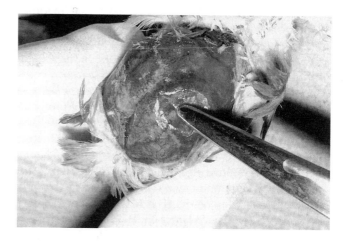

9.18.   Severe osteopenia leading to bone deformation with pressure. This female bird had produced numerous eggs and was eggbound at the time of death.

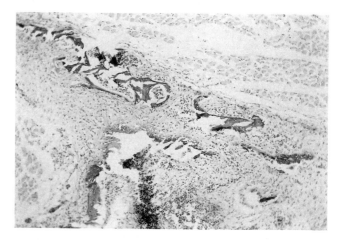

9.19.   Severe osteopenia illustrating marked loss of continuity of the cortical bone.

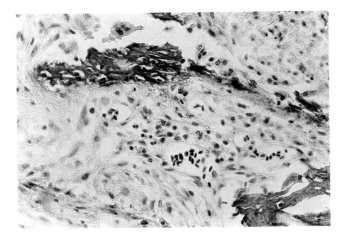

9.20.   Detail of cortical bone remnant in a case of osteopenia.

flared. Curving deformities of long bones and folding fractures are common. The histologic lesion will depend on the cause of the rickets and the duration of the dietary imbalance. The following descriptions are based on work done in chickens and on cases we have seen in other avian species.

The bone lesions of calcium-deficient rickets are characterized by disorganization and thickening of the zone of proliferation with poor physeal vascularization. Thick seams of unmineralized osteoid surround trabeculae, and metaphyseal fibroplasia may occur. The zone of proliferation is unchanged in hypophosphatemic and excessive-calcium rickets, but the hypertrophic zone is elongated, and there is defective mineralization of the hypertrophic cartilage cells resulting in long columns of cartilage, surrounded by wide unmineralized osteoid seams extending into the primary spongiosa (Fig. 9.21). Vitamin D_3-deficiency rickets results in a lengthening and disorganization of the proliferating zone and variable lengthening and dysplasia of the mineralizing zone. The primary spongiosa is initially lengthened with unmineralized cartilage and

subsequently becomes short with short, thick cartilage columns.

Angular limb deformities of the legs are a common problem in hand-raised chicks and, to a lesser extent, in parent-raised chicks. Underlying nutritional deficiencies are often present in these birds. Other birds, however, will have an adequate diet but improper bedding. As a result, their feet slide out from under them, and bending of the bones occurs.

Osteodystrophy Fibrosa. Increased osteoclastic resorption of bone and replacement of the bone with fibrous tissue characterize this condition. It is the result of persistently elevated parathyroid hormone, which can be a physiologic response to persistently low blood calcium or the result of unregulated release of parathyroid hormone from a neoplasia of the parathyroid.

Nutritional secondary hyperparathyroidism, which is a disease of birds that are no longer growing, is caused by a diet that is either deficient in calcium or contains excessive phosphorus or both. All seed diets fall into this last category. Excessive phosphorus interferes with intestinal absorption of calcium, resulting in hypocalcemia.

Renal secondary hyperparathyroidism occurs when the kidney is so severely damaged that it is unable to excrete excess phosphorus and unable to produce sufficient 1,25-dihydroxycholecalciferol. Phosphate retention leads to hyperphosphatemia, hypocalcemia, and increased parathormone (parathyroid hormone or PTH) excretion. This condition has not been documented in pet birds.

Birds with secondary hyperparathyroidism have soft bones that may bend, fracture, or become deformed due to increased osteoclastic resorption of cancellous bone and fibroplasia (Fig. 9.22).

Vitamin C Deficiency. Dietary requirements for vitamin C in birds are species dependent. No requirement has been demonstrated for common pet birds. For those that cannot synthesize the vitamin, a clinical deficiency is pos-

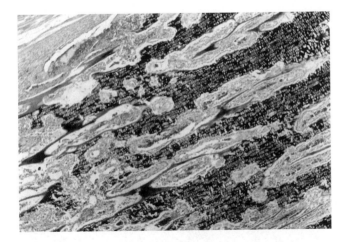

9.21.   Marked lengthening of the zone of hypertrophy in rickets.

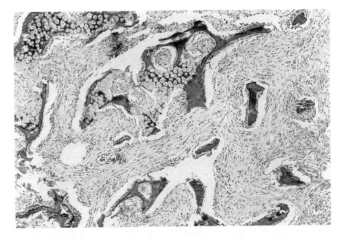

9.22.   Loss of normal bone and proliferation of fibrous connective tissue in osteodystrophy fibrosa.

sible. A deficiency leads to arrested osteoblastic activity. Since spicules of calcified cartilage remain as the only support for the metaphysis, fractures and hemorrhage may result and can be seen grossly and histologically.

Vitamin A Deficiency. Vitamin A is needed for osteoclast function. With a deficiency, osteoclast production is reduced, resulting in an imbalance between modeling and remodeling of bone. The failure of bone remodeling causes bone thickening and irregularity, with compression of adjacent soft tissue. The condition is infrequent but seems to involve the vertebrae rather than long bones. Histologically, excessive amounts of dense, mature bone are seen (Fig. 9.23). Birds deficient in vitamin A may also have squamous metaplasia in other organ systems.

Polyostotic Hyperostosis. This is the development of medullary bone in bones such as the femur, ulna, and radius, bones of the pectoral girdle, and vertebrae that would not normally develop medullary bone. This condition is thought to be associated with reproductive disorders such as ovarian tumors and ovarian cysts that cause prolonged estrogen secretion. However, these diseases are not always present in birds with polyostotic hyperostosis. Radiographically, increased medullary bone will be visible. The extent of bone involvement will depend on the duration of the underlying disease process. Affected bones are hard and difficult to break. Histologically, excessive medullary bone is present. It has trabecular architecture and is qualitatively similar to normal bone.

Degenerative Bone Disease/Trauma

Osteochondrosis. This is a focal area of disordered endochondral ossification in an area of growth that was previously normal. It can occur in the epiphysis (articular or nonarticular) and the growth plate. Nonarticular sites include areas of tendon and ligament attachment. Articular cartilage sites are associated with chondrocyte necrosis and cartilage dissection.

Osteochondrosis may be a dyschondroplasia that leads to degenerative changes, or it may be secondary to biomechanical forces and associated with ischemia, trauma, or improper nutrition. Three forms are recognized: osteochondritis dissecans, physitis, and subchondral bone cysts. Although these lesions are seen primarily in poultry, bone cysts have been reported in an ostrich and a cockatoo.

Osteochondritis dissecans develops when fractures of the epiphyseal cartilage extend to the articular surface. Ossified cartilage and free cartilage fragments may be present in the joint. Physitis usually results in widening of the physis associated with resorption of damaged bone. Subchondral bone cysts may be a sequel to linear defects in weight-bearing cartilage, possibly due to the accumulation of synovial fluid in the lesion and impairment of the cartilage vasculature.

Fractures (see the previous section) can result in severe hemorrhage in the surrounding tissue (Fig. 9.24). Healing is similar to that in mammals, and poor fracture healing leads to fibrous and chondroid callus formation (Fig. 9.25). Underlying causes include malnutrition, loss of blood supply, excessive movement, and infection.

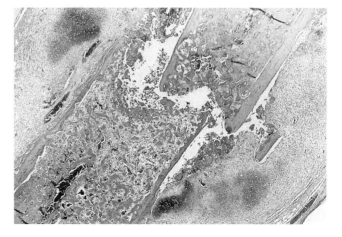

9.24. Severe hemorrhage associated with a fracture of the zygomatic process.

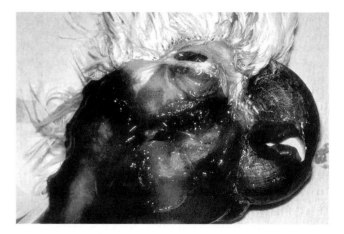

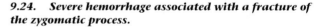

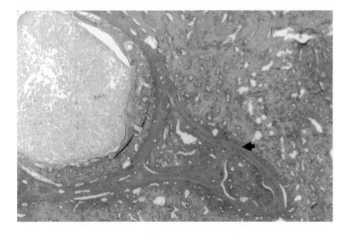

9.23. Marked osteosclerosis/bone proliferation associated with chronic vitamin A deficiency. Older cortex is indicated by the arrow.

9.25. Nonunited fracture with marked fibrous and cartilagenous callus associated with movement.

Ischemic necrosis of bone may be caused by neoplastic interruption of vascular supply, primary vascular disease, infection, or trauma with or without fracture. Bone that has undergone aseptic necrosis has a dry chalky appearance grossly. Histologically there is necrosis and loss of osteocytes, the marrow cells stain poorly, and vascular fibrous tissue invades the area.

Bone cysts apparently secondary to trauma have been seen in a cockatoo and in cockatiels. Grossly the lesion contained hemorrhagic fluid covered by an osseous shell. Histologically there were areas of new bone formation and connective tissue stromal proliferation.

Toxic Bone Disease

Although an excessive intake of vitamin D_3 leading to soft tissue damage has been documented in pet birds, effects on the bone, as seen in mammals, with prolonged uptake of small amounts of vitamin D_3, have not been reported in birds.

We have seen histologic bone changes suggestive of toxicity in a few cases. The lesion results from persistent hypercalcemia that depresses parathormone production and stimulates calcitonin secretion by C cells. Calcitonin lowers serum calcium levels by encouraging redeposition of calcium salts in the linings of the canalicular-lacunar system within bone and by depressing bone resorption by osteoclasts. Elevated calcitonin levels also stimulate osteoblasts to deposit woven bone having a basophilic matrix on preexisting bone surfaces. In our cases, there has been a minimal amount of osteosclerosis, rather than osteopenia.

Lead is bound to the mineral phase of bone leading to a "lead line," which is a growth retardation lattice secondary to lead-induced malformation of osteoclasts. The osteoclasts may contain acid-fast inclusion bodies in some species, but this is not documented in pet birds.

Vitamin A excess leads to lesions in the cartilagenous growth plates, thinning of the osteogenic layer of the periosteum, and osteoporosis. These changes have not been reported in pet birds.

Chronic fluorine toxicity results in osteopetrosis. The cortexes of the bones become thicker, obliterating the marrow cavity. Bone trabeculae are dense, and the periosteum is thickened at lower doses, whereas there may be osteoporosis at higher doses. Although not documented in pet birds, the microscopic appearance is similar to vitamin A deficiency and vitamin D toxicity and should be considered as a possible differential diagnosis.

Inflammatory Bone Disease: Osteomyelitis

The condition is usually infectious and may be caused by a variety of aerobic and anaerobic bacteria, *Mycobacteria,* fungi including *Aspergillus,* and *Candida.* The infection can be localized or be part of a generalized disease. Osteomyelitis may also be secondary to trauma or neoplastic disease. Grossly osteomyelitis is characterized as a swelling of soft tissue and irregularity of the affected bone. There may be an associated fracture that may be dif-

ficult to differentiate from a primary fracture. Caseous material is present in the lesion. Histologically, early lesions will have large numbers of heterophils with increasing numbers of plasma cells, macrophages, and giant cells seen with time (Fig. 9.26). Organisms are usually, but not always, found. Abscesses may form, and the lesion may become encapsulated (Fig. 9.27). If secondary to a fracture, there is interference with healing. Bacterial toxins and ischemia can lead to bone necrosis, and sequestra may form.

Proliferative Bone Disease
Exostosis/Enostosis/Osteophytes. Deposition of woven bone can occur on periosteal or medullary surfaces of cortical compacta as well as on the surfaces of cancellous bone. A variety of causes have been identified, including infection, trauma, and metastatic neoplasia. These lesions are single or multiple hard masses affecting any bone. They are comprised of trabeculae of mature woven bone. There may be associated soft tissue damage due to pressure from the proliferative bone.

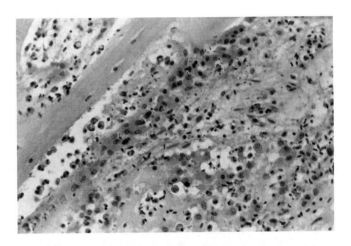

9.26.   Early bacterial osteomyelitis with necrosis and a pleocellular inflammatory infiltrate.

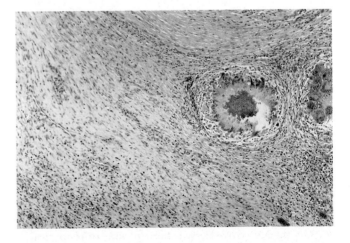

9.27.   Chronic bacterial osteomyelitis. Note the multiple microabscess formation and severe connective tissue proliferation.

Osteopetrosis. In chickens, osteopetrosis can be caused by retroviruses that lead to increased osteoblastic proliferation or decreased osteoclastic resorption. There is a marked diaphyseal swelling of long bones due to massive growth of subperiosteal bone. Although the histologic appearance and numbers of osteoclasts are unremarkable, there is what appears to be a neoplastic proliferation of osteoblasts. This condition has not been reported in pet birds.

Neoplastic Disease

Neoplasia can be of bone, cartilage, or marrow origin, as well as metastatic.

Osteomas are benign neoplasms of bone. They are seen sporadically in pet birds. They present as large hard swelling in any location but are most common in the skull or vertebrae (Fig. 9.28). Histologically they are comprised of normal-appearing cancellous bone with marrow spaces (Fig. 9.29).

Osteosarcomas, which are the most common primary tumor of bone, usually appear as a firm mass that replaces normal bone (Fig. 9.30). Histologically osteosarcomas are comprised of fusiform or stellate-shaped cells forming

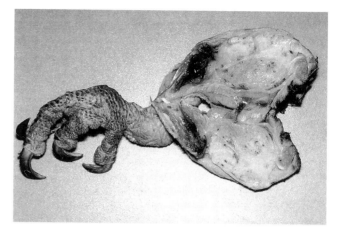

9.30.   Bone destruction associated with osteosarcoma of the femur.

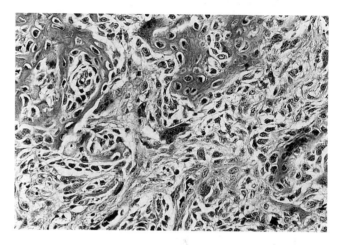

9.31.   Osteosarcoma with formation of osteoid and immature bone.

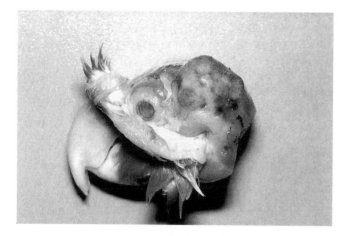

9.28.   Severe skull deformation due to osteoma formation.

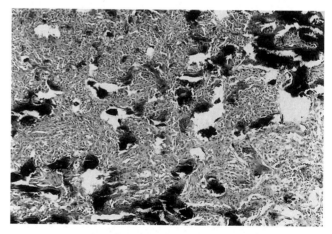

9.32.   Cellular and productive osteosarcoma with large amounts of mineralized bone.

bundles and sheets. There is variable osteoid and/or bone production (Figs. 9.31 and 9.32). Considerable superficial reactive bone often surrounds the osteosarcoma. Therefore a deep biopsy is necessary in order to reach the actual tumor (Fig. 9.33).

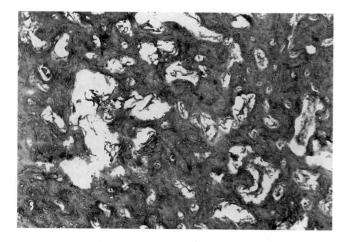

9.29.   Typical histologic appearance of avian osteoma.

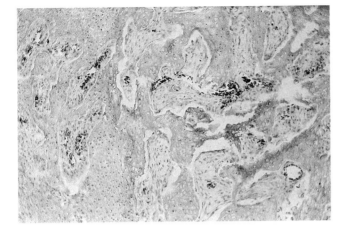

9.33. Marked reactive new bone formation on the surface of an osteosarcoma. If the biopsy is not deep enough, this may be the only material sampled.

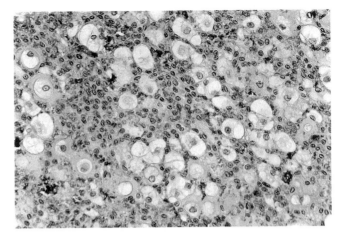

9.35. Cellular chondrosarcoma. Some attempt at lacunar formation is noted.

Parosteal osteosarcomas arise from the surface periosteum of bone, with no marrow involvement. In mammals, they may contain osseous, fibrous, and cartilagenous elements. These rare avian tumors are histologically difficult to differentiate from osteosarcoma (Fig. 9.34).

Chondromas are firm masses comprised of well-differentiated cartilage. They are infrequently seen and have no particular site predilection. Chondrosarcomas are comprised of poorly differentiated cartilage and have a high mitotic index. They are more cellular than chondromas, and there may be minimal matrix formation (Fig. 9.35). In our experience, they are more common than chondromas.

Osteochondroma is infrequently reported in pet birds; however, we have seen one tumor that was comprised of bone trabeculae covered by a cartilage cap in a cockatiel (Fig. 9.36). It was a solitary nodule. An osteochondroma was also reported in the tracheal wall of a bird.

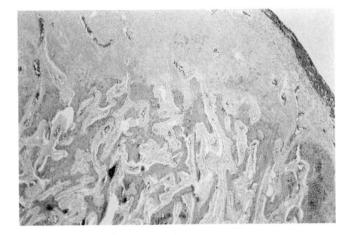

9.36. Lesion consistent with osteochondroma. The cartilagenous cap overlies an area of trabecular bone formation.

Giant cell tumors of bone are unusual and have no specific gross features. Histologically, numerous multinucleated giant cells are present (Fig. 9.37).

Fibrosarcoma can arise in the medullary space and may be difficult to differentiate from nonproductive osteosarcoma histologically in some cases. They may also be more typical, containing interlacing bundles of fusiform cells with vesicular nuclei.

Hemangiosarcoma may also be seen in the medullary cavity. There may be associated fractures. The tumors are usually reddish brown, and there may be excessive associated hemorrhage. Their histologic appearance is described in chapter 1.

Metastases/Secondary Tumors. Air-sac carcinomas may involve pneumatized bones by extension. Grossly they are firm masses often involving the shoulder or upper wing. Histologically moderately undifferentiated to poorly differentiated mesothelial cells form tubules, trabeculae, and papillary structures. There is variable stromal

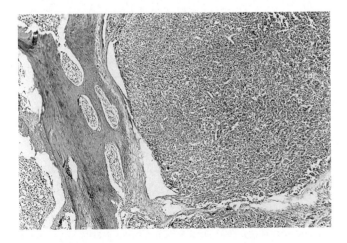

9.34. Parosteal osteosarcoma. Note the poorly differentiated tumor cells arising from the bone surface.

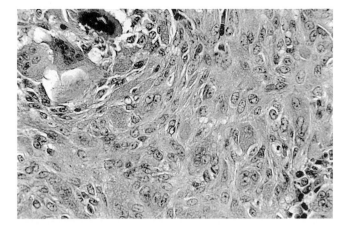

9.37.   Large multinucleated cells seen in giant cell tumor of bone.

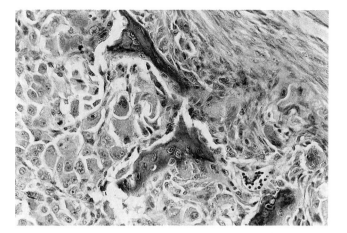

9.39.   Proventricular carcinoma metastatic to bone. Poorly formed nests of large anaplastic tumor cells are seen.

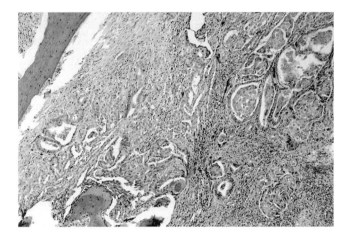

9.38.   Air-sac carcinoma. Tubular structures and cords are seen infiltrating bone.

proliferation, and bone spicules may be present interspersed with neoplastic tissue (Fig. 9.38). When located near joints, these tumors may be confused with synovial sarcomas, and immunohistochemistry may be necessary for differentiation.

Other carcinomas may metastasize to bones. Grossly there is usually proliferative new bone formation and associated soft tissue swelling. The neoplastic tissue is usually infiltrative within trabecular bone, and there may be associated bone necrosis and fibroplasia (Fig. 9.39).

DISEASE OF THE JOINTS

Congenital Disease
Congenital dysplasia, luxation, or subluxation are seen in many avian species. The causes are often multifactorial, including genetics, nutrition, and trauma.

Inflammatory Disease
Infectious arthritis in birds may be due to bacteria, including *Streptococcus, Chlamydiophila psittaci, Mycoplasma* sp.,

and *Reovirus.* Infectious arthritis of the elbow and hock joints is a common manifestation of salmonellosis in pigeons. In other species, any synovial membrane may be involved. Grossly, in acute cases, there is exudate and fibrin in the joint. Histologically an infiltration of heterophils and a few macrophages is common whether the condition is bacterial, viral, or due to mycoplasma (Fig. 9.40). Inflammatory cells variably infiltrate the synovium. The synovial membrane of the chronically inflamed joint is lined by hypertrophic synoviocytes and forms villi while the joint capsule becomes fibrotic due to organization of edema by fibrous tissue that limits the normal range of joint motion (Fig. 9.41). Lymphocytes and plasma cells predominate in the reaction. Eventually there is granulation tissue formation.

A common disease of raptors and waterfowl is "bumble foot," which is caused by physical damage to the bottom of the foot, resulting in bacterial penetration of the

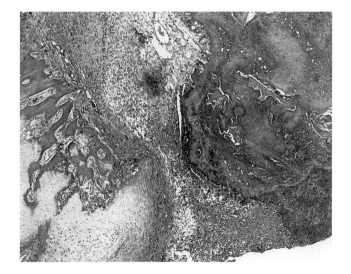

9.40.   Bacteria-caused arthritis. Severe necrosis, cellular proliferation, and exudate formation are noted.

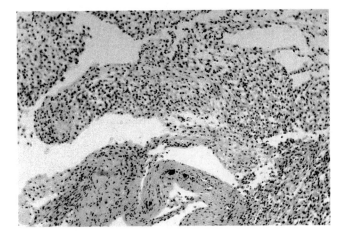

9.41. Chronic arthritis/synovitis with marked villar formation.

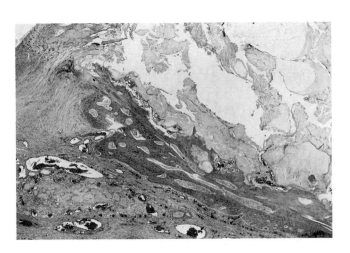

9.43. Amorphous urates typical of articular gout.

skin. Infection spreads to adjacent tendons, joints, and ultimately, bone. The disease in raptors is usually due to the use of improper perches and improper substrate in waterfowl.

Microfilaria have been found in inflamed joints, particularly in cockatoos, but their role in the pathogenesis of the lesion is difficult to determine. This is a rare disease of wild cockatoos and is not seen in hand-raised birds in North America and Europe.

Noninfectious arthritis is most often secondary to articular urate deposition (gout). Affected joints are swollen, and when incised there is chalky- or caseous-appearing material within the joint and adjacent soft tissue (Fig. 9.42). Histologically the urates are usually amorphous, although crystalline urates may be seen. A pleocellular inflammatory infiltrate, including giant cells, is present. There is variable tissue necrosis (Fig. 9.43).

Trauma, with or without foreign-body penetration, may also lead to arthritis. If the joint does not become septic, the reaction is usually mononuclear, with giant cells seen in more chronic cases. There may be variable hemorrhage.

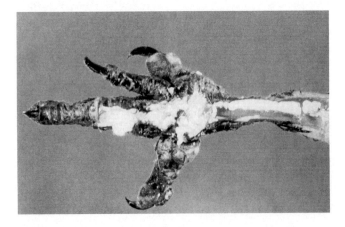

9.42. Severe articular urate deposition (gout) with extension into tendon sheaths and surrounding soft tissue.

Joint hemorrhage without any inflammatory component is usually from trauma; in conures, however, the possibility of "conure bleeding syndrome" is a differential diagnosis.

Degenerative Joint Disease

In pet species, degenerative lesions of the joints are usually found in older psittacine birds. Causes include previous trauma or infection, or metabolic conditions such as gout. Grossly affected joints are enlarged, and there may be cartilagenous erosions. Also noted are cartilagenous flaps and free cartilage in the joint cavity. Eventually there is formation of osteophytes and fibrosis in the joint capsule and periarticular soft tissue.

Neoplastic Disease

Synovial sarcoma is occasionally reported in birds. The tumor is similar to that seen in mammals and is characterized by gross destruction of the joint and bone associated with a proliferative mass. Histologically there are mucin-containing and fusiform cells. Spaces or clefts may be seen. The tumor can be difficult to distinguish from air-sac carcinoma of bone, since synovial sarcomas of birds may have two populations of cells, one of which is an epithelial type that will have some of the same immuno-histochemical staining properties as carcinomas.

Multiple foci of cartilagenous proliferation (chondromatosis) involving the synovium and perisynovial soft tissue have been reported in raptors. The lesion may be an example of metaplasia of unknown cause rather than neoplasia.

ADDITIONAL READING

Back WJ. 1974. The avian skeletomuscular system. In: Farner DS, King JR, Parkes KC, eds. Avian biology, vol 4. New York: Academic Press, pp 120–250.

Banks WJ. 1993. Applied veterinary histology, 3rd edition. St. Louis: CV Mosby, pp 163–181.

Baumgartner R, Hatt J-M, Dobeli M, Hauser B. 1995. Endocrinologic and pathologic findings in birds with polyostotic hyperostosis. J Avian Med Surg 9:251–254.

Brown R. 1990. Sinus, articular and subcutaneous *Mycobacterium tuberculosis* infection in a juvenile red-lored parrot. In: Proceedings of the American Association of Zoo Veterinarians, Seattle, WA, pp 305–308.

Droual R, Chin RP, Rezvani M. 1996. Synovitis, osteomyelitis and green liver in turkeys associated with *Escherichia coli*. Avian Dis 40:417–442.

Foutz TL, Rowland GN, Evans M. 1997. An avian modeling of analyzing bone loss due to disuse. Trans ASAE 40:1719–1725.

George JC, Berger AS. 1966. Avian myology. New York: Academic Press, pp 6–18.

Giddings RF, Richter AG. 2000. Multiple exostoses in a black-masked blue lovebird (*Agapornis personata*). J Avian Med Surg 14:59–58.

Grone A, Swayne DE, Nagode LA. 1995. Hypophosphatemic rickets in rheas (*Rhea americana*). Vet Pathol 32:324–327.

Harvey AL, Marshall IG. 1986. Muscle. In: Sturkie PD, ed. Avian physiology, 4th edition. New York: Springer-Verlag, pp 74–86.

Hillyer EV, Anderson MP, Greiner E, et al. 1991. An outbreak of *Sarcocystis* in a collection of psittacines. J Zoo Wildl Dis 22:434–445.

Knott L, Whitehead CC, Fleming RH, Bailey AJ. 1995. Biochemical changes in the collagenous matrix of osteoporotic avian bone. Biochem J 310[Part 3]:1045–1051.

Kogekar N, Spurgeon TL, Simon MC, Smith RE. 1987. Proliferative fibromatosis in avian skeletal muscle caused by cloned recombinant avian leukosis viruses. Cancer Res 47:2083–2091.

Labat ML. 1986. Retroviruses, immunosuppression and osteopetrosis. Biomed Pharmacother 40:85–90.

Law AS, Burt DW, Alexander I, Thorp BH. 1996. Expression of the gene for transforming growth-factor beta in avian dyschondroplasia. Res Vet Sci 61:120–124.

Martin HD, Kabler R, Sealing L. 1989 The avian coxofemoral joint. J Assoc Avian Vet 23:22–30.

Newton CD, Berger AS. 177. Avian fracture healing. J Am Vet Med Assoc 170:620–625.

Nie DT, Genge BR, Wu LNY, Wuthier RE. 1995. Defect in formation of functional matrix vesicles by growth-plate chondrocytes in avian tibial dyschondroplasia: Evidence of defective tissue vascularization. J Bone Miner Res 10:1625–1634.

Norman AW, Hurwitz. 1993. The role of the vitamin-D endocrine system in avian bone biology. J Nutr 123[Suppl 2]:310–316.

Orth MW, Cook ME. 1994. Avian tibial dyschondroplasia: A morphological and biochemical review of the growth-plate lesion and its causes. Vet Pathol 31:403–414.

Powers LV, Merrill CL, Degernes LA, et al. 1998. Axillary cystadenocarcinoma in a Moluccan cockatoo (*Cacatua moluccensis*). Avian Dis 42:408–412.

Riddell C. 1987. Avian histopathology. Lawrence, KS: Allen, pp 19–30.

Schmidt RE. 1992. Morphologic diagnosis of avian neoplasms. Semin Avian Exotic Pet Med 1:73–79.

Smith JH, Neill PJ. 1989. Pathogenesis of *Sarcocystis falcatula* (Apicomplexa: Sarcocystidae) in the budgerigar (*Melopsittacus undulatus*). III. Pathologic and quantitative parasitologic analysis of extrapulmonary disease. J Parasitol 75:270–287.

Smith JH, Neill PJ, Dillard EA, Box ED. 1990. Pathology of experimental *Sarcocystis falcatula* infections of canaries (*Serinus canarius*) and pigeons (*Columba livia*). J Parasitol 76:59–68.

Squire BT, More SJ. 1998. Factors on farms in eastern Australia associated with the development of tibiotarsal rotation in ostrich chicks. Aust Vet J 76:110–117.

Stark JM. 1996. Comparative morphology and cytokinetics of skeletal growth in hatchlings of altricial and precocial birds. Zool Anz 235:53–75.

Stone EG, Walser MM, Redig PT, et al. 1999. Synovial chondromatosis in raptors. J Wildl Dis 35:137–140.

Takechi M, Itakura C. 1995. Ultrastructural and histochemical studies of the epiphyseal plate in normal chicks. Anat Rec 242:29–39.

Torrella JR, Fouces V, Palomeque J, Viscor G. 1998. Comparative skeletal muscle fiber morphometry among wild birds with different locomotor behavior. J Anat 192[Part 2]:211–222.

Thorp BT. 1994. Skeletal disorders in the fowl: A review. Avian Pathol 23:203–236.

Tully TN Jr, Pechman RD, Cornick J, Morris JM. 1995. A subchondral cyst in the distal tibiotarsal bone of an ostrich (*Struthio camelus*). J Avian Med Surg 9:41–44.

Tully TN Jr, Hodgin C, Morris JM, et al. 1996. Exertional myopathy in an emu (*Dromaius noveahollandiae*). J Avian Med Surg 10:96–100.

Tully TN, Mitchell MA, Heatly JJ, et al. 2000. Trauma-induced periosteal bone cysts in psittacine species. In: Proceedings of the American Association of Zoo Verterinarians, International Association for Aquatic Animal Medicine Conference, New Orleans, LA, p 311.

Van den Horst H, Van der Hage M, Wolvekamp P, Lumej JT. 1996 Synovial cell sarcoma in a sulphur-crested cockatoo (*Cacatua galerita*). Avian Pathol 25:179–186.

Weissengruber G, Loupal G. 1999. Osteochondroma of the tracheal wall in a Fischer's lovebird (*Agapornis fischeri*, Reichenow 1887). Avian Dis 43:155–159.

Wilson S, Thorp BH. 1998. Estrogen and cancellous bone loss in the fowl. Calcif Tissue Int 62:506–511.

10 Nervous System

NORMAL STRUCTURE

The avian brain is covered by the semiopaque and relatively tough meninges. The cerebral hemispheres are lissencephalic (there are no sulci or gyri), tapered to a point rostrally, and rounded caudally. The telencephalon and diencephalon developed in a divergent path than those of mammals and have few homologous structures. The mesencephalon and rhombencephalon are derived from reptile brain as they are in mammals and contain structures homologous with the mammalian brain. The prominent features of the mesencephalon are the paired optic lobes, which project laterally under the ventral surface of the cerebral hemispheres. The optic nerves are short and thick and cross on the ventral surface of the brain just cranial to the optic lobes. The cerebellum is relatively large and has the characteristic folia seen in other animals. However, it only has a middle lobe; the lateral lobes found in mammals are absent. Birds have four ventricles in their brain. The villous choroid plexus projects into the lateral ventricles along their walls and from the roof of the third and fourth ventricles. Pathologists who are used to the microscopic anatomy of mammalian brains will find the avian cerebral hemispheres to be far more cellular. Many more glial cells are found in close proximity to the bodies of neurons in birds. The cerebellum, however, contains the molecular, Purkinje, and granular cell layer seen in other animals.

Unlike in mammals, the spinal cord is the same length as the spinal canal and extends to the last caudal vertebra. Therefore, birds do not have a cauda equina, and spinal nerves pass laterally to the adjacent intervertebral foramina. There are cranial and caudal enlargements in the area of the brachial and lumbosacral plexi. In the dorsal midline of the lumbosacral enlargement is the rhomboidal sinus, which is unique to birds. The rhomboidal sinus separates the left and right dorsal columns, leaving a cleft occupied by the gelatinous (or glycogen) body. This structure is comprised of glial cells rich in glycogen and innervated by unmyelinated fibers. The ventral part of the gelatinous body encloses the spinal canal. The function of the gelatinous body is unknown. The structure of the peripheral nervous system is similar to that of mammals.

CENTRAL NERVOUS SYSTEM

Congenital Anomalies

A variety of sporadic defects has been reported in birds, particularly poultry. Documented anomalies in pet birds are less frequent. A meningomyelocele has been reported in association with a spinal column defect in a scarlet macaw. The bird presented with a tract that extended from the skin over the thoracic spine to the spinal cord. Portions of the cord and meninges were herniated into the area of the spinal defect. Histologic changes were confined to distortion of normal architecture and mild degeneration.

Hydrocephalus is seen in a variety of psittacine birds. It seems to be more prevalent in older birds, indicating a possible acquired, rather than congenital, lesion. It usually involves the lateral ventricles, which are grossly distended, and leads to compression of the overlying cortex. If ruptured, the cortical tissue collapses and becomes flaccid, and excessive fluid will drain from the area of rupture. There is often herniation of the cerebellum into the foramen magnum. Histologically there is distortion and degeneration of nerve tissue in what was the cerebral cortex. Cerebellar hypoplasia has been reported in Fig parrots.

Lafora body neuropathy has been reported in psittacine birds, probably as a result of a congenital defect in intracellular metabolism. There is no gross lesion, and histologically glycoprotein-containing cytoplasmic inclusion bodies are seen in neurons.

A genetic defect leading to lysosomal storage disease is described in emus but is not seen in companion birds. It is a GM_1 and GM_3 gangliosidosis. Birds are typically 6 to 10 months old at the onset of the disease and have a history of slowed growth, poor weight gain, and upper motor neuron signs. Gross lesions are not seen, but histologically there is neuronal distension and enlargement with vacuolation of the cytoplasm. Neurons of the brain,

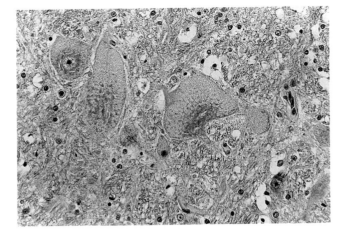

10.1. *Enlarged neurons with vacuolated cytoplasm typical of lysosomal storage disease in emus.*

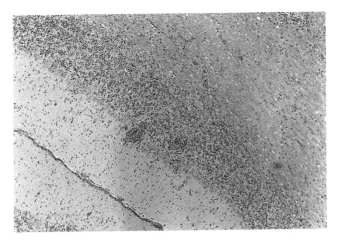

10.2. *Perivascular cuffing and mild hypercellularity in the brain of a bird with paramyxovirus-3 infection.*

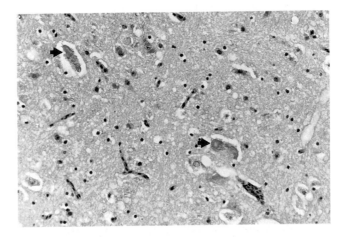

10.3. *Shrunken neurons with cytoplasmic inclusion bodies (arrows) in avian paramyxovirus-3 infection.*

spinal ganglia, and autonomic ganglia may be affected. Neuronal cytoplasm has a foamy appearance and may have a slight tan color, but no other staining is seen in hematoxylin-eosin sections (Fig. 10.1). Ultrastructurally there are numerous membranous cytoplasmic bodies.

Toxins can cause problems in the developing brain. Exposure to dioxin and dioxin-like compounds can lead to asymmetric brain formation in birds. The forebrain and tectum are most commonly affected. This problem is seen primarily in wildlife.

Inflammatory Disease

Inflammatory disease of the central nervous system (CNS) can be noninfectious or infectious. Noninfectious diseases that can cause inflammatory lesions include some toxins, autoimmune disease, and immune-mediated conditions, none of which have been well documented in pet birds. Viruses, bacteria, fungi, protozoa, and metazoan parasites all can cause inflammatory disease of the CNS.

Viral Disease. A variety of viruses cause nervous system disease. In general, perivascular cuffing, gliosis, and neuronal degeneration characterize lesions. Inclusion bodies may or may not be present.

Paramyxovirus. A number of paramyxoviruses (PMVs) cause neurologic disease in birds, and PMV-1, 2, 3, and 5 have been documented in pet birds. PMV-1 is the cause of Newcastle disease in domestic poultry. Exotic Newcastle disease has been extirpated from the United States, but in the past has entered this country in smuggled nestling double-yellow head and yellow-naped Amazon parrots and in fighting cocks. A closely related PMV-1 is a common cause of encephalitis in racing pigeons. This virus has a worldwide distribution. PMV-3 is the most common cause of encephalitis in psittacine and small passerine birds. PMV infections rarely cause gross lesions, and histologically the disease process is variable. Some birds have no inflammatory changes, whereas others have perivascu-

lar cuffing by lymphocytes and plasma cells, minimal necrosis, gliosis, and endothelial hypertrophy (Fig. 10.2). Hemorrhage is occasionally seen, and syncytial cells may be found in some cases. Intracytoplasmic inclusion bodies are usually not seen but may be present (Fig. 10.3). Australian grass parakeets (*Neophema* sp.) and cockatiels are birds that are most frequently affected by PMV-3. Chronic pancreatitis is a manifestation of this disease in *Neophema* (chapter 3).

Togavirus. Eastern equine encephalitis (EEE) and western equine encephalitis (WEE) are seen in emus, and EEE is considered to be the cause of avian viral serositis in psittacine birds. Gross CNS lesions, other than variable hemorrhage, are not seen with EEE or WEE. Histologic changes include nonsuppurative encephalitis, neuronal degeneration, and meningitis. Gross lesions of viral serositis are limited to parenchymal organs and will be discussed with the appropriate system. Histologic changes in the brain of birds with avian viral serositis include nonsuppurative meningitis and encephalitis. Lymphocytes are the primary cell type seen in the reaction.

Proventricular Dilatation Disease. Proventricular dilatation disease (PDD) appears to be caused by an as yet uncharacterized virus that affects both the autonomic nerves, particularly those of the digestive system (chapter 3), and the CNS. Most commonly, signs of this disease relate to the digestive system. However, CNS disease often accompanies the disease of the nerves of the digestive tract, and CNS lesions may be the predominant feature of some infections. PDD does not cause gross lesions in the CNS. Histologic changes are of a typical nonsuppurative inflammatory process most severe in the brain stem and spinal cord (Fig. 10.4). Gliosis and neuronophagia are occasionally seen. Between 60% and 100% of the birds in various case surveys have microscopic brain lesions. Spinal cord lesions are also common, but most pathologists rarely evaluate the spinal cord.

Picornavirus. This has been implicated as a cause of encephalitis, but there is minimal documentation. Histologic lesions are typical of nonsuppurative encephalitis.

Influenza A. This has occasionally been isolated from psittacine birds including African grey parrots, cockatoos and budgerigars, mynahs, and passeriformes. There are occasional reports of influenza virus-induced neuronal disease. The virus is reported to cause gross hemorrhage and histologic changes varying from no lesion to mild nonsuppurative encephalitis.

West Nile Virus. This virus, which causes systemic disease as well as CNS lesions, has infected a variety of pet and wild birds. Grossly, meningeal and brain congestion and hemorrhage are found. Histologically the hemorrhage is most severe in the cerebellar folia (Fig. 10.5). There is lymphoplasmacytic meningitis and variable encephalitis. In mild cases, lesions are more common in the cerebellum and brain stem but may be generalized in the more severe

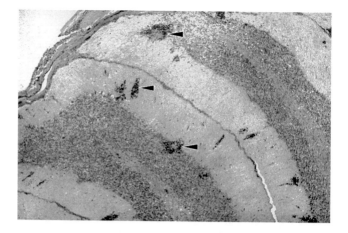

10.5. Multiple foci of hemorrhage and necrosis in a bird with West Nile virus infection (arrowheads).

disease. Cuffing of vessels by lymphocytes and plasma cells, gliosis or glial nodule formation, and neuronal necrosis are seen. Purkinje cells may be completely lost, and degenerative changes are common in the molecular layer of the cerebellum.

Lesions are also seen in the heart, intestine, spleen, pancreas, lung, and kidney. Grossly there may be pale foci or streaks. Splenic and renal enlargement, and hemorrhage in all affected organs, are seen. Histologically a lymphoplasmacytic and histiocytic inflammatory infiltrate, necrosis, and hemorrhage characterize the lesions. Adenitis of the adrenal gland can also occur.

Adenovirus. Neurologic signs associated with adenovirus infection are most common in cockatiels and budgerigars. No gross lesion is present, and histologic changes include degeneration of small blood vessels, endothelial necrosis, and intranuclear inclusion bodies in endothelial cells (Fig. 10.6). Inflammation is usually minimal or absent, but a nonsuppurative encephalitis is reported in budgerigars. Adenovirus inclusions have also been

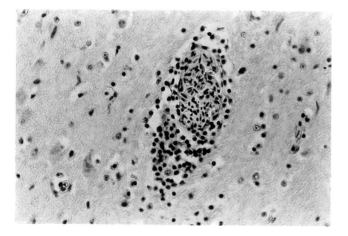

10.4. Perivascular inflammation in the brain of a bird with proventricular dilatation disease (PDD).

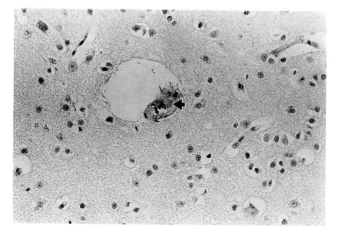

10.6. A degenerating endothelial cell with an intranuclear inclusion body consistent with adenovirus infection (arrow). There is usually no associated inflammation.

reported in the brain of a Moluccan cockatoo with a progressive CNS disease.

Avian Polyomavirus. In some outbreaks in budgerigars, significant cerebellar lesions may be seen. Affected chicks will have prominent intention tremors. Characteristic intranuclear inclusion bodies with karyomegaly are abundant in the molecular layer of the cerebellum. Two cases of a progressive fatal neurologic disease caused by avian polyomavirus have been reported in cockatoos.

Lesions in these birds were confined to the gray matter. They included hemorrhage and degeneration of astrocytes and neurons, with characteristic intranuclear inclusions found in some of these cells (Figs. 10.7 and 10.8). Inflammation was not seen in these birds. The second case was concurrently infected with the psittacine beak and feather disease virus, suggesting that immunosuppression may play a role in this disease.

Bacterial Infection. Numerous bacteria, including *Staphylococci* sp., *Salmonella* sp., *Escherichia coli*, *Pseudomonas* sp., and *Klebsiella* sp., are possible causes of meningitis, encephalitis, and myelitis. Inflammation of the brain and meninges can be from direct extension of an infection from the sinuses, nasal cavity, or inner ear, or may be the result of a bacteremia or septicemia. Gross lesions are absent in many cases, but exudate can occasionally be seen in the meninges, and in chronic cases, abscesses can be found in the brain.

Infiltrating inflammatory cells and fibrin deposition thicken the leptomeninges (Fig. 10.9). Malacia and a pyogranulomatous inflammatory lesion with the presence of intralesional bacteria characterize bacterial-induced lesions (Fig. 10.10). In some cases, septic thrombi are present in blood vessels.

Chlamydophila psittaci will affect serous membranes throughout the body and can induce a nonsuppurative meningitis.

Mycobacterial infection of the CNS is usually part of a systemic process. Gross lesions are proliferative and gray-

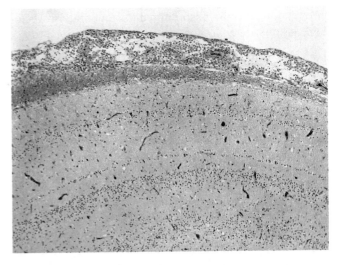

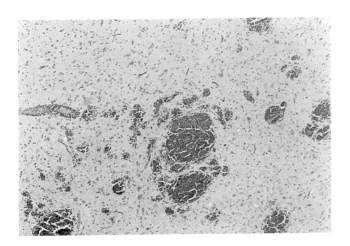

10.7. Multifocal brain hemorrhage in a bird with polyomavirus infection.

10.9. Severe leptomeningitis due to bacteria. Heterophils and macrophages are present, and there is minimal edema and fibrin deposition.

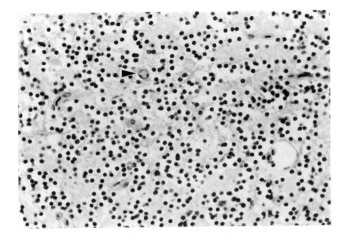

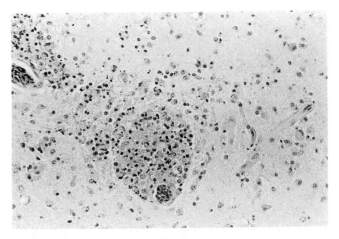

10.8. Chromatin margination and clear intranuclear inclusion body (arrowhead) occasionally seen in the brain of birds with polyomavirus infection.

10.10. Bacteria-caused encephalitis. Note the necrosis and numerous large macrophages containing bacteria in their cytoplasm.

white or yellow. Early microscopic changes are similar to those seen in mycobacteriosis in other organs and contain heterophils, lymphocytes, and small macrophages. As the lesion progresses, large macrophages containing organisms are seen. There may be variable necrosis (Figs. 10.11 and 10.12).

Fungal Infection. As with bacterial disease, fungal infections can be blood-borne or may occur secondary to extension from the nasal cavity or sinuses. The brain, spinal cord, and meninges all may be affected. Gross changes depend on the chronicity of the lesion and vary from none to the presence of granulomas. Microscopically, pyogranulomatous inflammation and fungal hyphae are noted in the lesion and in blood vessel walls (Figs. 10.13 and 10.14).

Parasitic Infection. Several protozoa, including *Sarcocystis falcatula*, *Toxoplasma gondii*, and *Leukocytozoon* sp., may cause brain lesions. The most common in pet species is *S. falcatula*. Encephalitis usually occurs as a part of systemic disease and seems to be more prevalent in birds that have

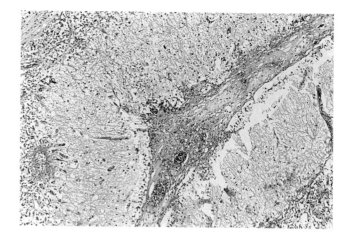

10.13.   Meningoencephalitis due to fungal infection. At a lower magnification, the lesion is morphologically similar to a bacterial infection.

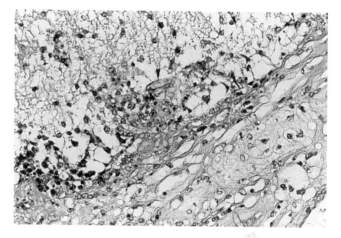

10.14.   Fragment of a fungal hypha (arrowhead) within the lesion illustrated in Fig. 10.12. The exact organism cannot usually be determined based on its microscopic appearance.

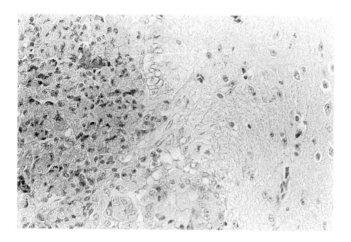

10.11.   Mycobacterial encephalitis. The primary infiltrate is comprised of large macrophages with slightly granular cytoplasm.

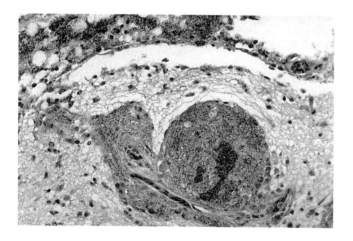

10.12.   Acid-fast stain to illustrate intracytoplasmic organisms in mycobacterial encephalitis.

had prolonged natural disease or survived for some time due to aggressive therapeutic regimens. Gross lesions are usually absent.

Histologic changes include a necrotizing encephalitis and a pleocellular reaction that may include giant cells. Schizonts and merozoites are present in the lesion but can be few and difficult to find in some cases. Associated blood vessels have variable endothelial swelling and are cuffed by plasma cells, lymphocytes, and macrophages (Figs. 10.15 and 10.16).

Toxoplasmosis causes similar histologic lesions. Immunochemistry or electron microscopy may be needed to differentiate the lesions. Toxoplasmosis is infrequently seen in pet birds in the North America.

Leukocytozoon infection may lead to the formation of megaloschizonts in the brain. On careful gross examination, these may present as small white foci, but they are difficult to see. Histologically they are similar to megaloschizonts in other organs, and there is minimal cellular

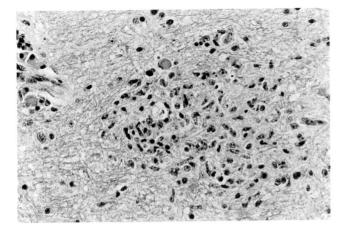

10.15. *Focus of gliosis in the brain of a bird with systemic sarcosporidiosis.*

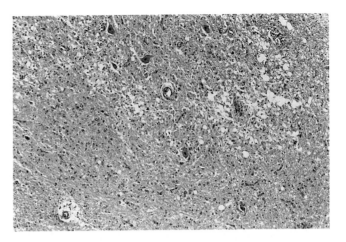

10.17. *Encephalomalacia following nematode migration in the brain.*

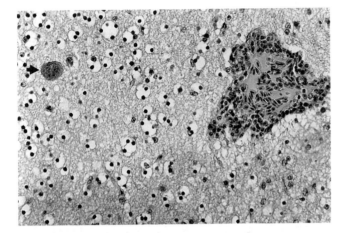

10.16. *Sarcosporidial encephalitis. Note the perivascular cuffing and one protozoal cyst (arrow).*

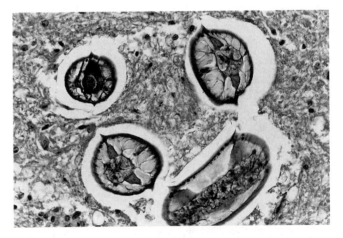

10.18. *Nematodes, probably* **Baylisascaris** *sp., in the brain due to aberrant migration.*

reaction unless they rupture. These lesions are found in pigeons and some species of wild birds.

Wandering nematode parasites can cause severe lesions in the avian brain. *Baylisascaris procyonis* is the most common and is the result of ingestion of food contaminated with raccoon feces. The condition is more prevalent in zoos and outdoor aviaries. In severe cases, there is grossly noticeable malacia and hemorrhage. Microscopic malacic tracts are seen, and fragments of parasites may be found. A nonsuppurative inflammatory reaction is present, and there can be gitter cell accumulation. Cuffing of associated blood vessels by lymphocytes and plasma cells is common (Figs. 10.17 and 10.18).

Chandlerella quiscali is a filarial parasite of grackles. The adult worm lives in the ventricles of the brain, and microfilaria are readily demonstrated in the blood. Emus, 2 to 6 months old, can be devastated by this parasite. Birds have a history of ataxia and torticollis. Many larval forms of the parasite are found in the spinal cord and brain. They elicit a lesion similar to that caused by *Baylisascaris proyconis*.

Microfilariasis with plugging of the small vessels in the brain, ischemia, and clinical disease is a condition that is most prevalent in wild or wild-caught cockatoos but could be found in any bird with subcutaneous or peritoneal cavity filariasis. Microscopically, in addition to the microfilaria, there may be small areas of malacia and variable congestion. There is usually no inflammatory response (Fig. 10.19).

Noninflammatory Disease

Infectious Disease. Spongiform encephalopathy results from an abnormal conformational change in brain glycoprotein that creates infections proteins called prions. A condition resembling bovine spongiform encephalopathy is reported to occur in psittacine birds. Gross lesions are not seen. Histologically there is vacuolar degeneration of neurons in specific nuclei of the cerebellar peduncles and brain stem (Fig. 10.20). There may be single or multiple discrete cytoplasmic vacuoles in affected neurons. Mild spongiosis of white matter and gliosis are also seen. A prion has yet to be isolated from these birds.

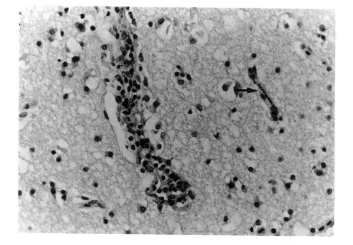

10.19.   *Minimal perivascular inflammation associated with microfilariasis involving capillaries in the brain (arrow).*

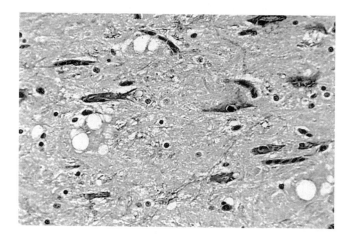

10.20.   *Multiple neuronal vacuolation typical of spongiform encephalopathy due to possible infection.*

Physical/Traumatic Head Injuries. One of the most common causes of traumatic brain damage is aggression from cage mates or attack by wild predatory birds on unprotected captive birds. There is often, but not always, associated bruising and hemorrhage of the skin and subcutis over the skull, and, in severe cases, there may be damage to the external portion of the skull.

When there has been trauma, the meninges and brain will be hemorrhagic, and the hemorrhage will extend into the brain parenchyma (Figs. 10.21 and 10.22). If there is only severe congestion, either antemortem or postmortem, no hemorrhage will be noted when the brain is incised. Histologically the hemorrhage is accompanied by variable malacia (Fig. 10.23).

Head injuries must be differentiated from postmortem pooling of blood in venous sinuses of the calvarium. This postmortem artifact is very common and will not be associated with damage to the skin or brain or with meningeal hemorrhage.

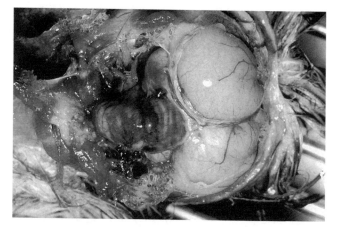

10.21.   *Trauma-induced hemorrhage of the brain and meninges.*

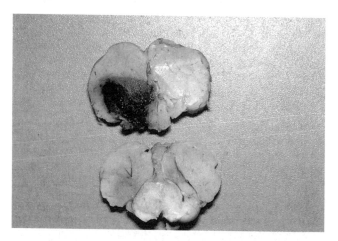

10.22.   *Hemorrhage deep within the brain following severe trauma.*

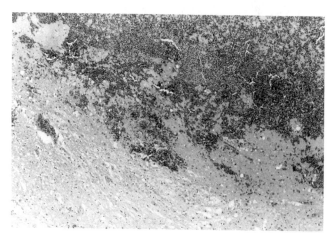

10.23.   *Severe malacia and hemorrhage within the brain parenchyma.*

Thrombosis can lead to acute ischemia and hemorrhage. A common cause of thrombosis in female birds is yolk emboli. Parenchymal changes are similar to those just described, but yolk emboli are found in affected arteries (Fig. 10.24). In more chronic lesions, there may be an

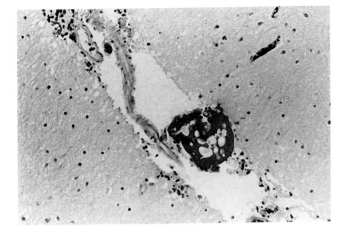

10.24. *Embolus of yolk material in a cerebral vessel. Some of the separation of brain parenchyma is artifactual.*

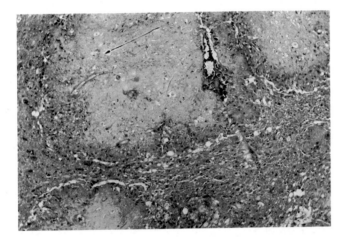

10.25. *Malacia, gitter cells, and amorphous material within the brain following yolk embolization.*

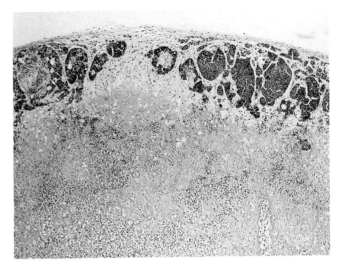

10.26. *Infarct of the brain. This type of lesion can be seen in vascular disease, but often no specific cause is determined.*

accumulation of gitter cells and amorphous yellow-brown material (Fig. 10.25).

Cases of brain hemorrhage and malacia without any identifiable cause are sporadically seen. Morphologically they resemble the traumatic lesion described (Fig. 10.26). Hemorrhage into the brain and spinal cord may also occur in cases of conure bleeding syndrome, a problem of conures whose etiology and pathogenesis are not well understood.

Toxic Neuropathy. Toxins known to cause problems in the avian brain include lead, zinc, sodium, poisonous plants, mycotoxins, and insecticides. Gross changes are not usually seen. Neuronal degeneration and variable edema are noted in cases of lead poisoning. Edema and hemorrhage are seen with sodium intoxication, and neuronal degeneration may be found in zinc toxicity. The latter can be histologically similar to infectious spongiform encephalopathy as previously described, and electron microscopy will be necessary to make a definitive diagnosis.

Mycotoxins cause encephalomalacia, which may be grossly visible if severe. Organic phosphate and carbamate insecticides can lead to demyelination in the spinal cord and peripheral nerves.

Nutritional Deficiencies. Vitamin E deficiency affects several organ systems including cardiac, ventricular, and skeletal muscle and skin. It may cause encephalomalacia in poultry, emus and, occasionally, psittacine birds. Grossly there may be hemorrhage and edema of the brain, but often no lesion is seen. Histologic changes include malacia, gliosis, and neuronal necrosis primarily involving the cerebellum.

Brain lesions believed to be associated with vitamin E deficiency occur in great-billed parrots. There is degeneration and loss of Purkinje cells and a spongiform degeneration of the white matter of the cerebellum and, in severe cases, of the cerebrum. Prominent myocardial and skeletal muscle lesions are also present in these birds

Degenerative Lesions. Cerebellar degeneration of unknown cause was seen in a turquoise parrot (*Neophema pulchella*). No gross change was noted, but histologically the granular layer was small and there was neuronophagia and necrosis.

Mineralization is an occasional incidental finding in the brain, as is lipofuscin deposition in neurons (Figs. 10.27 and 10.28). Lipofuscin is a common finding in the neural cell bodies of older parrots. Generally the lesion is mild, but in some birds, the lesion is prominent. It is suspected that in most cases this pigment accumulation does not have a functional significance.

Hemosiderin-containing macrophages may accumulate in the brain of birds (particularly toucans and mynahs) with severe iron metabolic problems (Fig. 10.29).

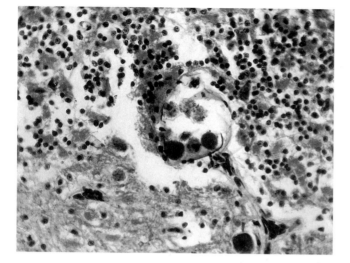

10.27.   Foci of cerebellar mineralization. This is an occasional incidental finding. The tissue separation is artifact.

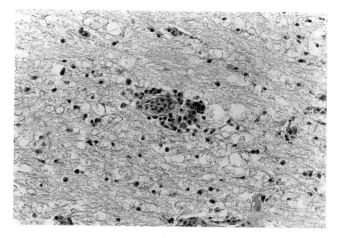

10.29.   Perivascular accumulation of iron pigment-containing macrophages in a toucan with a generalized iron storage.

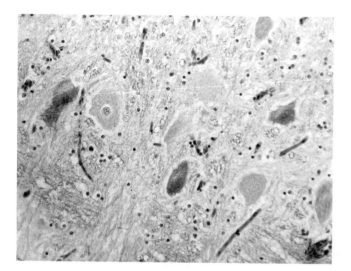

10.28.   Scattered neuronal lipofuscin accumulation. Although considered an incidental finding in most birds affected, lipofuscin accumulation may indicate inadequate dietary antioxidants.

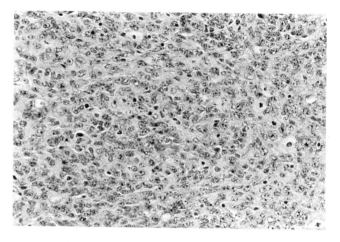

10.30.   Meningeal tumor consistent with possible sarcoma. The exact cell of origin may not be apparent morphologically.

Proliferative Lesions. A variety of primary and metastatic tumors are reported in the avian brain and spinal cord. Although much of the literature concerns domestic poultry, most tumors are found in pet birds.

Meningioma. These tumors are usually solitary within the meninges and are of variable shape. They are firm and gray-white to yellow. If there has been any hemorrhage, they may be slightly reddened. Microscopically, tumor cells usually have abundant cytoplasm and are fusiform. Whorls and bundles of neoplastic cells are the most common pattern. These tumors grow by expansion, and some compression of adjacent brain may be seen.

Avian meningeal tumors not morphologically typical are also occasionally seen. They appear to be undifferenti-

ated sarcomas with pleomorphic cells arranged in sheets (Fig. 10.30). There may also be minimal invasion of the brain (Fig. 10.31).

Choroid Plexus Papilloma. These tumors present as well-defined papillary structures within ventricles. They are gray-white to red. Histologically the tumors have a vascular connective tissue stroma covered by epithelial cells that are cuboidal or columnar and resemble normal choroid plexus.

Primary Tumors of Glial Cells. Glioblastoma multiforme, astrocytoma, and oligodendroglioma are all seen in birds. Grossly these tumors may be difficult to detect, particularly in early stages. There may be some enlargement and distortion or dislocation of normal structures. Asymmetry can be noted on coronal sections of brain. If there is necrosis or hemorrhage, the area of tumor may resemble an abscess or infarct.

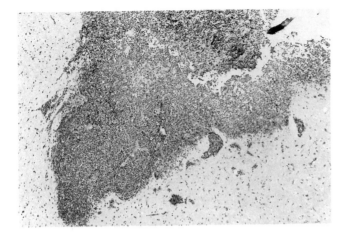

10.31. Undifferentiated tumor arising in the lep-tomeninges with extension into the brain.

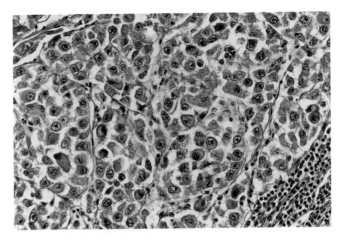

10.33. Adrenal carcinoma (interrenal cell origin) metastatic to the spinal cord.

Glioblastoma multiforme is cellular and has a pleomorphic histologic appearance. Some cells resemble differentiated astrocytes, whereas others are elongated and fusiform with numerous mitotic figures (Fig. 10.32).

Astrocytomas are usually fairly uniform, with hyperchromatic nuclei and abundant cytoplasm. Cell process can be seen with silver stains. Few mitotic figures are present. Oligodendrogliomas are cellular and comprised of sheets of small cells with hyperchromatic nuclei and poorly staining cytoplasm. Mitoses are infrequent.

Medulloblastoma and Neuroblastoma. These primary tumors of neuronal cells have not been documented in companion bird species. Medulloblastoma is considered an embryonic neoplasm that grossly is well defined and histologically is composed of anaplastic cells that may form rosettes.

Metastatic Tumors of the Brain. Metastatic carcinomas, various sarcomas including lymphosarcoma and hemangiosarcoma, and malignant melanoma have been seen in

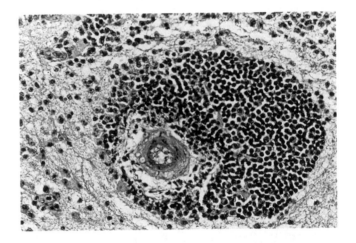

10.34. Lymphosarcoma in the brain. Multiple cuffs of neoplastic cells are present.

the avian brain. These will be described with their primary system (Figs. 10.33–10.35).

PERIPHERAL NERVOUS SYSTEM

Inflammatory Disease

Peripheral nerves can be involved in a variety of infectious and noninfectious diseases. In many conditions, the histologic changes are similar due to the limited responses of peripheral nerves.

Viral Disease. Proventricular dilatation disease was mentioned previously as a primary disease of the nervous system, and its lesions are more prevalent in the peripheral nervous system. Gross changes are usually referable to the heart (chapter 1) or to the gastrointestinal tract (chapter 3). Histologic lesions are seen in peripheral nerves and nerve ganglia. The most prevalent change is a lympho-plasmacytic inflammatory infiltrate around and within nerves and ganglia (Fig. 10.36). In some early cases, there may also be a heterophilic component.

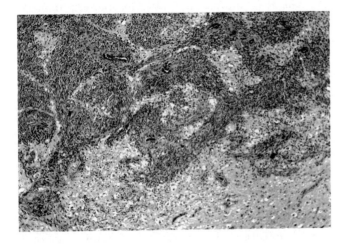

10.32. Glioblastoma multiforme replacing brain parenchyma.

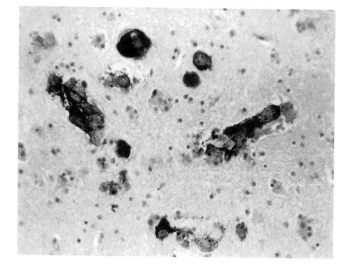

10.35. Malignant melanoma. Multiple small accumulations of neoplastic melanophores are present in the brain parenchyma.

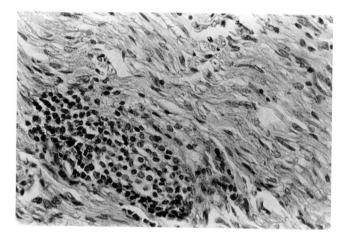

10.36. Peripheral neuritis typical of proventricular dilatation disease. Note the localized accumulation of lymphocytes and a few plasma cells.

West Nile virus also can cause a peripheral neuritis that is morphologically similar to PDD (Fig. 10.37). The species of bird and the characteristics of other lesions must be evaluated in making a distinction between the two diseases.

Other Infections. Bacterial, mycobacterial, and fungal infections can involve adjacent peripheral nerves, with lesions typical of the primary problem.

Noninfectious Disease. Inflammation of nerves is also seen in some cases of trauma. Nerves are involved in the reaction, as are other tissues in the affected area.

Noninflammatory Disease
Toxins. Arsenic toxicity can lead to a peripheral neuropathy. Gross lesions are not seen. Histologic changes include axonal fragmentation, demyelination, and Schwann cell proliferation.

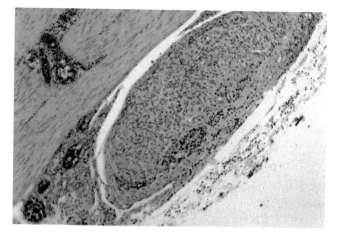

10.37. Mild lymphoplasmacytic inflammatory infiltrate into the peripheral nerve of a bird with West Nile virus infection. Note the morphologic similarity to proventricular dilatation disease infection (Fig. 10.35).

Trauma. Many cases of trauma lead to noninflammatory nerve degeneration, associated with direct nerve involvement or secondary to compression. There is no gross change, and microscopically demyelination and axonal loss are noted (Fig. 10.38).

Nutritional Deficiencies. Riboflavin (Vitamin B$_2$) deficiency leads to classic "curled toe paralysis" in chickens and can cause polyneuritis and degeneration in a variety of birds. Grossly there may be slight swelling and discoloration of large nerves such as the sciatic. Histologic changes consist of Schwann cell proliferation, demyelination, and axonal degeneration. Similar changes are occasionally reported in birds with thiamine deficiency.

Neoplastic Disease. Schwannomas are sporadically seen in pet birds. They can be single or multiple white, firm nodules. Storiform patterns, whorls and bundles of cells

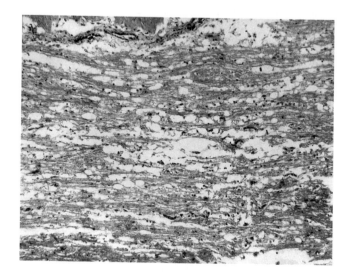

10.38. Peripheral nerve demyelination and degeneration secondary to trauma.

with fibrillar cytoplasm, and spindle-shaped nuclei are seen. Mitotic figures are rare, and there is a loose myxoid stroma. Basic myelin protein can be demonstrated with immunohistochemistry. In more malignant tumors, the cells are less well differentiated, and there is an increase in the mitotic index.

Ganglioneuromas are also seen in pet birds, particularly involving the adrenal gland and associated ganglia. These tumors are comprised of large ganglion cells, glial elements, and unmyelinated axons (Fig. 10.39).

Idiopathic Lesions. Sporadic cases of peripheral nerve degeneration of undetermined cause are seen in pet avian species. There is no gross lesion, and microscopic changes consist of axonal degeneration and demyelination (Fig. 10.40).

ADDITIONAL READING

Aguilar RF, Shaw DP, Dubey JP, Redig P. 1991. *Sarcocystis*-associated encephalitis in an immature northern goshawk (*Accipiter gentilis atricapillus*). J Zoo Wildl Med 22:466–469.

Aye PP, Morishita TY, Grimes S, et al. 1998. Encephalomalacia associated with vitamin-E deficiency in commercially raised emus: Case report. Avian Dis 42:600–605.

Bermudez AJ, Freischutz B, Yu RK, et al. 1997. Heritability and biochemistry of gangliosidosis in emus (*Dromaius novaehollandiae*). Avian Dis 41:838–849.

Bicknese EF. 1993. Review of sarcocystosis. In: Proceedings of the Association of Avian Veterinarians, Nashville, TN, pp 52–58.

Bossart GD. 1983. Neurofibromas in a Macaw (*Ara chloroptera*): Morphologic and immunocytochemical diagnosis. Vet Pathol 20:773–776

Cheville NF, Stone H, Riley J, Ritchie AE. 1972. Pathogenesis of virulent Newcastle disease in chickens. J Am Vet Med Assoc 161:169–179.

Garnham PCC, Duggan AJ, Sinden RE. 1979. A new species of *Sarcocystis* in the brain of two exotic birds. Ann Parasitol Hum Comp 54:393–400.

Gaskin JM, Homer BL, Eskelund KH. 1991. Preliminary findings in avian viral serositis: A newly recognized syndrome of psittacine birds. J Assoc Avian Vet 5:27–34.

Gregory CR, Latimer KS, Niagro FD, et al. 1994. A review of proventricular dilatation syndrome. J Assoc Avian Vet 8:69–75.

Henshel DS. 1998. Developmental neurotoxic effects of dioxin and dioxin-like compounds on domestic and wild avian species. Environ Toxicol Chem 17:88–98.

Jones MP, Orosz SE. 1996. Overview of avian neurology and neurological diseases. Semin Avian Exotic Pet Med 5:150–164.

Kwiecien JM, Smith DA, Key DW, et al. 1993. Encephalitis attributed to larval migration of *Baylisascaris* species in emus. Can Vet J 34:176–178.

Latimer KS, Niagro FD, Steffens III WL, et al. 1996. Polyomavirus encephalopathy in a Ducorps' cockatoo (*Cacatua ducorpsii*) with psittacine beak and feather disease. J Vet Diagn Invest 8:291–295.

Leach MW, Higgins RJ, Lowenstine LJ, Shor B. 1988. Paramyxovirus infection in a Moluccan cockatoo (*Cacatua moluccensis*) with neurologic signs. AAV Today 2:87–90.

Quist CF, Ritchie BR, McClure H, et al. 2000. Spongiform encephalopathy in three psittacine birds. In: Proceedings of the Association of Avian Veterinarians, Portland, OR, pp 205–206.

Rae M. 1995. Hemoprotozoa of caged and aviary birds. Semin Avian Exotic Pet Med 4:131–137

Reece RL, Butler R, Hooper PT. 1986. Cerebellar defects in parrots. Aust Vet J 63:197–198.

Schmidt RE, Goodman GJ, Higgins RJ, Fudge AM. 1987. Morphologic identification of papovavirus in a Moluccan cockatoo (*Cacatua moluccensis*) with neurologic signs. AAV Today 1:107–108.

Smit TH, Rondhuis PR. 1976. Studies on a virus isolated from the brain of a parakeet (*Neophema* sp.). Avian Pathol 5:21–30.

Steele KE, Linn MJ, Schoep RJ, et al. 2000. Pathology of fatal West Nile virus infections in native and exotic birds during the 1999 outbreak in New York City, New York. Vet Pathol 37:208–224.

Suedmeyer WK. 1992. Diagnosis and clinical progression of three cases of proventricular dilatation syndrome. J Assoc Avian Vet 6:159–163.

Teglas MB, Little SE, Latimer KS, Dubey JP. 1998. *Sarcocystis*-associated encephalitis and myocarditis in a wild turkey (*Meleagris gallopavo*). J Parasitol Hum Comp 84:661–663.

Woods LW, Plumlee KH. 1999. Avian toxicoses: Veterinary diagnostic laboratory perspective. Semin Avian Exotic Pet Med 8:32–35.

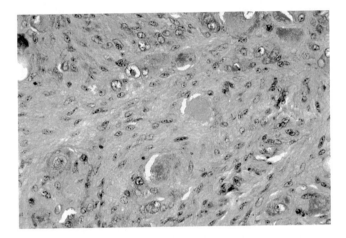

10.39. *Ganglioneuroma comprised of large ganglion cells and neurofibrils.*

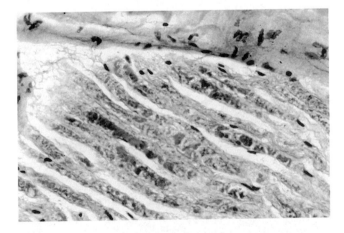

10.40. *Swollen, degenerating axons seen in idiopathic peripheral neuropathy.*

11 Integument

THE NORMAL ANATOMY OF THE SKIN AND FEATHERS

All feathers are composed of a hollow central shaft that ends in a quill or calamus, the tip of which anchors the feather to the feather follicle. The vane, which emanates from both sides of the shaft, is composed of long slender barbs and small hooklike barbules that project from the leading and trailing edges of the barbs. The barbules of the leading edge of the barbs interlock with the barbules of the trailing edge of its adjacent barb, causing the vane of the feather to act as a single flexible membrane. These elements of the feathers are modified to varying degrees at the base of the contour feathers, in down feathers, and in filoplumes. Birds typically molt once or twice a year. During the molt, old feathers fall out one at a time, and new feathers grow in their place. The base of the growing feather contains a vascular core and is surrounded by a partially opaque sheath. The bird breaks off the sheath, exposing the vane as the feather grows out. Powder-down feathers are specialized feathers that occur in dense tracts in a band cranial and dorsal to the legs. These feathers grow continuously. They are present in cockatoos and cockatiels.

An axial artery enters the growing feather through the centrally located proximal umbilicus. The dermal papilla surrounds the proximal apex of the feather and fills the proximal umbilicus. The developing calamus is filled with a loose vascular mesenchymal reticulum (pulp). Surrounding the pulp is a thin layer of inner sheath cells: a broad layer of cells developing into the barbs and barbules (the zone of differentiation), the relatively thin, keratinized feather sheath, and the epidermis of the follicle wall. Surrounding the proximal umbilicus and forming the collar of the growing feather, from medial to lateral, is a thin layer of regenerative cells that are continuous with the follicular epithelium, a thicker layer of inner sheath cells that are continuous with the feather sheath, and the intermediate cell layer that is continuous with the layer of inner sheath cells. Feather follicles are surrounded by the dermis and attached to several bundles of muscle.

The epidermis of the bird is very thin, except on the beak and scales of the legs. The stratum germinativum has only two layers. Superficially there is a transitional layer and finally one or more layers of keratinized epithelium (stratum corneum). The stratum germinativum and corneum of the scales are markedly thickened. Lipogenesis takes place in the epidermis, which functions as a holocrine sebaceous gland.

Birds have a single skin-associated gland: the uropygial gland. The remaining skin is devoid of glands. The uropygial gland, which is found at the base of the dorsum of the tail, is bilobed and pear shaped. From its caudally directed nipplelike apex protrude short down feathers. The uropygial gland is a holocrine tubuloalveolar gland. Although present in most birds, it is larger in aquatic species. It is absent in most parrots, ratites, and pigeons.

EXTERNAL EXAMINATION: SKIN AND SUBCUTIS

The necropsy begins with an examination of the skin and feathers. Diseases of the skin and feathers can indicate either a primary disorder of the integument or an underlying systemic disorder. Skin and feather problems are common in pet avian species. Since the skin has a limited range of response to insults, a variety of causes will lead to similar clinical signs and, in many cases, similar lesions. The skin may vary from grossly normal to severely inflamed to necrotic. Feather disease or damage may occur with or without skin disease. Both skin and feather damage are commonly the result of, or at least complicated by, some degree of self-trauma. The distribution of the skin and feather disease and the presence of plaques, ulcers, or exudates on the skin may assist pathologists in reaching a diagnosis.

CONGENITAL AND ACQUIRED MALFORMATIONS

True genetic disorders are poorly documented in pet birds. Occasionally feather cysts are seen in all species. Norwich and crested canaries have an apparent inherited predisposition to the development of feather cysts. Feather cysts grossly are oval or elongated swellings of the feather follicle. If the cyst is incised, it contains yellow-white dry layered material (keratin) (Fig. 11.1). The gross lesion must be differentiated from a follicular abscess.

Histologically, proliferated stratified squamous epithelium lines the keratin-filled cyst (Fig. 11.2). If there is secondary infection, inflammatory cells and possibly microorganisms may be seen. Although the cause of acquired cyst formation is usually not determined, infection, trauma, or any condition that interferes with normal growth of the feather may be responsible.

Abnormalities of the beak or claws can result from a variety of problems that interfere with growth of the germinal epithelium of the beak or claw keratin. Vitamin deficiency, toxicity, and improper incubation temperatures all may lead to asynchronous growth or incomplete keratinization. Excessive growth of the beak is often associated with chronic liver disease (Fig. 11.3). History, physical examination, and laboratory profiles are necessary to try to determine the etiology of each individual case.

Constricted-toe syndrome is seen in nestling parrots. The etiology of this disease in not known. An annular

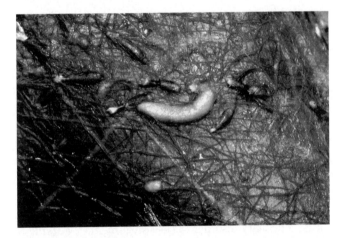

11.1. Typical appearance of follicular (epidermal inclusion) cyst.

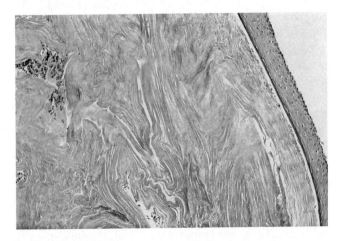

11.2. Follicular cyst containing keratin.

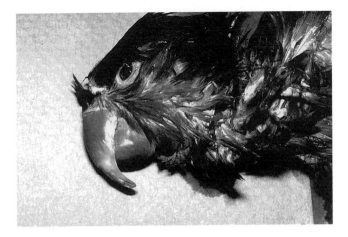

11.3. Overgrown beak secondary to chronic liver disease.

band of what appears to be scar tissue completely surrounds a segmental section of the toe. The distal toe then becomes swollen, and, if constriction is not surgically repaired, the distal toe will undergo necrosis.

True genetic disorders are poorly documented in pet birds. So-called feather-duster disease is seen in budgerigars. There is continued, excessive growth of feathers, and the birds cannot fly. Several types of inherited beak malformation have also been described in budgerigars, including straight rhinotheca, abnormally curved rhinotheca, and excessively broad upper and lower beaks.

Color mutations of the feathers are highly sought after by aviculturists. As a result, species of birds that have been kept in aviculture for many years, such as the budgerigar, cockatiel, ring-necked parrot, and lovebird, are now available in many different colors. More recently color mutations have been selected for in other species such as the Quaker parrot and parrotlet. Many of these birds are, at least initially, highly inbred and often smaller, less robust, and possibly more susceptible to disease than the wild-type birds.

INFECTIOUS DISEASE

Parasitic Disease

Knemidokoptic mites are found in budgerigars, canaries, and occasionally other species of companion birds. The cere and legs are commonly affected (Fig. 11.4), but feathered portions of the skin may also be involved in severe cases. Severe hyperkeratosis and acanthosis lead to variable gross thickening, irregularity, and flaking. Malformations of the beak can result in chronic cases. Mites are either superficial or deep, and with magnification may be seen moving in open spaces that occur in some extensive lesions. They are abundant and are readily seen in skin scrapings. *Dermanyssus* and *Ornithonysis* mites are uncommon to rare in cage birds and, in our experience, are most likely to been seen on finches and birds that are housed outside. *Dermanyssus* only feeds on birds at night, and therefore diagnosis depends on finding the mite in the cage environment.

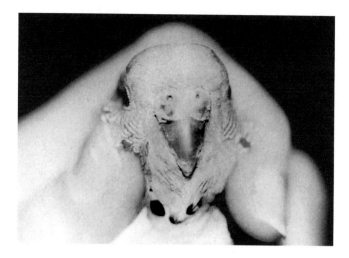

11.4. Roughened beak and cere due to Knemidocoptes infection.

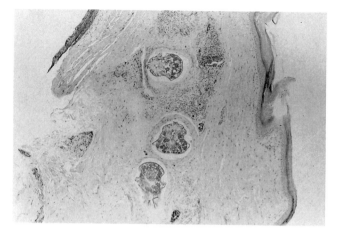

11.6. Deep mite infection with organisms in the dermis. Fibroplasia and a variable inflammatory infiltrate are seen.

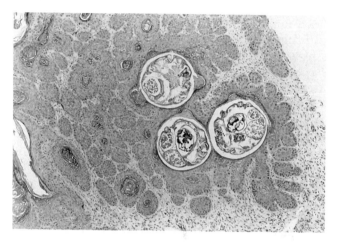

11.7. Deep mite infection with marked secondary acanthosis.

Histologically mites are associated with a variable inflammatory infiltrate, including heterophils, macrophages, plasma cells and, occasionally, giant cells (Figs. 11.5 and 11.6). Deep mite infection is often accompanied by markedly proliferative epidermis (Fig. 11.7). Occasionally numerous mites are seen in large cystic structures (Fig. 11.8).

Filarid nematodes, both adults and microfilaria, can be found in the subcutis. Gross congestion and/or hemorrhage may be noted, and adult nematodes may be found. Microfilaria are usually found in the superficial subcutis, with essentially no inflammatory response.

Cysts of *Leukocytozoon* may be found in the feather pulp in disseminated infections. A pleocellular inflammatory response is seen (Fig. 11.9).

Lice are uncommon in well-cared-for companion birds but are relatively common in domestic gallinaceous birds, pigeons, and wild birds. Unless the infestation is severe, no gross lesion is seen.

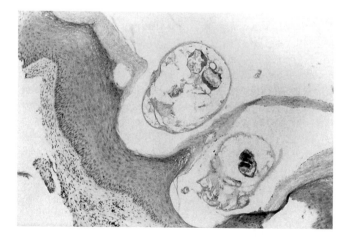

11.5. Superficial mite infection. The mites are present within the epidermis. There is hyperkeratosis and a mild dermal inflammatory response.

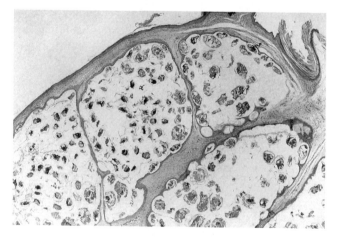

11.8. Large numbers of mites within a raised dermal mass.

Mycotic Disease

There is relatively little in the literature about the types of fungi that may cause feather disease in companion birds. This issue is complicated by the fact that many fungi are found on the feathers and skin of healthy birds, and

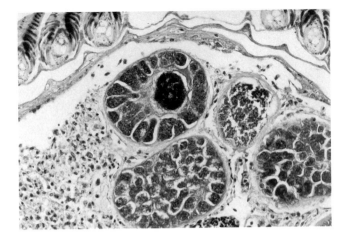

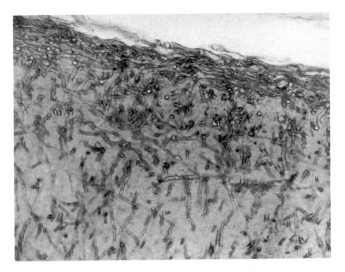

11.9. *Megaloschizonts of* **Leukocytozoon** *within the feather pulp.*

11.11. *Periodic acid-Schiff stain to demonstrate fungal hyphae in the keratin.*

heavy fungal growth may occur on old and soiled feathers without causing disease. Fungal organisms associated with skin or feather disease in companion birds include *Trichophyton* sp., *Microsporum gypseum*, several species of *Aspergillus*, *Mucor circinelloides*, *Rhizopus arrhizus*, *Penicillium chrysogenum*, *P. cyclopium*, and *Candida* sp.

Folliculitis due to dermatophytes appears to be less common in birds than is its counterpart in mammals, based on biopsy material. *Microsporum* sp. and *Trichophyton* sp. have been identified. When present, there may be gross swelling of follicles, with variable hyperkeratosis and crust formation. There is a pleocellular inflammatory infiltrate associated with necrosis and fungal hyphae, the latter giving the lesion its specificity (Figs. 11.10 and 11.11). Hyphae are also present in the follicular and surface keratin.

In some unusual cases of fungal infection, necrotizing lesions are seen not associated with feather follicles. These may appear as nodules with caseous centers, and there is a pleocellular response. Fungal hyphae are found in the necrotic centers (Fig. 11.12).

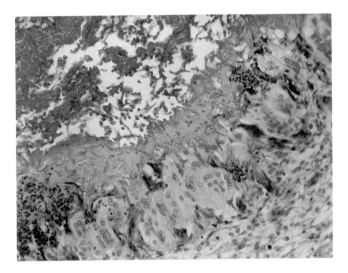

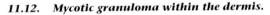

11.12. *Mycotic granuloma within the dermis.*

Occasionally birds are seen with superficial infections by yeasts morphologically resembling *Malassezia* (*Pityrosporum*).

The organisms, which are present in superficial and follicular keratin, may cause problems due to inflammation or possibly due to a hypersensitivity response. Gross changes are usually not seen in psittacine birds, and, in small passerines, they are nonspecific, with some flaking, thickening of the skin, and possible reddening, particularly if there is pruritis and self-trauma.

In psittacine birds, there is usually a minimal perivascular dermal inflammatory infiltrate comprised primarily of lymphocytes and plasma cells, with organisms found in the keratin (Fig. 11.13). Small passerine birds may have significant superficial dermatitis, with a pleocellular infiltrate (Fig. 11.14).

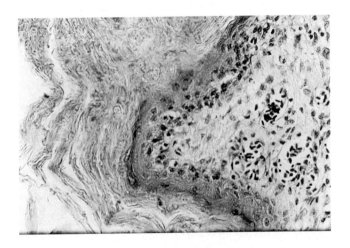

11.10. *Acanthosis and severe hyperkeratosis due to fungal infection. Organisms are present in the keratin but may be difficult to see on routine stains.*

Bacterial Disease

Bacterial skin disease in pet birds may either be confined to the feather follicle or be generalized. *Staphylococcus* sp.

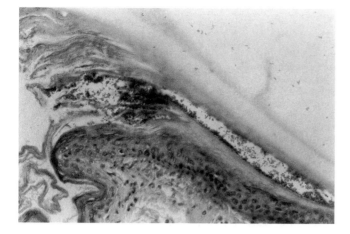

11.13. *Hyperkeratosis associated with small yeasts consistent with Malassezia sp. in the keratin in a psittacine bird.*

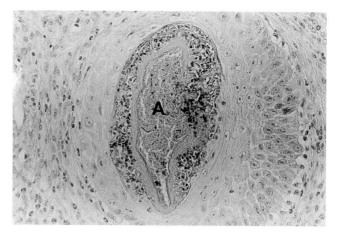

11.15. *Bacterial folliculitis. Large numbers of organisms (A) within a necrotic, inflamed follicle.*

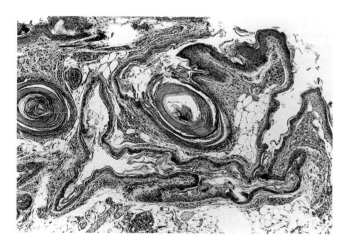

11.14. *Hyperkeratosis, acanthosis, and diffuse dermatitis in a passerine bird with Malassezia sp. infection.*

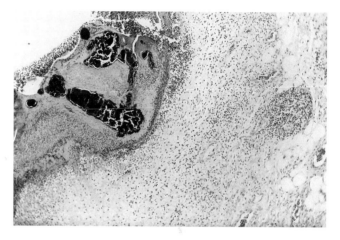

11.16. *Severe superficial bacterial dermatitis with necrosis of the epidermis and large bacteria colonies.*

is the most common bacteria associated with folliculitis. Grossly they cause a swelling of the perifollicular skin, with a variable amount of reddening. Follicular abscessation and feather pulp inflammation may also occur (Fig. 11.15). Generalized bacterial dermatitis (pyoderma) may be pruritic, leading to self-trauma that results in a more severe lesion. Reddening, induration, and crust formation are grossly associated with necrosis.

Histologically a diffuse infiltration of heterophils and lesser numbers of plasma cells and macrophages are present. Necrosis extends through the epidermis into the dermis in severe cases (Fig. 11.16). Bacteria, usually gram-positive cocci, may present.

Secondary bacterial infections may follow skin trauma. If untreated, these usually result in abscess formation. Gross changes include localized swelling and necrosis, and a yellow, caseous exudate may be seen. The necrotic center of the abscess is usually surrounded by heterophils, lymphocytes, and macrophages, and giant cells are seen in some cases. Organisms are not always present.

Pododermatitis is usually secondary to trauma, with subsequent dermatitis and cellulitis leading to swelling and abscessation of the foot and toes (Fig. 11.17). Birds of prey and waterfowl are highly prone to disease of the plantar surface of the feet (bumble foot). Disease occurs secondary to the use of improper perches in raptors and improper substrate in waterfowl. Injury to one leg that results in increased weight bearing on the other leg may also predispose some raptors to bumble foot. Damaged skin is infected with a *Staphylococcus* sp. that results in ulceration and infection of the underlying tissues. Secondary infections with *Escherichia coli* are common.

Improper perch size and texture is a common cause of lesions of the bottom of the feet of parrots. Flattened patches of skin characterize these lesions. Additionally the roughened texture of the foot is lost, and the skin becomes pink to red and smooth. Birds that are housed on perches that are too large will bear weight on their hocks, and similar flat smooth skin lesions will develop on the ventral surface of the hocks. It is rare for the affected skin to become ulcerated.

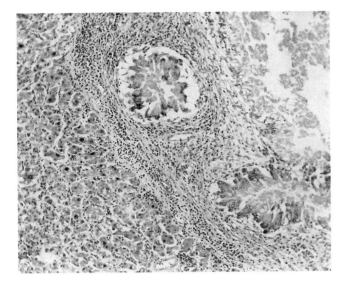

11.17. *Chronic pododermatitis with granuloma formation and fibroplasia.*

Mycobacterial infections of the skin and subcutis may be primary due to localized invasion but also may indicate systemic mycobacterial disease. The condition may present as single or multiple granulomas and grossly can resemble abscesses due to other bacteria or fungi, although in some birds nonpainful and nonpruritic nodules may be seen. It may also present as an area of localized thickening and induration (Fig. 11.18). Although *Mycobacterium avium* may be the cause, *M. genavense* must be included as an etiologic differential in cutaneous mycobacteriosis.

The histologic lesion is characterized by the accumulation of numerous large macrophages with pale basophilic cytoplasm (Fig. 11.19). The cytoplasm of these cells contains acid-fast bacteria. Scattered heterophils and small macrophages will also be seen. Necrosis and caseation is minimal in most pet birds.

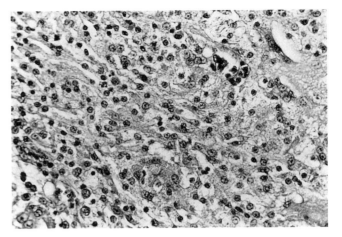

11.19. *Mycobacterial dermatitis. There is diffuse infiltration of large macrophages with abundant cytoplasm. The cytoplasm is filled with organisms that are difficult to identify with routine stains.*

Viral Disease

Papillomaviruses. These viruses are thought to cause cutaneous lesions in European finches, canaries, and the African grey parrot. Lesions in finches are found on the feet, the lesions in canaries are reported to be at the corner of the beak, and the lesions on African grey parrots are widely disseminated on the face. Virus particles consistent in size and shape with a papillomavirus have been reported in the lesions of these birds, and a protein immunologically cross-reactive to the major capsid protein of a human papillomavirus has been reported to occur in cutaneous papillomas from an African grey parrot. Grossly this disease is characterized by the presence of multiple proliferative skin lesions that superficially resemble those caused by mite infestations and by poxvirus infections.

Histologically the lesions are fronds of hyperplastic epithelial cells supported by a vascular stroma (Fig. 11.20). Epidermal nuclei are often enlarged and homogeneous,

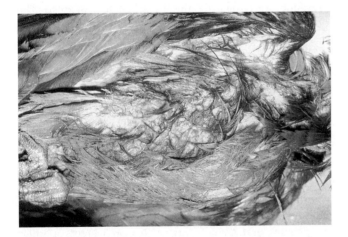

11.18. *Mycobacterial skin infection. Note the thickening and nodularity of the skin in areas of feather loss.*

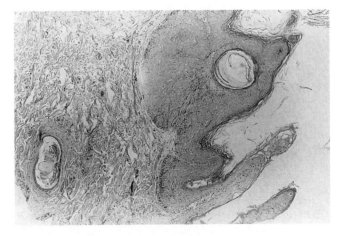

11.20. *Virus-induced papilloma in an African grey parrot. Multiple fronds are seen.*

suggestive of inclusion body formation. Well-defined inclusion bodies usually are not seen, but viral particles are demonstrated by electron microscopy. Similar lesions are seen in cockatiels but have not been characterized.

Polyomavirus. Polyomavirus was originally reported as a disease of budgerigars, with feather loss one of the primary clinical signs.

Feather dysplasia is a common finding in fledgling budgerigars raised in large commercial aviaries. Breeders often call these birds runners or creepers (Fig. 11.21). Grossly, primary wing feathers and tail feathers are either absent entirely or have thick sheaths, and there may be hemorrhage in their shafts. These birds are typically infected with avian polyomavirus, psittacine beak and feather disease virus (PBFDV), or both. We have seen birds with these feather abnormalities that did not have either infection. It is speculated that giardiasis may also cause this type of lesion, but that has not been proved, and giardiasis is very common in budgerigars with and without feather disease.

Feather disease may be the only manifestation of avian polyomavirus in budgerigars, or it may accompany the systemic form of the disease seen in nestlings. Affected nestlings may have dysplasia of contour feathers, down feathers, flight feathers, or a combination of all of them. Within the growing feather, there is often massive infection of the cells in the zone of differentiation, with nearly every cell showing karyomegaly and containing the characteristic intranuclear inclusion bodies (Figs. 11.22 and 11.23). Inclusions in the epidermis of the skin are usually also present but are infrequent.

Feather changes are rare in larger psittacine birds with avian polyomavirus. In some cases, however, these birds will have hemorrhage within the shaft of affected feathers. Subcutaneous hemorrhage is a common feature of avian polyomavirus disease in nonbudgerigar parrots (Fig. 11.24). Nonpsittacine birds with polyomavirus infection rarely have gross feather changes.

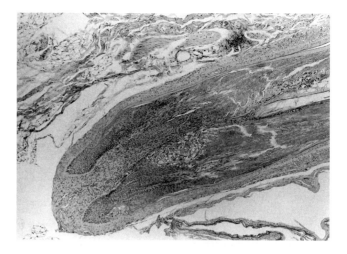

11.22. Polyomavirus-induced karyomegaly and intranuclear inclusion body formation in the epidermal collar.

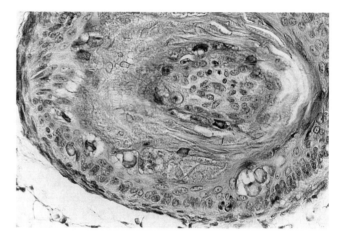

11.23. Detail of polyomavirus intranuclear inclusions. They are clear or lightly granular and basophilic.

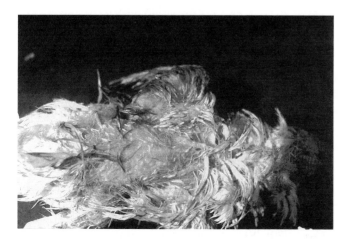

11.21. Feather loss and dystrophy due to polyomavirus infection.

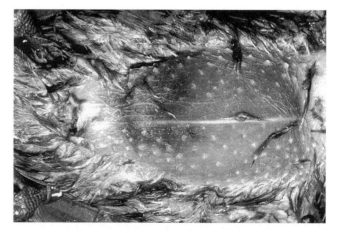

11.24. A psittacine bird with polyomavirus infection. With no history available, the lesion would have to be differentiated from trauma-induced hemorrhage.

Poxviruses. Poxviruses are large, enveloped DNA viruses. The biology of the poxviruses is complex. They have been isolated from many species of birds, but each virus has the ability to infect only a limited range of species. Disease is transmitted in most cases by biting insects; therefore, most affected birds are housed out of doors. Domestic birds that are commonly affected are the chicken, the ostrich, and the canary.

Historically this disease was a major problem in wild-caught blue-fronted Amazon and Pionus parrot nestlings held in quarantine. Some of these birds would be infected with the virus prior to capture, and then the use of common feeding instruments between birds would result in its dissemination. Since the end of the importation of wild-caught parrots, this disease is no longer seen in these birds.

Poxvirus infections are very common problem in nestling and fledgling wild birds, particularly doves, grackles, and mockingbirds. The so-called dry or cutaneous form of the poxvirus infection is confined predominantly to the skin. Lesions are common on the head, face, and feet but can also be present in feather tracts in severe infection. The lesions are proliferative, presenting as papules, pustules, and nodules. These lesions may ulcerate and crust over.

Grossly the lesions can have rough or smooth surfaces, depending on the duration of the lesion, self-trauma, and the degree of secondary bacterial infection (Fig. 11.25). The lesions may be massive, causing the eye to close and interfering with prehension. Severe lesions may be mistaken for neoplasia.

Histologically there may be epidermal ulceration and superficial bacterial infection. There is severe hyperplasia of the epidermis, with intraepithelial vesicle formation, ballooning degeneration, and large eosinophilic intracytoplasmic inclusion bodies (Bollinger bodies) that may cause the nucleus to have a crescent shape and be displaced to the side of the cell. Inclusion bodies are often abundant but in some cases are uncommon (Figs. 11.26

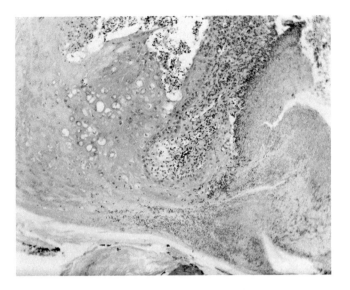

11.26. *Typical poxvirus lesion with marked epidermal hyperplasia and associated necrosis and hemorrhage.*

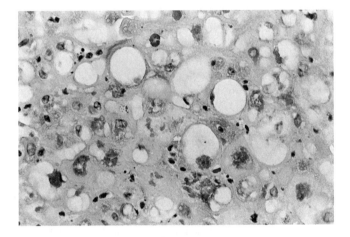

11.27. *Detail of poxvirus infection illustrating ballooning degeneration and eosinophilic, intracytoplasmic inclusion bodies.*

and 11.27). Ultrastructurally virus particles are present in the inclusions (Fig. 11.28).

Herpesvirus. Pacheco's disease typically causes systemic infection that can occasionally include involvement of the epidermis of the skin or feather, leading to necrosis. Inclusion bodies can be seen in cells surrounding the necrosis. Since the generalized disease is usually catastrophic, little attention is paid to what may be grossly minimal skin lesions.

Proliferative lesions of the lower legs and feet are seen in a number of species of psittacine bird, particularly cockatoos and macaws. A cytomegalic herpesvirus is thought to cause these lesions, because virus particles can be seen with electron microscopy of this tissue.

In cockatoos, this disease presents as solitary proliferative nodule or as multiple proliferative nodules. The lesion in macaws is typically a roughening of the skin

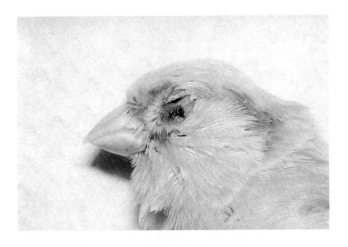

11.25. *Proliferative and hemorrhagic lesion due to poxvirus infection. The face and feet are common locations.*

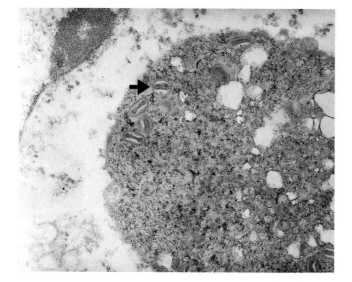

11.28.   Electron photomicrograph of poxvirus particles (arrow) within an inclusion body.

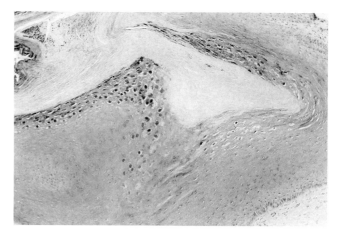

11.30.   Cytomegalic herpesvirus infection. Marked parakeratosis is seen, and basophilic inclusion bodies fill the nucleus, which is surrounded by a clear halo.

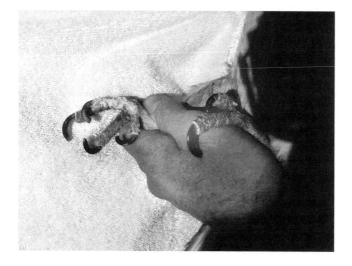

11.29.   Cytomegalic herpesvirus infection. The skin of the feet is typically affected, being thickened and depigmented.

and/or a flat, raised plaque. Depigmentation of the diseased tissue is common (Fig. 11.29). These lesions are very dry, and the thickened skin is readily scraped away.

Microscopically there is epidermal hyperplasia and marked acanthosis, with large intranuclear inclusion bodies that fill the nucleus, which is often surrounded by a clear halo (Fig. 11.30).

Circovirus. PBFDV is one of several avian circoviruses (chapter 8). This virus is enzootic in many species of wild Australian parrots and has also been found in wild African parrots. It causes an acute fatal infection in nestling cockatoos and, less frequently, nestlings of other species and a chronic disease in young adult birds, including cockatoos, lovebirds, African grey parrots and, rarely, New World parrots. The disease in nestlings is acute in onset and generalized so that it affects all growing feathers. Flight feathers

take longer to develop than contour feathers; therefore, if nestlings are somewhat older when infected, only the flight feathers may be involved.

Affected birds typically die within 2 weeks of the onset of the disease. The chronic form of disease is generally seen in birds 8 months to 3 years old and is first recognized when birds go through their first molt. Dystrophic feathers replace normal ones during the molt. Powder-down feathers may be the first affected in cockatoos.

Currently PBFDV is most commonly seen in lovebirds, budgerigars, lories, lorikeets, and eclectus and African grey parrots. Feather lesions in lovebirds are rarely as florid as those seen in cockatoos. Many affected lovebirds show only dull plumage or have an increased number of broken or worn feathers. Advanced cases may show some feather dysplasia, or new feathers may simply not develop, leaving portions of the bird unfeathered. A significant percentage, perhaps the majority of lovebirds infected with PBFDV, show no signs of disease at all.

A generalized feather disease is seen in African grey parrots, but often it is confined to the tail feathers, or there may be no feather involvement at all. Eclectus parrots do not show typical feather lesions of PBFDV, but affected birds may have a delayed molt and poor-quality feathering.

A variant of the originally sequenced PBFDV appears to be widespread in lories and lorikeets in North American collections. Many birds with this infection do not show signs of disease, but a certain percentage develops characteristic feather lesions.

Grossly there is necrosis and annular constriction of the base of the feather shaft and hemorrhage in the feather pulp. There may be severe shedding of affected feathers (Fig. 11.31). Affected feathers are stunted and may have thickened, hyperkeratotic sheaths, pulp hemorrhage, annular constrictions of the calamus, curling, or stress lines on the vanes (Fig. 11.32). The apex of the sheath and the ensheathed feather may be necrotic. Affected feathers may only grow out partially and may be

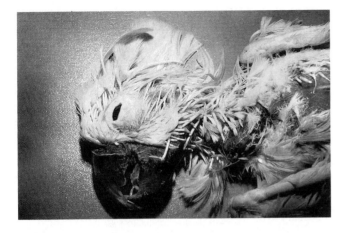

11.31. Severe feather loss due to circovirus infection.

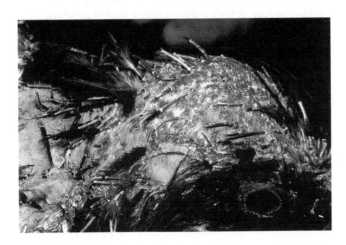

11.32. Dystrophic feathers in a bird with circovirus infection.

clubbed. Discoloration of feathers may be the initial sign in some birds. African grey parrots may develop red feathers, and yellow feathers have been seen to replace green feathers in other species of parrots.

Beak lesions are less common than feather changes but are a prominent feature of this disease in sulfur-crested, umbrella, and Moluccan cockatoos (chapter 3). Variable necrosis and loss of keratin can be seen. Although this form of the disease is still common in Australia, since the importation of wild-caught birds has ceased, it is uncommon in captive-raised parrots. External gross lesions are usually not seen in nonpsittacine birds. Feather dystrophy similar to that seen in psittacines has been reported in pigeons, doves and finches.

Follicular epidermal hyperplasia, hyperkeratosis, and degeneration of germinal cells are seen histologically. There is ballooning and patchy degeneration of cells of the epidermal collar. Although considered to be an example of necrosis, the process may actually be apoptosis. The feather-shaft constriction noted grossly is secondary to the necrosis in the epidermal collar. An associated infiltration of macrophages, which may contain large, globular, basophilic, cytoplasmic inclusion bodies, is seen. Similar

cells are seen in the pulp, and there may also be hemorrhage and a heterophilic infiltrate, particularly if there has been self-trauma. In chronic cases, small granulomas with keratin fragments and giant cells are seen (Figs. 11.33–11.36). Multifocal to confluent inflammation may be present in the superficial dermis, with lymphocytes and plasma cells predominating. A few epithelial cells of the epidermis or epidermal collar may contain structures resembling intranuclear inclusion bodies.

With electron microscopy, non-membrane-bound paracrystalline arrays representing the small 12- to 26-nm virus are seen (Fig. 11.37). Definitive diagnosis can also be done with polymerase chain reaction assays, DNA in situ hybridization, and immunoperoxidase staining.

In some psittacine birds, mixed infections with polyomavirus and circovirus are found. Grossly there are a variety of feather and skin changes as previously described (Fig. 11.38). Histologic changes consistent with both diseases are seen.

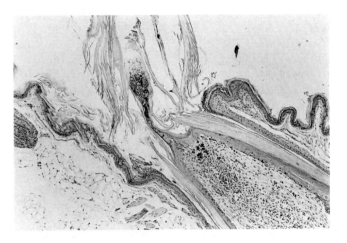

11.33. Circovirus-induced epidermal collar necrosis leading to constriction of the feather shaft.

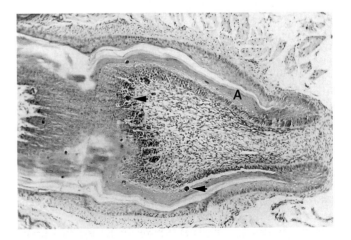

11.34. Epidermal collar (A) necrosis and scattered intracytoplasmic inclusion bodies (arrowheads) in circovirus infection.

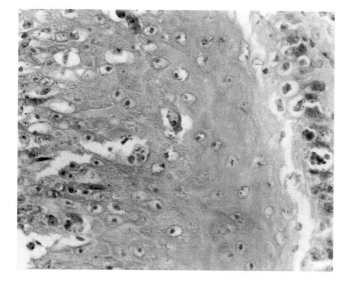

11.35.   Detail of epidermal collar necrosis or possible apoptosis.

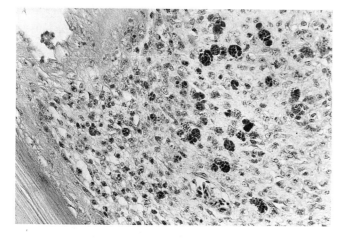

11.36.   Numerous globular intracytoplasmic inclusion bodies in circovirus infection.

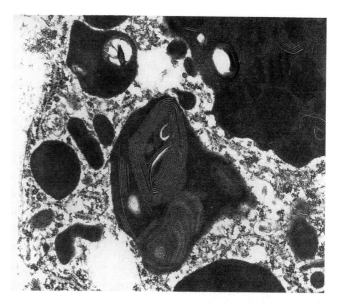

11.37.   Electron photomicrograph of circovirus intracytoplasmic inclusion bodies. Note the non-membrane-bound paracrystalline arrays.

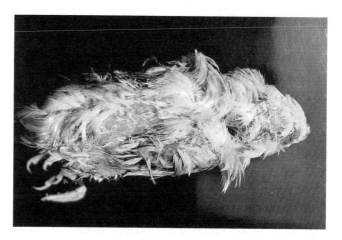

11.38.   Severe feather loss associated with mixed infection by polyomavirus and circovirus.

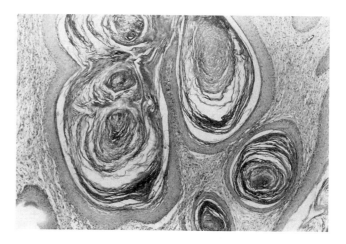

11.39.   Squamous metaplasia and hyperkeratosis of the uropygial gland due to vitamin A deficiency.

NONINFECTIOUS DISEASE

Nutritional/Metabolic Disease

Specific and nonspecific nutritional problems that can result in poor feathering and skin disease include vitamin, mineral, and amino acid deficiencies, as well as generalized malnutrition. Depigmentation, altered pigmentation, improper molting, and poor-quality feathers can be seen. Gross changes are rarely specific, and, in many cases, mild hyperkeratosis and acanthosis may be the only histologic changes noted.

Vitamin A deficiency may lead to scaly skin, poor feather quality, and focal hyperkeratosis, particularly of the feet. The uropygial gland may become enlarged, with yellow caseous-appearing material present instead of the typical secretion product. Squamous metaplasia is seen microscopically, with hyperkeratosis a primary contributor to the gross appearance (Fig. 11.39).

African grey parrot nestlings fed a diet that was misformulated to contain no vitamin A had pronounced transverse ridges develop on their beaks. The lesions resolved once the diet was corrected.

Lack of carotenoids in the diet can lead to dilution of skin and feather color, because carotene is a component of yellow, orange, red, and green feather colors. Tyrosine deficiency can lead to poor melanin production and color changes. Protein or specific amino acid imbalances can result in alterations in feather structure leading to color changes due to changes in light scattering.

Horizontal, 1- to 2-mm, dark, dysplastic bands are a common lesion seen in hand-fed nestling birds. These bands are segmental sections of the vane that did not form barbules. Empirically it appears that these bands are the result of a short period of stress that occurs while the feather is growing in. In this case, stress is broadly defined to include such things as being chilled, not eating, and illness. A few dysplastic bands are a common finding on the feathers of most nestling parrots. However, multiple bands suggest that the bird suffered from a prolonged illness or an extended period of improper husbandry. Dysplastic bands are particularly obvious on young birds, because all their feathers grow in simultaneously and, thus, if one feather is affected, most others will be also. After the first molt, dysplastic bands will generally be confined to only a few feathers.

Physical/Environmental Agents

Trauma, burns, excessive cold, and other physical factors often cause skin lesions. Loss of feathers, varying degrees of hemorrhage, necrosis, and superficial crust formation are seen (Fig. 11.40). Severe necrosis and sloughing of epidermis and possibly portions of dermis can be seen in injuries due to both heat and cold. Discoloration of the lesions is variable. Severe frostbite may lead to complete loss of digits.

Histologically there is severe coagulative necrosis, with an active, well-defined inflammatory margin between necrotic and live tissue. Traumatic injuries are characterized by variable amounts of hemorrhage, edema, and

inflammation, depending on severity of the insult and time elapsed prior to examination.

Self-trauma of the feathers and the skin is a common problem in parrots and may occur in other species. Self-trauma may be due to a primary disease of the skin or feathers, a multisystemic disease, or it may be psychogenic in nature. In these birds, typically the head feathers are unaffected, and there are varying degrees of damage to other feathers. There are many patterns of feather picking. Some birds confine their attention to wing feathers and some to contour feathers, whereas others will damage both. Some birds will chew only on the feathers; others will pull them out entirely. Some birds will even pull out growing feathers or bite them off at the level of the feather follicle.

Self-trauma to the skin is less common and often associated, initially, with an underlying disease. As birds damage the skin, the problem escalates to the point that large areas of skin are destroyed, sometimes including underlying muscle (Fig. 11.41). Traumatic wounds over the sternum are often aggravated by self-trauma and may result in osteomyelitis of the keel of the sternum.

Endocrinopathies

Hypothyroidism is the only described endocrine disease affecting pet birds, and there is only one published report of this disease. In this bird and those seen by us, there is no specific pattern of feather disease or feature lesions that are specific for endocrine disease. Instead, these birds have a generalized loss of feathers, a failure of new feathers to grow in, and the absence of observable skin lesions (Fig. 11.42).

Histologic changes can be poorly defined, with generalized follicular inactivity and atrophy associated with epidermal thinning and atrophy of dermal collagen (Fig. 11.43). In some cases of hypothyroidism, excessive mucus deposition is seen in the dermis. To confirm a diagnosis of endocrine-related skin disease, appropriate clinical laboratory testing is necessary. Confirmation can also result

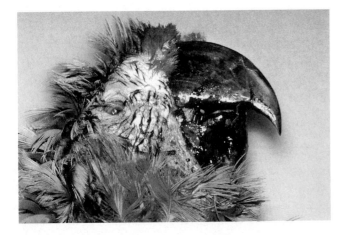

11.40. Traumatic hemorrhage and beak damage.

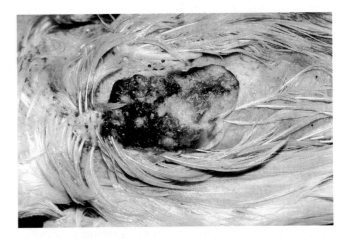

11.41. Severe focal ulceration and hemorrhage due to self-trauma.

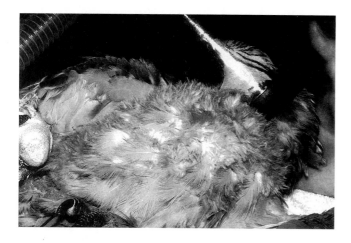

11.42. *Loss of mature feathers in a bird with clinical hypothyroidism.*

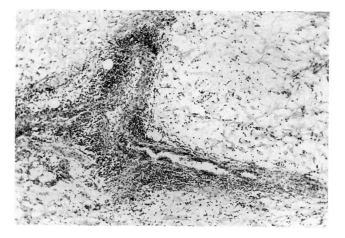

11.44. *Severe angiocentric dermatitis consistent with hypersensitivity.*

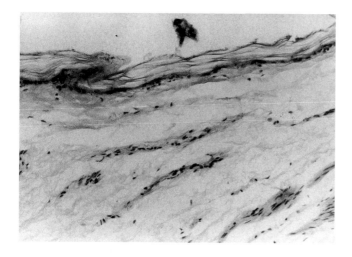

11.43. *Mild hyperkeratosis associated with epidermal atrophy and dermal edema in a hypothyroid bird.*

from finding appropriate endocrine gland lesions at necropsy.

Hypersensitivity

Allergic skin disease in birds is occasionally reported but is not well documented, and confirmation can be difficult. Gross changes that may be associated with allergic skin disease include feather loss, reddening of the skin and, occasionally, surface exudates. Some of the gross lesions may be secondary to self-trauma.

Histologic lesions are not definitive, because there are still an insufficient number of cases with follow-up information. Perivascular inflammatory cell foci are seen in the dermis and subcutis. These foci usually consist primarily of mononuclear cells, with a few granulocytes in some cases (Fig. 11.44). In severe lesions in some species, large numbers of granulocytes and a variable amount of degranulation have been noted. A pleocellular inflammatory infiltrate is often present in the feather pulp. Severe superficial necrosis, variable acanthosis, and dermal fibrosis are often associated with self-trauma. Secondary infection is possible.

A condition known as "Amazon foot necrosis" is seen in Amazon parrots. Affected birds suddenly begin chewing at their feet and lower legs. The pathogenesis of this lesion is not known, but there is speculation that it represents a delayed hypersensitivity reaction following staphylococcal dermatitis. Owners of many of these parrots smoke cigarettes, and it is also postulated that nicotine or some element in tobacco smoke may initiate this disease. Gross lesions are seen in unfeathered skin of the leg and foot and begin as erythematous areas. There is usually severe self-trauma leading to ulceration. In some cases, staphylococci are found in the lesion.

Chronic Internal Disease

Feather loss and poor-quality feathering are nonspecific findings in many cases of chronic internal disease, including infectious, degenerative, and neoplastic conditions.

Miscellaneous Conditions

Calcinosis circumscripta, which is an unusual condition in birds, presents as nodular lesions that may have a white, chalky appearance grossly. Histologically a chronic inflammatory reaction and variable fibrosis surround mineralized foci (Fig. 11.45).

Follicular malformations and dystrophy are occasionally seen. The most recognized is the so-called polyfolliculitis, which is a misnomer, as in many cases there is no inflammation. The condition is seen in budgerigars, cockatiels, and lovebirds. Multiple feather shafts appear to grow from a single follicle. Feathers are thick and short and may have retained sheaths. Histologically the feather follicles appear to coalesce due to an atrophy of the skin between the follicles, leading to what appear to be multiple shafts and epidermal collars within a dilated follicle (Fig. 11.46).

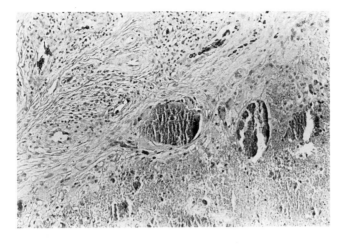

11.45. *Calcinosis circumscripta. Multiple foci of dermal mineralization and a variable inflammatory reaction are seen.*

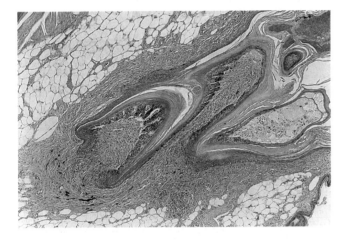

11.46. *Feather dystrophy typical of polyfollicle formation. Several feather shafts appear to be arising in an area of one feather follicle.*

Occasionally structures morphologically consistent with adventitial bursa formation are found. Grossly they present as fluctuant subcutaneous swellings that contain slightly viscid fluid. Histologically, synovial-like cells usually line the structures. The wall is usually chronically inflamed with an infiltrate of macrophages, heterophils, and plasma cells.

Collagen necrosis associated with a severe granulocytic response is occasionally seen in dermal lesions. Although many of the granulocytes may be eosinophils, they are difficult to distinguish from heterophils histologically. The lesion is similar to idiopathic collagenolytic inflammation seen in several mammalian species.

Autoimmune skin disease has not been documented in birds, but several cases with intraepidermal pustule formation and acantholysis have been seen. Unfortunately these few cases were lost to follow-up.

Perifollicular lymphoid aggregates and perivascular lymphoid cuffing are common findings in birds with specific feather disease and in birds that are self-mutilating.

This may be a nonspecific finding associated with antigen stimulation when there is inflammatory skin disease. However, it is not clear why these lesions are commonly seen in birds that are damaging their feathers but do not have other obvious skin disease.

PROLIFERATIVE DISEASE

Neoplastic Disease

Epithelial Tumors. Papillomas of the skin are not common and may be virally induced in African grey parrots (see the section on viral disease). In other birds, particularly cockatiels, these tumors usually present as papillary growths on the face. Histologically the lesions are similar, but viral causation has not been proved. They are comprised of fronds covered by proliferative, hyperkeratotic epidermis (Fig. 11.47). There is a delicate vascular stroma.

Squamous cell carcinomas are often ulcerated and hemorrhagic as well as infiltrative. They tend to grow slowly and can become large if not treated (Fig. 11.48). They can arise anywhere in the skin and also within the

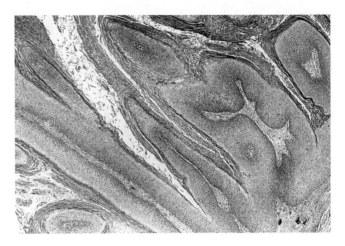

11.47. *Squamous papilloma. Multiple epithelial fronds are seen. Other than in African grey parrots, viral causation has not been proven.*

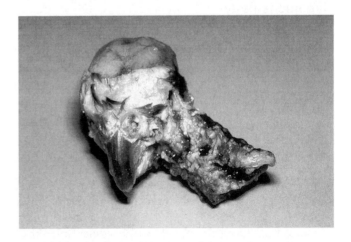

11.48. *Squamous cell carcinoma involving a large area of the face and neck.*

uropygial gland, where they must be differentiated from primary tumors of the gland.

The microscopic appearance of squamous cell carcinomas is variable. Many are fairly well differentiated, with cells forming nests and cords that may contain keratin centers (Fig. 11.49). Others are poorly differentiated, with no keratin differentiation. The cells will form diffuse sheets that are infiltrative (Fig. 11.50). Metastasis is possible but seldom reported.

Basal cell tumors can present as solitary nodules, may also originate in feather cysts, and, although expansile, are histologically benign, forming sheets, cords, or nests. Basal cell tumors associated with attempted feather formation have been called "feather folliculomas" and may be the avian equivalent of trichoepitheliomas. The proliferative basal cells form nests and ridges that grow by expansion in the wall of the cyst (Fig. 11.51).

Basal cell carcinoma is rare but can be invasive, with a high potential for recurrence or possible metastasis.

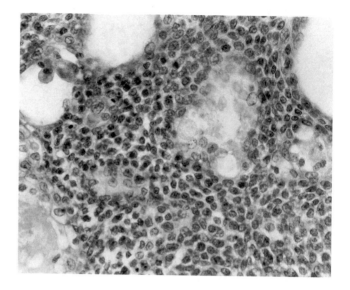

11.51. Sheet of neoplastic cells in basal cell tumor.

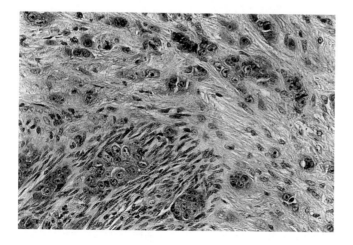

11.49. Squamous cell carcinoma with keratin pearls that is invasive into bone.

Uropygial gland tumors can be either adenomas or carcinomas, and gross differentiation is difficult. Grossly there is an enlarging mass in the region of the uropygial gland. The mass is ulcerated in some cases.

Adenomas are usually well circumscribed and encapsulated, and are comprised of fairly well differentiated glandular epithelial cells (Fig. 11.52). Carcinomas contain less well differentiated cells that are infiltrative into surrounding tissue (Fig. 11.53). Carcinomas are more likely to be necrotic, hemorrhagic, and secondarily inflamed.

Mesenchymal Tumors. Mesenchymal tumors include those of vascular origin, fibrous and adipose connective tissue, and myxomas. In addition, lymphosarcoma and mast cell tumors may be found. Gross differentiation can be difficult with malignant tumors.

Lipomas are common and have the gross appearance of a mass of normal fat. Histologically the typical lipoma is comprised of a sheet of well-differentiated adipose cells

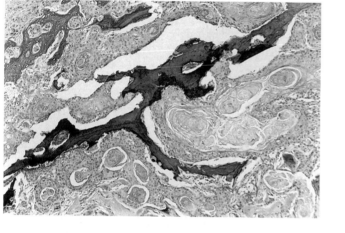

11.50. Poorly differentiated squamous cell carcinoma with individualization of tumor cells and a scirrhous response.

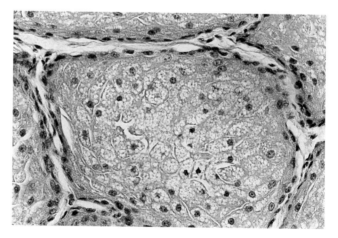

11.52. Uropygial gland tumor with a lobule of well-differentiated epithelial cells.

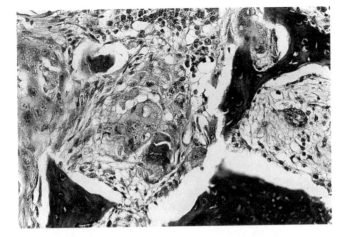

11.53. *Poorly differentiated cells of uropygial gland carcinoma invasive into bone.*

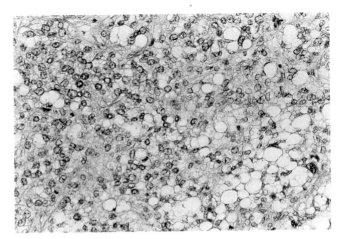

11.55. *Liposarcoma. Moderately undifferentiated to poorly differentiated adipose cells and minimal stroma.*

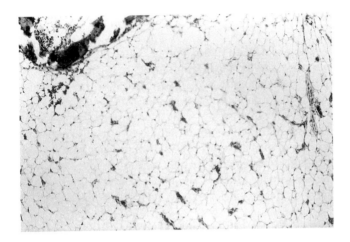

11.54. *Typical subcutaneous lipoma comprised of a sheet of well-differentiated adipose cells.*

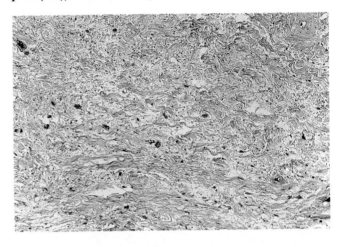

11.56. *Bundles of well-differentiated collagen typical of fibroma.*

(Fig. 11.54). At least three variants have been noted on histologic examination. Myelolipomas, in addition to the adipose cells, contain multiple foci of extramedullary hematopoiesis. Sections of these tumors resemble normal bone marrow.

Osteolipomas and hemangiolipomas have also been identified. They are characterized respectively by the formation of either normal bone spicules or numerous well-differentiated capillaries.

Liposarcomas are less common. They are usually fatty-appearing, poorly demarcated masses (Fig. 11.55).

Hemangiomas and hemangiosarcomas occur in the skin and subcutis with essentially the same frequency in pet birds. Lymphangiomas are rarely seen. These tumors are described in chapter 1.

Fibrosarcomas are common tumors of the skin of pet birds, but fibromas are infrequently diagnosed. Both tumors present as firm nodules or masses. Benign tumors are encapsulated, but sarcomas may have indistinct margins. These tumors present as firm nodules or masses.

Histologically fibromas are comprised of interlacing bundles of well-differentiated collagen (Fig. 11.56).

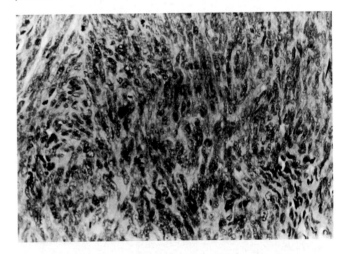

11.57. *Highly cellular fibrosarcoma common in pet birds. Numerous mitotic figures are seen.*

Fibrosarcomas are very cellular, with fusiform cells forming interlacing bundles and sheets (Fig. 11.57). Numerous mitotic figures are usually seen.

Tumors morphologically similar to mammalian hemangiopericytoma are occasionally diagnosed. They

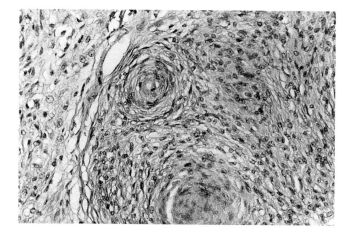

11.58. *Pattern of fusiform cells consistent with probable hemangiopericytoma. These tumors are uncommon in birds.*

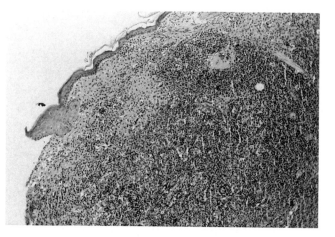

11.60. *Dermal lymphosarcoma comprised of a sheet of neoplastic lymphoid cells.*

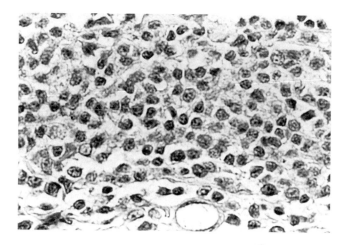

11.61. *Dermal lymphosarcoma. The cells have indistinct cytoplasmic boundaries and are minimally pleomorphic.*

are comprised of whorls of fusiform cells that appear to surround blood vessels (Fig. 11.58).

Some connective tissue tumors contain large amounts of extracellular mucin and morphologically are called myxofibromas or myxomas, depending on the cell-to-ground substance ratio. Mitotic activity is usually minimal.

Undifferentiated sarcomas are occasionally found at the site of skin tattoos. Histologically tattoo ink is present in the lesion (Fig. 11.59).

Dermal lymphosarcoma can present as solitary or multiple masses or as diffuse thickening of the skin with loss of feathers. Neoplastic lymphoid cells form diffuse sheets, and there is variable mitotic activity (Figs. 11.60 and 11.61). Multifocal infiltration of feather follicles, similar to Marek's disease in chickens, occurs sporadically in pet birds. An etiologic agent has not been identified.

Melanocytic Tumors. Melanoma has been diagnosed in several psittacine birds. The tumor is not common and is usually malignant. These tumors, which often occur on

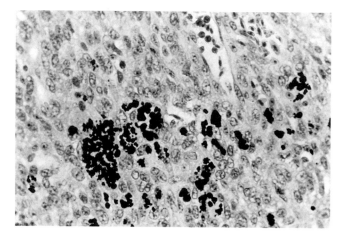

11.59. *Undifferentiated sarcoma associated with the site of a skin tattoo. The dark pigment is tattoo ink.*

the face and may involve the beak, are brown-black, raised masses with poorly defined margins. Histologically they are comprised of pleomorphic melanocytic cells that form nests and sheets (Fig. 11.62).

Tumors of Uncertain Origin. Granular cell tumors are infrequent in birds and are seen primarily in psittacine birds, particularly Amazon parrots. They are small, smooth nodules comprised of pleomorphic cells with abundant pale eosinophilic cytoplasm containing distinct granules (Fig. 11.63). The granules are periodic acid-Schiff positive and, in one bird, were histochemically positive for muscle actin. Although they are morphologically distinct, the cells may not have a distinct histogenesis.

NONNEOPLASTIC PROLIFERATIVE LESIONS

Xanthomatosis is a condition of uncertain etiology. Xanthomas are seen most commonly in cockatiels and budgerigars and usually present on the wing as a variably

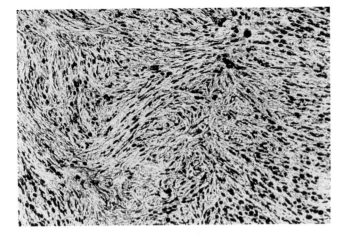

11.62. Malignant melanoma comprised of primarily fusiform cells.

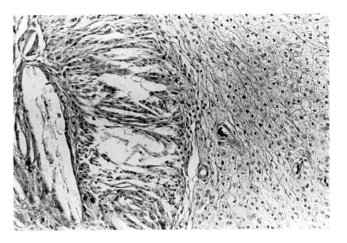

11.65. Large macrophages with abundant foamy cytoplasm and cholesterol cleft formation typical of avian dermal and subcutaneous xanthoma.

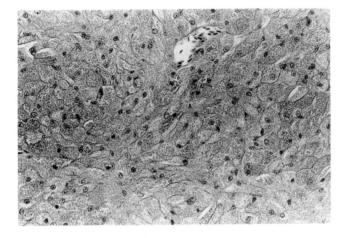

11.63. Granular cell tumor with distinct granules seen on periodic acid-Schiff-stained section.

plasmic material is lipid, and there may also be free lipid and cholesterol cleft formation (Fig. 11.65). There can be variable inflammation and necrosis, with infiltration of heterophils and lymphocytes as well as giant cell formation. Superficial ulceration may occur.

ADDITIONAL READING

Andre JP, Delverdier M, Cabanie D, Bartel G. 1993. Malignant melanoma in an African grey parrot. J Am Vet Med Assoc 7:83–85.

Brush AH. 1993. The origin of feathers: A novel approach. In: Farner DS, King AS, Parkes KC, eds. Avian biology, vol 9. New York: Academic Press, pp 121–162.

Ferrer L, Ramis A, Fernandes J, Majo N. 1997. Granulomatous dermatitis caused by a *Mycobacterium genavense* in 2 psittacine birds. Vet Dermatol 8:213–219.

Garcia A, Latimer KS, Niagro FD, et al. 1993. Avian polyomavirus infection in three black-bellied seed crackers (*Pyrenestes ostrinus*). J Am Vet Med Assoc 7:79–82

Graham DL. 1985. The avian integument. In: Proceedings of the American Veterinary Medical Association, Boulder, CO, pp 33–52.

Hadley NF. 1991. Integumental lipids of plants and animals: Comparative function and biochemistry. Adv Lipid Res 24:303–320.

Jacobson ER, Mladinich CR, Clubb S, et al. 1983. A papilloma-like virus infection in an African grey parrot. J Am Vet Med Assoc 183:1307–1308.

Latimer KS, Niagro FD, Rakich PM, et al. 1992. Comparison of DNA dot-blot hybridization immunoperoxidase staining and routine histopathology in the diagnosis of psittacine beak and feather disease in paraffin-embedded cutaneous tissues. J Am Vet Med Assoc 6:165–168.

Latimer KS. 1994. Oncology. In: Ritchie BW, Harrison GJ, Harrison LR, eds. Avian medicine: Principles and application. Lake Worth, FL: Wingers, pp 640–672.

McDonald SE, Lowenstine LJ, Ardans AA. 1981 Avian pox in blue-fronted Amazon parrots. J Am Vet Med Assoc 179:1218–1222.

Pass DA. 1989. Pathology of the avian integument: A review. Avian Pathol 18:1–72.

Patnaik AK. 1993. Histologic and immunohistochemical studies of granular cell tumors in 7 dogs, 3 cats, one horse and one bird. Vet Pathol 30:176–185.

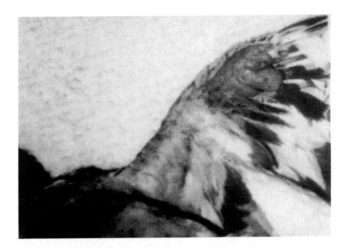

11.64. Typical nodular appearance of xanthoma.

sized, yellow mass (Fig. 11.64). The lesion is often extensive and often bothers the bird, causing it to self-mutilate, resulting in a further increase in lesion size.

Xanthomas are comprised of numerous large macrophages with abundant foamy cytoplasm. The cyto-

Pizarro M, Villegas P, Rodriques A, Rowland GN. 1994. Filariasis (*Pelecitus* sp.) in the cervical subcutaneous tissue of a pigeon with trichomoniasis. Avian Dis 38:385–389.

Pye GW, Carpenter JW, Goggin JM, Bacmeister C. 1999. Metastatic squamous cell carcinoma in a salmon-crested cockatoo (*Cacatua moluccensis*). J Avian Med Surg 13:192–200.

Quist CF, Latimer KS, Goldade SL, et al. 1999. Granular cell tumor in an endangered Puerto Rican Amazon parrot (*Amazon vittata*). Avian Pathol 28:345–348.

Raidal SR. 1995. Viral skin diseases of birds. Semin Avian Exotic Pet Med 4:77–82.

Raidal SR, Riddoch PA. 1997. A feather disease in Senegal doves (*Streptopelia senegalensis*) morphologically similar to psittacine beak and feather disease. Avian Pathol 26:829–836.

Ramis A, Latimer KS, Niagro FD, et al. 1994. Diagnosis of psittacine beak and feather disease (PBFD) viral infection, avian polyomavirus infection, adenovirus infection and herpesvirus infection in psittacine tissues using DNA in-situ hybridization. Avian Pathol 23:643–657.

Ramis A, Latimer KS, Gilbert X, Campagnoli R. 1998. A concurrent outbreak of psittacine beak and feather disease virus and avian polyomavirus infection in budgerigars (*Melopsittacus undulatus*). Avian Pathol 27:43–50.

Rece RL. 1992. Observations on naturally occurring neoplasms in birds in the state of Victoria, Australia. Avian Pathol 21:3–32.

Ritchie BW, Niagro FD, Lukert PD, et al. 1989. A review of psittacine beak and feather disease. J Am Vet Med Assoc 3:143–150.

Schmidt RE. 1992. Morphologic diagnosis of avian neoplasms. Semin Avian Exotic Pet Med 1:73–79.

Schmidt RE. 1996. Pathologic aspects of the skin and feathers. In: Rosskopf WJ Jr, Woerpel RW, eds. Diseases of cage and aviary birds, 3rd edition. Baltimore: Williams and Wilkins, pp 387–396.

Spearman RFC, Hardy J. 1989. Integument. In: King AS, McLelland J, eds. Form and function in birds, vol 3. New York: Academic Press, pp 1–52.

Tell LA, Woods LW, Mathews KG. 1997. Basal-cell carcinoma in a blue-fronted Amazon parrot (*Amazona aestiva*). Avian Dis 41:755–759.

Trinkaus K, Wenisch S, Leiser R, et al. 1998. Psittacine beak and feather disease infected cells show a pattern of apoptosis in psittacine skin. Avian Pathol 27:551–561.

Tsai SS, Chang SF, Chi YC, et al. 1997. Unusual lesions associated with avian poxvirus infection in rosy-faced lovebirds (*Agapornis roseicollis*). Avian Pathol 26:75–82.

Wheeldon DB, Culbertson MR Jr. 1982. Feather folliculoma in the canary (*Serinus canarius*). Vet Pathol 19:204–206.

Woods LW, Latimer KS. 2000. Circovirus infection of nonpsittacine birds. J Avian Med Surg 14:154–163.

12 Special Sense Organs

EYE

Normal Structure

Relative to most other animals, birds have large eyes. They are recessed in the skull and fill most of the space in the rostral skull. The shape of the eye varies significantly between species but in most companion birds is spherical with an anterior to posterior flattening. The eye is surrounded dorsally, rostrally, ventrally, and medially to some extent by the infraorbital sinus. Two muscular eyelids and the third eyelid cover the eye. The lower eyelid contains a fibroelastic tarsal plate. There are no meibomian glands. A harderian gland is present at the base of the third eyelid. The eyelash-like filoplumes of the upper lids are modified feathers. Avian eyelids close mostly in sleep, as the nictitating membrane is responsible for blinking. Two striated muscles move the nictitating membrane, which in diurnal birds is usually transparent.

The lacrimal apparatus includes a gland of the nictitating membrane (harderian gland) that is a compound tubular or tubuloalveolar gland located on the ventromedial surface of the eye. It contains plasma cells derived from the bursa of Fabricius that produce specific antibodies to local antigenic stimulation. The lacrimal gland, which is smaller than the harderian, is located in the area of the caudal or lateral temporal commissure and is attached to the orbital ring. Secretions drain via lacrimal ostia of upper and lower eyelids to a lacrimal canaliculus and finally to a nasolacrimal duct that extends to the nasal cavity.

The cornea and sclera comprise the fibrous tunic of the eye. The cornea is composed of an outer stratified squamous epithelial layer, and a thick inner lamina propria comprised of collagen fibers. Both Bowman's and Descent's membranes are present in some birds, but in others the anterior limiting membrane is not differentiated. At the junction of the anterior and posterior chambers, the sclera is reinforced by ring of overlapping bones called the scleral ossicles. Their number varies from 10 to 18 depending on species. The sclera surrounding the posterior chamber is thick and has two layers: a cartilage layer and a thick fibrous layer. In some species, the scleral cartilage around the optic nerve is ossified.

The vascular tunic is comprised of the choroid, ciliary body, and iris. The choroid is very vascular and pigmented. A tapetum lucidum is seen in only a few nocturnal birds. The choroid continues as the ciliary body and iris. The lens is suspended by the zonular fibers of the ciliary body. Small folds—ciliary processes—produce the aqueous humor and are pressed against the rim of the lens by the ciliary muscles. In birds, these muscles are striated rather than smooth.

The avian lens is softer than the mammalian lens, having a fluid-filled lens vesicle between the annular pad and body of the lens. The anterior surface of the lens is flatter in diurnal species than in nocturnal and aquatic birds. In diurnal birds, the cornea and lens are clear and will transmit wavelengths of light to about 350 nm, making near-ultraviolet radiation visible.

The neural tunic (retina) is relatively thick and, unlike in mammals, does not contain blood vessels. As in mammals, it is comprised of inner optic fiber layer, the ganglion cell layer, the inner plexiform layer, the bipolar (inner nuclear) layer, the outer plexiform layer, the neuroepithelial layer (outer nuclear and rod and cone layers), and the pigment epithelium. Visual cells of the avian retina include rods that lack oil droplets, cones, and double cones. Avian cones contain oil droplets that may be red, yellow, yellow-green, or multiple colors. Oil droplets are comprised of one or more stable carotenoid pigments. There are thin chief cones and short, broad accessory cones. Oil droplets are consistently found in the chief cone but are not present in the accessory cones of all species. Diurnal birds have far more cones than rods, and the rods are confined to the periphery of the retina. The retina of nocturnal birds contains mostly rods. The central portion of the retina may have a fovea whose depth may increase visual acuity. Some birds have patches where the retina is thickened by densely packed cells (foveas). These areas are thought to be locations of improved visual acuity. Birds that pursue moving prey or feed in flight have both central and temporal areas.

The pecten, which projects from the retina into the vitreous at the exit of the optic nerve, is markedly vascular and may be active in nutrition of inner retinal layers. Its size and morphology vary by species. Conical pectens are seen only in the kiwi; vaned pectens are found in rheas, ostriches, and tinamous; and pleated pecten are present in most other birds.

Three striated muscles control the eyelids: the levator of upper eyelid (third cranial nerve), depressor of lower lid (fifth cranial nerve), and sphincter muscles that encircle the lids. Extraocular muscles in birds include the dorsal and ventral oblique, and dorsal, medial, ventral, and lateral rectus. Eye movements are independent (unlike in mammals).

Disease of the Eye and Adnexa

Developmental anomalies include cryptophthalmos (continuous skin over the globe with no evidence of lid formation) and agenesis of eyelids, symblepharon, improperly draining nasolacrimal ducts, and corneal dermoids. Microphalmia is probably the most commonly reported anomaly, with a small globe being obvious grossly.

There may be anomalies of all segments of the eye, associated with disturbances of optic vesicle involution or embryonic fissure closure. Congenital cataracts are infrequent, and their underlying cause is not known. Retinal dysplasia results as a nonspecific altered response of the retina at certain stages of development. There are variable histologic changes and different etiologies. Coloboma is a focal absence of ocular tissue that can occur anywhere in the eye. Colobomas are secondary to defective differentiation of mesenchyme leading to problems in the choroid and iris.

Ocular Adnexa. Blepharitis is often an extension of periocular dermatitis due to a variety of causes. Viruses that may affect the eyelids include poxvirus, psittacine beak and feather disease virus (PBFDV), polyomavirus, and papillomavirus. Acute changes in poxvirus infection include mild inflammation and edema with a serous ocular discharge. With chronicity, there is ulceration of the lids and a proliferative mass may form (Fig. 12.1). The exudate may become purulent due to secondary bacterial infection. Histologic lesions are typical and are described in chapter 11.

Chemosis is a characteristic feature of poxvirus infections of canaries. PBFDV infection can lead to acute lesions in the periorbital skin that may be difficult to differentiate from poxvirus infection grossly. Histologic lesions are consistent with those previously described (chapter 11). Polyomavirus can cause blepharitis as part of generalized infection in budgerigars. Intranuclear inclusion bodies are seen. Papillomas, which are reported to be caused by a papillomavirus, are in rare instances found on the skin of the face and eyelids of African grey parrots (chapter 11).

Bacterial infection can be primary in the eyelid or secondary to dermatitis of the periorbital skin. Gross changes are variable, from reddening and swelling to ulceration. Histologic examination may be necessary to rule out underlying poxvirus infection.

Knemidokoptes sp. infections present as crusts and/or scales and commonly involve the periorbital skin. Histologically mites can be found in the chronic inflammatory response.

Fungi can cause nonspecific inflammation just as in any other location. Organisms are usually found on histologic examination. Deep lesions have been associated with *Cryptococcus* infection (Fig. 12.2).

Noninfectious Disease. Vitamin A deficiency may cause periorbital epidermal hyperplasia and hyperkeratosis, with secondary infections possible. Histologically the lesion is characterized by marked proliferation of keratin without an inflammatory response.

Neoplastic lesions of the eyelids potentially include all of the tumors reported in the skin of birds (chapter 11). Xanthomas are also seen in the eyelids, including the third eyelid (Fig. 12.3).

Lacrimal Glands. Lacrimal glands may become infected with bacteria, leading to swelling and abscess formation. The swelling must be differentiated from possible gland or

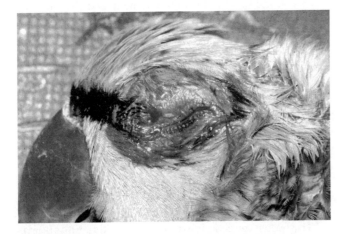

12.1. *Marked swelling and reddening of eyelids due to poxvirus infection.*

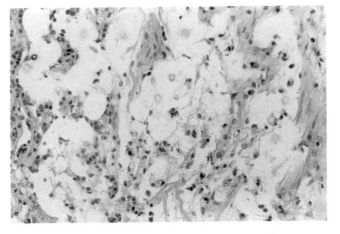

12.2. *Mycotic blepharitis due to Cryptococcus sp. Organisms with large mucinous capsules are present.*

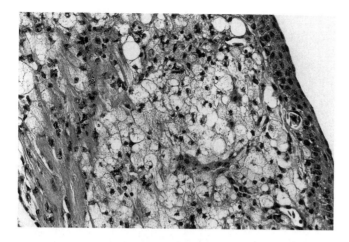

12.3. *Xanthoma of the eyelid. The mass is comprised of numerous large cells with foamy, granular cytoplasm.*

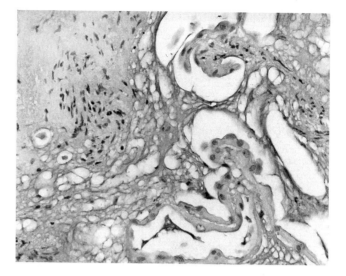

12.5. *Minimally infiltrative tubules and foci of necrosis in lacrimal gland carcinoma.*

periorbital neoplasia. Grossly the lesion is fluctuant, and purulent material may be expressed. Histologically, variable necrosis is seen associated with a pleocellular inflammatory infiltrate. Organisms must be found for etiologic specificity.

Lacrimal gland neoplasia is seen infrequently in birds. Based on our experience, carcinoma appears to occur the most commonly based. The tumors present as firm gray-white masses. Histologically there are acini, trabeculae, and tubular structures lined by moderately undifferentiated epithelial cells. There can be variable necrosis and inflammation (Fig. 12.4 and Fig. 12.5).

Conjunctiva. Lesions of the conjunctiva may be primary or associated with diseases of the lids and periorbital skin. They can involve palpebral or bulbar conjunctive or the nictitating membrane. Secondary lesions are most commonly associated with sinusitis and therefore may be due to a variety of infectious agents including viruses, bacteria, chlamydia, and mycoplasma. In some cases, conjunctival lesions may indicate a generalized infection or septicemia.

Primary disease may be infectious or noninfectious. Infectious disease may have similar gross signs, including reddening and ocular discharge, regardless of cause. Poxvirus infection causes lesions that are similar to those of the eyelids. The finding of intracytoplasmic inclusion bodies in proliferative conjunctival epithelial cells is diagnostic.

A cytomegalovirus is the cause of conjunctivitis in Gouldian finches. Grossly the conjunctiva is swollen due to edema and congestion. There is a serous exudate in the conjunctival sac.

Histologically, conjunctival epithelial cells are hypertrophied, hyperplastic, and variably necrotic. Karyomegalic nuclei contain basophilic inclusion bodies. A submucosal infiltrate consisting primarily of lymphocytes and plasma cells is seen. The lesions are usually associated with systemic disease.

Adenoviral conjunctivitis is occasionally seen as a part of generalized disease. Lesions are nonspecific unless intranuclear inclusions consistent with adenovirus are found. Conjunctivitis can also be caused by paramyxovirus 2. Inclusion bodies are not seen, and the lesions are nonspecific, with variable necrosis and a lymphoplasmacytic inflammatory infiltrate noted.

Bacterial conjunctivitis has been associated with a variety of organisms. Affected conjunctival surfaces are variably proliferative and reddened. In chronic cases, multifocal to confluent yellow-white foci are seen. Necrosis and a pleocellular infiltrate with numerous heterophils are histologic characteristics of acute inflammation. With chronicity, granulomatous foci containing macrophages and giant cells are seen associated with fibrin deposition, necrotic debris, and proliferation of the mucosa (Fig. 12.6). Organisms must be found to characterize the lesion definitively.

Mycobacterial infection leads to proliferative lesions that have necrotic centers surrounded by giant cells, macrophages, and heterophils. Mineralization may be

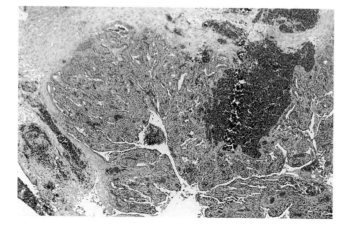

12.4. *Lacrimal gland carcinoma comprised of numerous trabecular and tubular structures.*

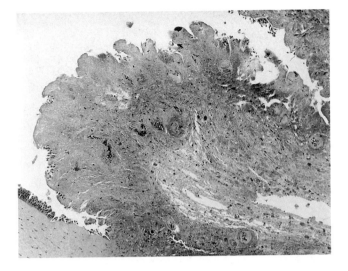

12.6. *Conjunctival necrosis and inflammation due to bacterial infection.*

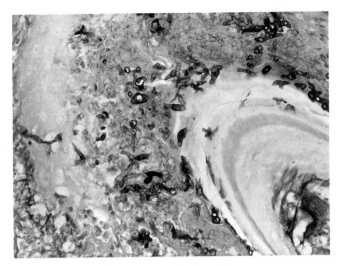

12.7. *Mycotic conjunctivitis with hyphal fragments in necrotic debris.*

present. Acid-fast bacteria are seen in giant cells and macrophages. The lesions are usually part of a systemic disease process.

Conjunctivitis is a fairly common feature of *Chlamydiophila psittaci* and *Mycoplasma* sp. infections in birds. *Chlamydiophila psittaci* causes conjunctival reddening with a serous or purulent exudate. Histologically there is necrosis associated with a lymphohistiocytic infiltrate. Unless organisms are found, a definitive diagnosis cannot be made based on the conjunctival lesion. Conjunctivitis may be the only clinical sign of *C. psittaci* infection in cockatiels.

Mycoplasmosis is seen occasionally in individual companion birds, and we have seen it flocks of commercial budgerigars. It is also suspected to be one of the causes of the chronic conjunctivitis seen in cockatiels, but this remains to be proven. *Mycoplasma gallisepticum* is widespread in wild house finches in North America. Several other species of native American birds are also reported to be susceptible to this organism. These house finches are potential sources of *M. gallisepticum* for companion birds housed outdoors. Affected birds have swollen conjunctival membranes and a serous to mucopurulent discharge. Histologically there is a chronic lymphoplasmacytic inflammatory infiltrate. Variable epithelial hyperplasia is noted. Similar lesions are often seen in the upper respiratory tract.

Fungi causing conjunctivitis include *Aspergillus* sp., *Candida* sp., and *Cryptococcus neoformans*. Gross lesions are similar to those of bacterial infections, and histologic changes include necrosis, pleocellular inflammation including giant cells, and the presence of intralesional organisms (Fig. 12.7).

Cryptosporidial conjunctivitis is occasionally seen. It may indicate an underlying immunosuppression and systemic disease. Gross changes are minimal and nonspecific. Histologically there is epithelial hyperplasia and a

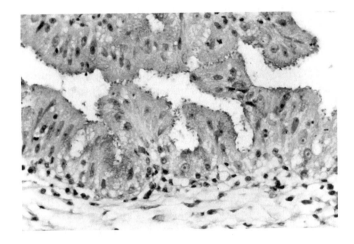

12.8. *Proliferative conjunctival epithelial cells with cryptosporidial organisms adhering to their surface.*

mild lymphoplasmacytic infiltrate. Organisms are found on the surface of epithelial cells (Fig. 12.8).

Nematodes that can cause conjunctivitis include *Oxyspirura mansoni*, which irritates the conjunctiva and may enter the lacrimal ducts, and *Thelazia* sp., which can be found in the conjunctival sac of birds with mild inflammatory changes. *Oxyspirura* has an indirect life cycle with cockroaches as intermediate hosts. Larvae travel from the crop to the esophagus and eventually up the nasolacrimal duct. Both of these parasites would be expected to be found only in wild-caught birds and are relatively rare findings.

Philophthamus gralli is a trematode that is the cause of severe chronic conjunctivitis, primarily in waterfowl. Gross lesions include swelling and reddening of the conjunctiva. Generally, multiple flukes are present, and they are large enough to be seen with the unaided eye (Fig. 12.9). A chronic inflammatory reaction with numerous macrophages, lymphocytes, and plasma cells is present

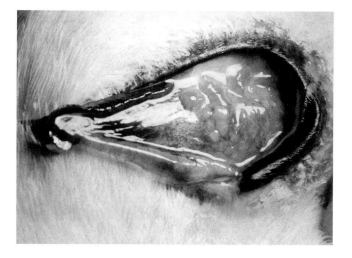

12.9. Numerous conjunctival swellings due to infection by Philophthalmus gralli.

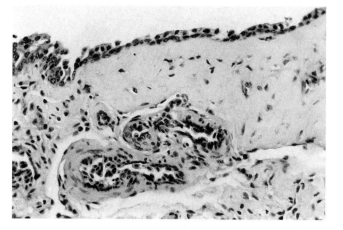

12.11. Conjunctival thickening due to diffuse amyloid deposition.

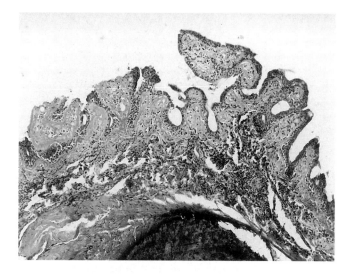

12.10. Conjunctivitis due to Philophthalmus gralli. Organisms are not seen, but there is marked proliferation and chronic inflammation.

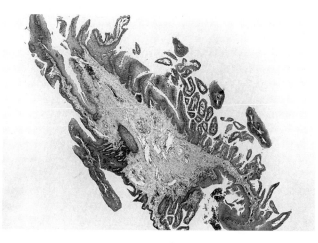

12.12. Conjunctival papilloma. The cause of these lesions has not been determined.

histologically. The conjunctival epithelium may be proliferative (Fig. 12.10).

Noninfectious causes of conjunctivitis include foreign bodies, which lead to reddening and discharge, which is generalized or localized. The latter may present as a focal swelling due to a granulomatous reaction. Physical irritants such as smoke aerosols or chemical fumes can cause nonspecific conjunctival inflammation. Vitamin A deficiency can result in metaplasia and hyperkeratosis of conjunctival epithelium. Advanced causes of vitamin A deficiency will result in the accumulation of large semicircular plaques of sloughed squamous cells in the ventral conjunctival recesses. Amyloid deposition is sometimes seen associated with systemic amyloid deposition (Fig. 12.11).

Proliferative lesions include conjunctival papillomas (Fig. 12.12) and tumors such as squamous cell carcinoma

and melanoma (Fig. 12.13). The papillomas are similar to those of the skin, and the possibility of a viral etiology has been considered but not proved.

Cornea. Keratitis will present grossly as corneal opacity, with possible reddening if there is vascularization. In severe cases, there may be ulceration. It can be associated with a variety of causes.

Infectious keratitis can be due to any of the agents described as causes of conjunctivitis. In birds, bacterial infection (Figs. 12.14 and 12.15) and mycotic infection are the most common. Gross changes are similar, but there may be yellow-white or greenish, fluffy exudate in mycotic infections (Fig. 12.16).

Histologically the lesion is comprised of a pleocellular infiltrate with varying proportions of heterophils, macrophages, lymphocytes, and giant cells, depending on the exact organism and duration. Finding organisms in the lesion gives specificity (Figs. 12.17 and 12.18).

Microsporidial keratitis is occasionally seen in psittacine birds. Gross changes include conjunctival reddening and corneal opacity. Histologically there is

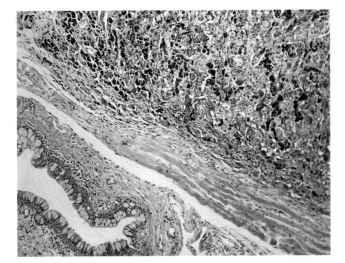

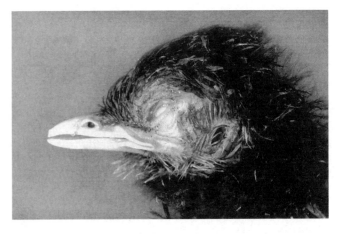

12.16.   Proliferative yellow exudate seen in mycotic conjunctivitis.

12.13.   Malignant melanoma infiltrating a portion of the conjunctiva.

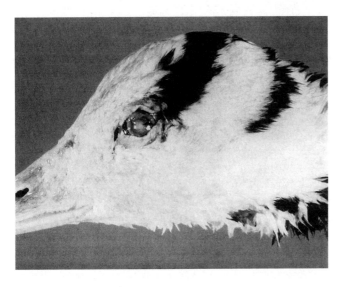

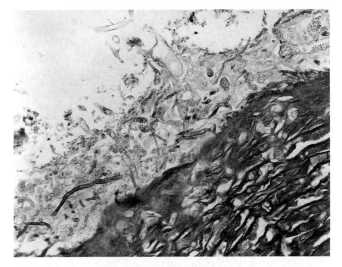

12.14.   Chronic bacterial keratitis leading to corneal opacity.

12.17.   Mycelial fragments present in mycotic keratitis. The exact organism cannot be determined histologically.

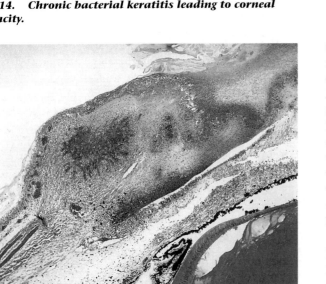

12.15.   Severe necrotic keratitis due to bacterial infection.

stromal infiltration by heterophils, lymphocytes, and macrophages associated with stromal necrosis. Protozoal organisms are found in the lesion (Fig. 12.19). *Microsporidia* stain best with Gram stains and trichrome stains. These birds may have a history of a chronic non-healing conjunctivitis that is refractory to traditional antimicrobial treatment. Organisms are more common on the cornea than they are in the adjacent conjunctiva, which will also be inflamed. Conjunctival smears stained with calcofluor MR2 and viewed with ultraviolet light is the most specific way to identify these organisms in live birds.

Noninfectious keratitis is usually secondary to trauma; however, unless there is foreign material found in the lesion, the cause is usually inferred due to a lack of any infectious agent. Chronic keratitis results in corneal epithelial hyperplasia and stromal hypercellularity (Fig. 12.20).

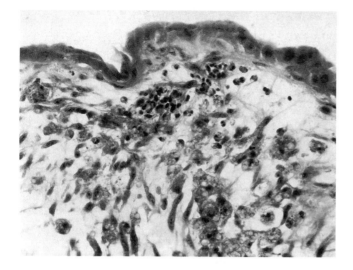

12.18. Deep mycotic keratitis. Numerous macrophages contain organisms morphologically consistent with Histoplasma sp.

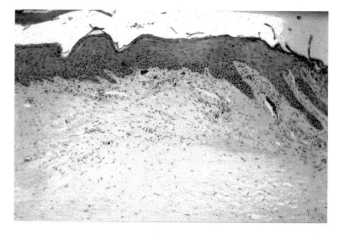

12.20. Chronic keratitis with marked epithelial hyperplasia and stromal fibroplasia.

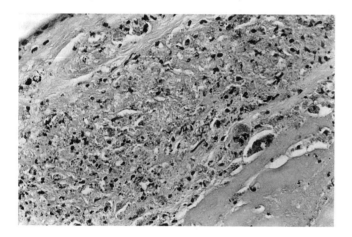

12.19. Necrosis and an infiltrate of macrophages in microsporidial keratitis. The small dark foci within many of the macrophages are organisms.

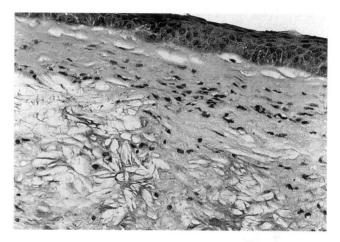

12.21. Corneal stromal degeneration with the formation of numerous cholesterol clefts.

Noninflammatory corneal lesions are infrequently seen. Stromal dystrophy would imply a primary inherited condition and is not documented in pet birds. Stromal degeneration secondary to previous inflammation is seen in a variety of pet species. Grossly there is corneal opacity, and histologically stromal inflammation associated with lipid deposition and cholesterol cleft formation are noted (Fig. 12.21).

Lens. Lens luxation may be secondary to trauma or inflammation leading to zonule lysis. Careful gross sectioning of the eye is necessary to be sure that the lens was not displaced artifactually.

Cataracts may be congenital or acquired. They are hereditary in some canaries (Yorkshire and Norwich). The condition appears to be caused by an autosomal recessive gene. Acquired cataracts have been associated with nutri-

tional deficiencies, trauma, toxins, infection and inflammation of the eye, and aging. Many older psittacine birds will have cataracts, and falcons appear to have a higher incidence than many other birds. Cataracts are opacities of the lens secondary to altered lens metabolism usually following some injury to lens epithelium and/or capsule (epithelial basement membrane). Cataracts can be classified according to age of onset or location within the lens. Morphologically the usual structure of the capsule and lens fibers is altered.

Grossly, cataracts present as lens opacities. Histologically, early changes may be limited to swelling of lens fibers with bladder cell formation. There may be epithelial hyperplasia and foci of capsular thinning. With progression, cystoid spaces can develop and lens protein will coagulate and fibers fragment (Figs. 12.22 and 12.23). The epithelium will become necrotic, and the capsule may rupture. Occasionally mineralized foci are noted. In some cases, the lens liquefies and lens fibers fragment (Fig.

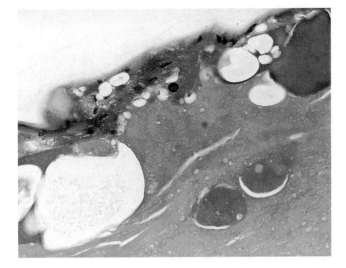

12.22. Early cataract formation. The capsule is irregular, and there is cystoid degeneration.

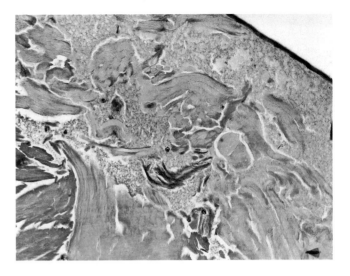

12.24. Morgagnian cataract with severe lens fragmentation and partial liquefaction.

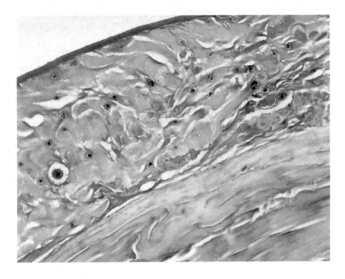

12.23. Bladder cell formation and lens fiber fragmentation in a cataract.

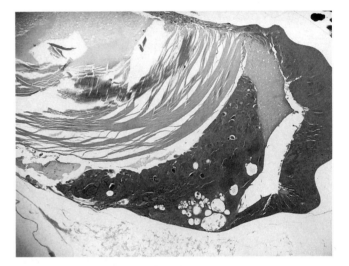

12.25. Hypermature cataract. A shrunken lens with a wrinkled capsule is noted.

12.24). Mature cataracts involve the entire lens. Hypermature cataracts develop when necrotic cortical material is lost, leading to a small lens with a wrinkled capsule. Fragments of lens material may be seen (Fig. 12.25).

Uveal Tract (Iris, Ciliary Body, and Choroid). Uveitis may be anterior, posterior, or diffuse, involving the entire uveal tract. Suppurative uveitis may be secondary to penetrating trauma, extension from the corneal or sclera, or the result of localization of systemic infections. Grossly there may be fibrin clots in the anterior chamber, hemorrhage, hypopyon, and hyphema.

Histologic lesions depend on the exact cause and location but will include fibrin deposition and a reaction that is primarily heterophilic initially. Eventually there may be typical granuloma formation. Nonsuppurative uveitis due to an immune-mediated reaction may occur in birds but is rarely seen.

Synechia is adherence of the iris to either the cornea (anterior) or the lens (posterior). It is a sequela to an inflammatory lesion in the anterior chamber. Histologically there will often be histologic evidence of the underlying cause.

Retina. Retinitis may be caused by a variety of infectious agents, be secondary to trauma, or be associated with diseases of the central nervous system. Gross lesions are usually not seen unless severe. Viral disease can lead to a nonsuppurative inflammatory infiltrate, but this is infrequent, possibly due to the avascularity of the retina. Bacterial infections that involve the retina result in inflammation that is primarily heterophilic. Specificity is associated with demonstration of specific etiologic agents (Fig. 12.26).

Retinal degeneration is potentially due to a variety of causes (toxins, nutrition, and hypoxia), but no specific

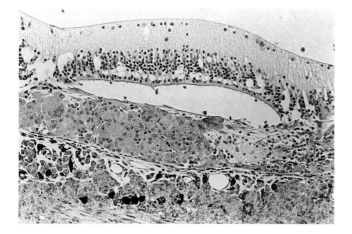

12.26. Chorioretinitis due to Mycobacterium *sp.* infection. Numerous large macrophages are infiltrating the tissues, leading to a partial retinal detachment.

conditions are reported in birds. In many cases, areas of degeneration are found incidentally on histologic examination of grossly normal eyes. The severity of the lesion may vary, but outer retinal segments seem to be more commonly affected (Figs. 12.27–12.29).

Congenital retinal dysplasia is sporadically reported, and the cause is usually not known.

Retinal detachment can also be secondary to trauma or inflammation of the retina and/or choroid. Depending on the duration of the detachment, there will be variable degeneration. The pigment epithelium is usually reactive, with hypertrophy and individualization of cells. Retinal tears, hemorrhage, and detachment are very common lesions in birds of prey that are struck by vehicles.

Optic Nerve. Lesions of the optic nerve are similar to those seen in the brain and are due to the same causes.

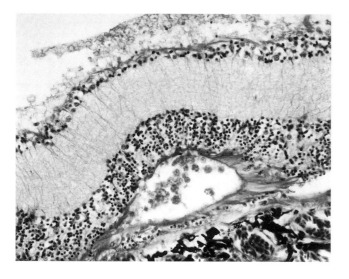

12.27. Focal area of retinal degeneration with loss of photoreceptor outer segments. The cells in the area of detachment may be reactive retinal pigment epithelial cells.

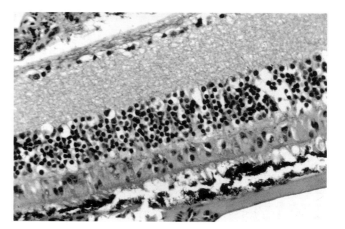

12.28. Retinal degeneration characterized by loss of photoreceptors and detachment.

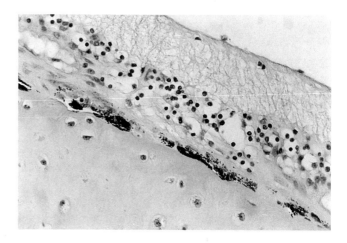

12.29. Severe retinal degeneration. The inner plexiform layer is present, but only scattered unidentified nuclei are seen in the remaining portion of the retina.

Optic neuritis can be seen in cases of proventricular dilatation disease, and birds with this disease may have a history of blindness. A lymphoplasmacytic infiltrate characterizes this lesion. Any cause of nerve fiber degeneration in the brain can also cause degeneration of the optic nerve. Pituitary tumors may cause pressure and secondary optic nerve degeneration at the chiasm. Optic nerve demyelination of unknown cause is seen sporadically (Fig. 12.30).

Eye as a Whole. Panophthalmitis may result from trauma or a variety of infectious agents as listed for the various segments of the eye. It represents spread of the infection and/or inflammatory process throughout the eye. A sequela of chronic panophthalmitis is phthisis bulbi. Affected eyes are shrunken, and histologically there is evidence of chronic inflammation, fibroplasia, and loss of normal components of the globe (Fig. 12.31).

Glaucoma. Glaucoma is occasionally reported in birds. It is usually secondary to trauma, but primary glaucoma is infrequently suspected. Grossly the affected eye is

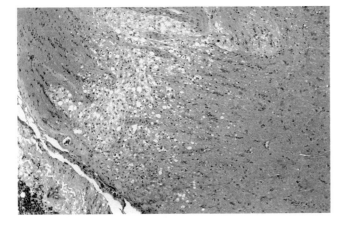

12.30. Focal demyelination of unknown cause affecting the optic nerve.

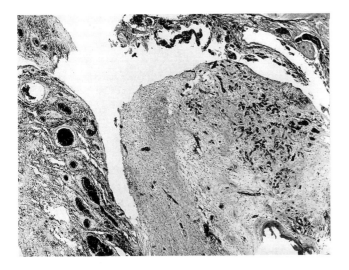

12.31. Unrecognizable mass of inflamed fibrous tissue and neovascularization consistent with phthisis bulbi.

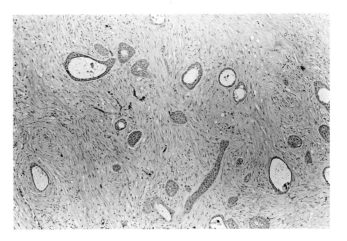

12.32. Infiltrative orbital squamous cell carcinoma. The centers of many of the nests and trabeculae are necrotic.

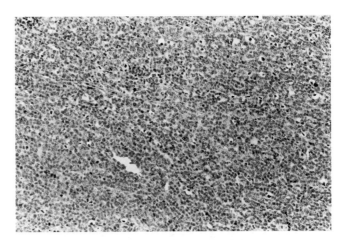

12.33. Lymphosarcoma obliterating the eye and orbit.

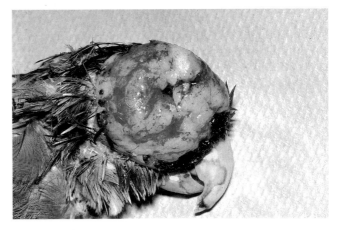

12.34. Typical appearance of lymphosarcoma.

enlarged. The lens may be luxated. Grossly and histologically there may be changes indicative of the underlying cause.

Ocular Neoplastic Disease. Tumors of skin and subcutis affecting the eyelids have been previously mentioned. Squamous papilloma, squamous cell carcinoma, malignant melanoma, and basal cell tumors are seen.

Adnexal tumors include adenomas and adenocarcinomas of the lacrimal gland and were previously described. Orbital neoplasia includes chondroma, infiltrative carcinoma (Fig. 12.32), lymphosarcoma (Figs. 12.33 and 12.34), and teratoma (Fig. 12.35). The gross appearance is of an orbital mass that displaces the eye. Histologically they are similar to the tumor type in any other location.

Intraocular malignant melanoma can arise in the uveal tract. These tumors may or may not be grossly pigmented and histologically are comprised of poorly differentiated cells that form an infiltrative sheet (Fig. 12.36).

Primary intraocular tumors are rarely reported in birds. Medulloepithelioma, an embryonic tumor of the central nervous system and retina, is reported in cockatiels. This tumor usually presents as an undiagnosed gray-white and somewhat friable intraocular mass. The tumor extends

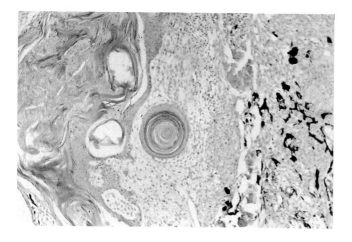

12.35. *Orbital teratoma with several tissue types present.*

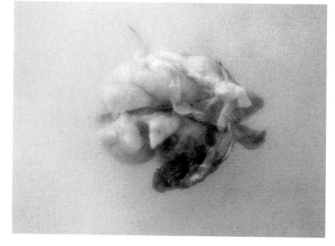

12.37. *Destruction of the cranial portion of the brain due to infiltration by medulloepithelioma.*

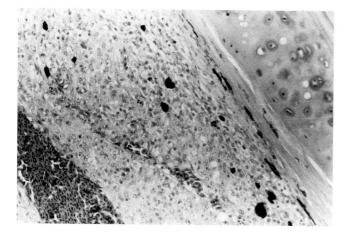

12.36. *Malignant melanoma diffusely infiltrating the choroid.*

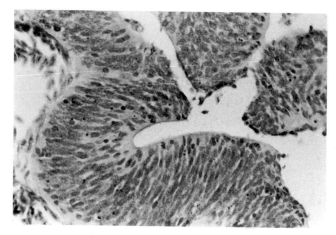

12.38. *Medulloepithelioma. Bands of poorly differentiated columnar epithelium resemble embryonic retina.*

through the orbit and impinges on the brain (Fig. 12.37). Histologically the tumor is comprised of tubular structures lined by tall neuroepithelial cells. Structures resembling rosettes are also seen. Less well differentiated areas are comprised of nests and sheets of neoplastic cells (Figs. 12.38 and 12.39).

Orbital Disease. Inflammation or neoplasia in the orbit can impact the eye even if the fibrous tunic is not penetrated. Trauma and localization of systemic disease can lead to retrobulbar abscess formation (Fig. 12.40).

EAR

Normal Structure

The avian external ear has a short canal extending vertically and caudally from the external acoustic meatus to the tympanic membrane. The external meatus is small, usually circular, and opens on the side of the head. In most birds, it is usually covered by specialized contour feathers called ear coverts that reduce drag caused by tur-

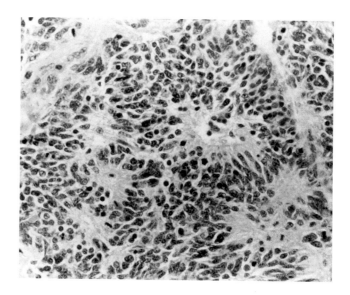

12.39. *A portion of medulloepithelioma with rosette formation.*

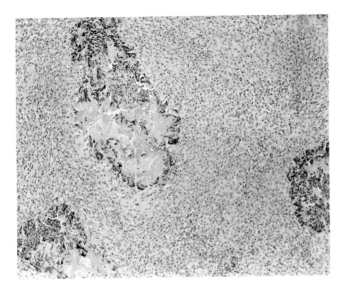

12.40.   Retrobulbar abscess with multifocal areas of necrosis surrounded by giant cells and numerous macrophages.

bulence and diminishes the masking of sound by noise from turbulence in the external ear.

The external surface of the tympanic membrane is covered by epidermis continuous with the external auditory meatus. The internal surface is covered by epithelium continuous with the tympanic cavity and pharyngotympanic tube. The tympanic membrane projects outward in birds rather than inward as in mammals.

The middle ear is the air-filled cavity between the tympanic membrane and the inner ear that transmits acoustically induced vibrations of the tympanic membrane to the vestibular window. It contains a single ossicle called the columella, which is the homologue of the mammalian stapes. The columella extends across the tympanic cavity to form a direct connection between the tympanic membrane and the perilymph of the inner ear. The paratympanic organ, which is within the dorsomedial wall of the tympanic cavity, is not present in owls or psittacine birds. It contains tall cells in contact with nerves from the geniculate ganglion, but its exact sensory function has not been determined.

The inner ear has two major portions and two functions. The bony labyrinth is formed by compact bone and is comprised of the vestibule, semicircular canals, and cochlea. It encloses the membranous labyrinth. Perilymph is present between the bony and membranous labyrinths, and endolymph is present within the cavities of the membranous labyrinth. The membranous labyrinth contains the utricle, saccule, and semicircular ducts concerned with position and movement of the head in space, and the cochlear duct involved in hearing.

Disease

External Ear. Otitis externa is uncommon in birds. Potential causes include bacteria, fungi, and arthropod

parasites. There may be problems associated with extension of skin disease. The gross appearance may be altered by self-trauma. Hemorrhage, necrosis, and exudate are seen (Fig. 12.41). A definitive etiologic diagnosis depends on finding an organism on histologic examination.

Carcinoma of the glands of the external ear canal is occasionally seen. It may present as a chronic condition with thickening of the ear canal, as well as a localized mass lesion (Fig. 12.42). Microscopically these tumors are comprised of moderately undifferentiated to poorly differentiated cells that form infiltrative nests and cords. There may be moderate amounts of fibrous stroma (Fig. 12.43). These tumors must be differentiated from carcinoma of nasal or sinus origin.

Middle Ear. Otitis media is rarely reported. A variety of infections are possible, and it may be secondary to

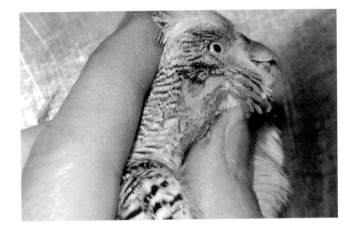

12.41.   Otitis externa. There is loss and discoloration of feathers and exudate on the skin surrounding the ear opening.

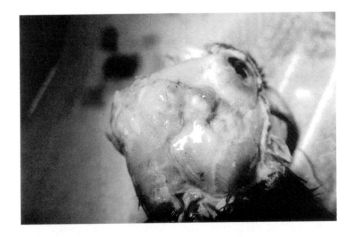

12.42.   Carcinoma of the glands of the external ear canal. An irregular lobular mass with destruction of surrounding tissue is seen.

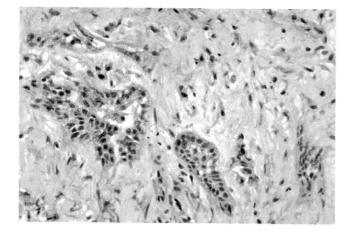

12.43. *Histologic appearance of infiltrative ear canal carcinoma. Abundant stroma is seen.*

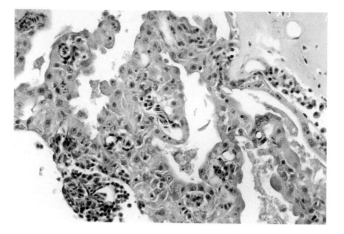

12.45. *Swelling, necrosis, and distortion of hair cells of the crista basilaris due to paramyxovirus infection.*

oral/pharyngeal disease with extension via the pharyngo-tympanic tube.

Inner Ear. Congenital lesions have been reported in Belgian Waterslager canaries. There are often multiple abnormalities associated with dysgenesis of the pars inferior of the otocyst. These include stunting of tall hair cells of the organ of Corti, loss of short hair cells, and narrowing of the tectorial membrane.

Otitis interna can be due to paramyxovirus infection, particularly in Australian grass parakeets (*Neophyma* sp.). Lesions can lead to "twisted neck," "stargazing," and similar syndromes. Inner ear disease can be associated with brain lesions but also may occur in the absence of central nervous system involvement. Gross changes are usually not apparent. Histologically there is nonsuppurative inflammation, loss of normal structures, and intranuclear inclusion bodies within hair cells of the crista basilaris in some cases (Figs. 12.44–12.46).

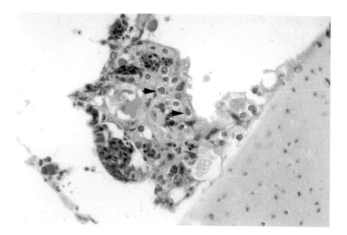

12.46. *Intracytoplasmic inclusion bodies of paramyxovirus in damaged hair cells of the inner ear (arrowheads).*

Poxvirus can also affect the inner ear. There may be ballooning degeneration of epithelial cells and intracytoplasmic inclusion body formation (Fig. 12.47).

Ototoxicity can be a problem in birds treated with aminoglycoside antibiotics. High doses lead to damage to the basilar papilla. At the cellular level, there are changes leading to loss of organelles and to cell necrosis. There is a linear increase in the levels of intracellular calcium and reactive oxygen species associated with the antibiotic dose. After loss of hair cells, macrophages and microglia-like cells infiltrate the sensory epithelium. There may be associated sensory epithelial cell proliferation.

Acoustic trauma can lead to transitory or permanent loss of sensory epithelium. The amount of damage is related to the level of, and duration of, the sound.

OLFACTORY/TASTE ORGANS

Normal Structure

The avian olfactory organ arises as an area of thickened ectoderm on the ventrolateral surfaces of the head. The

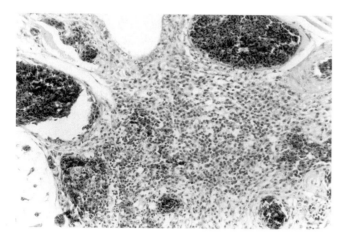

12.44. *Nonsuppurative otitis interna due to paramyxovirus infection. A diffuse cellular infiltrate is seen.*

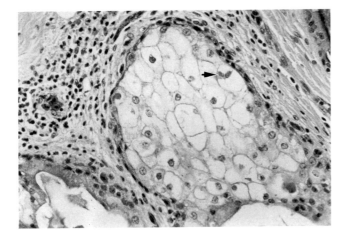

12.47. Poxvirus infection of the inner ear. Sensory epithelial cells are swollen with ballooning degeneration. Cytoplasmic inclusion bodies are small (arrowhead) and not seen in all affected cells.

epithelial lining of the developing nasal passages becomes the olfactory epithelium (bipolar nerve cells). Each cell tapers to an olfactory nerve fiber, which joins others and grows toward the olfactory bulb of the brain. Axons of the receptor cells form the olfactory nerve—cranial nerve I—and terminate in the olfactory bulb. The olfactory receptors are in the nasal mucosa of the caudal nasal concha.

Taste receptors vary by species. Many species have no interest in sweet substances, with nectar feeders and many parrots as exceptions. Most birds will consume salt and have a range of tolerance for acidity and alkalinity. Birds vary in regard to tolerance to bitter substances.

Disease

No specific avian disease syndromes are known that affect smell or taste, but there is no way to measure subjective changes. Lesions of the cranial nerves or brain could affect the senses of smell and taste. Infections, nerve degeneration, and neoplasia are all possible causes. Lesions of nasal or oral cavities may involve olfactory and taste organs.

SOMATOSENSORY RECEPTORS

Normal Structure

These organs give information about the physical condition of the internal and external environment. They respond to mechanical, thermal, or chemical stimuli. Afferent nerves transmit impulses to the central nervous system. Peripheral structures include Herbst corpuscles that are probably mechanoreceptors. They occur in the integument, tendons, muscles, and joint capsules. They have a central area and perineural capsule and are variable in size and shape. Other structures are Grandry corpuscles that occur in ducks and are velocity sensitive, Ruffini

nerve endings that detect amplitude components in mechanical stimuli, muscle spindles and tendon organs, and mechanoreceptors such as the bill-tip organ in parrots and other species, particularly those that use the beak for prehension. This organ is comprised of a dermal core and cornified epidermal covering.

Disease

Nothing specific is known. Any trauma, infectious disease, or tumor that damages one of the aforementioned structures could be the cause of a decrement in function. Inflammation of dermal receptors could cause sensation and lead to feather picking or self-trauma. The gross and histologic appearance depends on the particular disease process involved.

ADDITIONAL READING

Bang BG, Wenzel BM. 1985. Nasal cavity and olfactory system. In: King AS, McLelland J, eds. Form and function in birds, vol 3. New York: Academic Press, pp 195–225.

Brooks DE, Greiner EC. 1983. Conjunctivitis caused by *Thelazia* sp. in a Senegal parrot. J Am Vet Med Assoc 183:1305–1306.

Brooks DE. 1997. Avian cataracts. Semin Avian Exotic Pet Med 6:131–137.

Busch TJ. 1985. Corneal dermoids in a goose. NZ Vet 33:189–190.

Buyukmihci N, Murphy CJ, Schulz T. 1988. Developmental ocular disease of raptors. J Wildl Dis 24:207–213.

Desmidt M, Ducatelle R, Uyttebroeck E, et al. 1991. Cytomegalovirus-like conjunctivitis in Australian finches. J Assoc Av Vet 5:132–136.

Dukes TW, Fox GA. 1983. Blindness associated with retinal dysplasia in a prairie falcon. J Wildl Dis 19:66–69.

Canny CJ, Ward DA, Patton S, Orosz SE. 1999. Microsporidian keratoconjunctivitis in a double yellow-headed Amazon parrot (*Amazona ochrocephala oratrix*). J Avian Med Surg 13:279–286.

Fischer FP. 1994. General patterns and morphological specializations of the avian cochlea. Scanning Microsc 8:351–364.

Gilger BC, McLaughlin SA, Smith P. 1995. Uveal malignant melanoma in a duck. J Am Vet Med Assoc 206:1580–1582.

Graham DL. 1978. Poxvirus infection in a spectacled Amazon parrot (*Amazona albitrons*). Avian Dis 22:340–343.

Hirose K, Westrum LE, Stone JS, et al. 1999. Dynamic studies of ototoxicity in mature avian auditory epithelium. Ann NY Acad Sci 884:389–409.

Kern TJ, Paul-Murphy J, Murphy CJ, et al. 1996. Disorders of the third eyelid in birds: 17 cases. J Avian Med Surg 10:12–18.

Keymer IF. 1977. Cataracts in birds. Avian Pathol 6:335–341.

King AS, McLelland J. 1984. Birds: Their structure and function, 2nd edition. London: Bailliere Tindall, pp 284–314.

Kühne R, Lewis B. 1985. External and middle ears. In: King AS, McLelland J, eds. Form and function in birds, vol 3. New York: Academic Press, pp 227–271.

Leach MA. 1992. Survey of neoplasia in pet birds. Semin Avian Exotic Pet Med 1:52–64.

Luttrell MP, Stallknecht DE, Fischer JR, et al. 1998. Natural *Mycoplasma gallisepticum* infection in a captive flock of house finches. J Wildl Dis 34:289–296.

Pocknell AM, Miller BJ, Neufeld JL, Grahn BH. 1996. Conjunctival mycobacteriosis in 2 emus (*Dromaius novaehollandiae*). Vet Pathol 33:346–348.

Schmidt RE, Toft II JD. 1981. Ophthalmic lesions in animals from a zoologic collection. J Wildl Dis 17:267–275.

Schmidt RE, Hubbard GB. 1987. Special sense organs. In: Atlas of zoo animal pathology, vol 2. Boca Raton, FL: CRC, pp 125–133.

Slatter DH. 1983. Hereditary cataracts in conures. J Am Vet Med Assoc 183:872–874.

Stanz KM, Miller PE, Cooley AJ, et al. 1995. Mycobacterial keratitis in a parrot. J Am Vet Med Assoc 206:1177–1180.

Stillman AJ. 1973. Avian vision. In: Farner OJ, King JR, eds. Avian biology, vol 3. New York: Academic Press, pp 349–383.

Tudor DC, Yard C. 1978. Retinal atrophy in a parakeet. Vet Med Small Anim Clin 73:85.

Weisleder P, Lu Y, Park TJ. 1996. Anatomical basis of a congenital hearing impairment: Basilar papilla dysplasia in the Belgian waterslager canary. J Comp Neurol 369:292–301.

Willis AM, Wilkie DA. 1999. Avian ophthalmology. J Avian Med Surg 13:245–251.

13 Peritoneum and Mesenteries

STRUCTURE

The avian coelomic cavities are more complex than the peritoneal cavities of mammals. The best anatomic descriptions have been of the domestic fowl. In poultry, there are 16 cavities, eight of which are air sacs and eight pleuroperitoneal cavities. The caudal coelom is divided into five chambers or cavities: the intestinal, left and right ventral hepatic, and left and right dorsal hepatic peritoneal cavities. These chambers are separated by double-layered septa consisting of membranes formed by a thin band of fibrovascular stroma supporting a thin mesothelium with resident macrophages. Normally only a small amount of lubricating fluid is present. Passive diffusion of water and solutes of low molecular weight can occur between the peritoneal cavities and the subperitoneal vasculature. The remaining three cavities are present in mammals as well as avian species. They are the pericardium and left and right pleural cavities.

The intestinal peritoneal cavity, which is midline and elongated, encloses the gonads and intestines that are suspended by the mesenteries. The abdominal air sacs also penetrate into this cavity. The cavity is formed by the left and right posthepatic septa. The liver lobes protrude into the left and right ventral hepatic cavities. These are blind cavities along the lateroventral body wall. Nothing is suspended in these cavities. The left and right dorsal hepatic peritoneal cavities are smaller cavities in which project the craniodorsal left and right liver lobes. All these cavities are blind with the exception of the left dorsal hepatic peritoneal cavity that connects with the intestinal peritoneal cavity. The liver is essentially isolated from the rest of the viscera by the posthepatic septum.

Because of the arrangement of the peritoneal partitions, disease conditions may be confined to specific cavities. Inflammation or neoplasms of the reproductive or intestinal tracts tend to remain confined to the intestinal peritoneal cavity. Acute pulmonary distress can occur if fluid accumulating within the intestinal peritoneal cavity gains access to the abdominal air sacs that penetrate into this cavity. Any mass effect that expands the intestinal peritoneal cavity can also result in increased respiratory effort that is clinically described as a "tail bob." Ascitic fluid may accumulate primarily in the ventral hepatic peritoneal cavities secondary to chronic liver disease. The inflammation and contents from ruptures or perforations of the proventriculus or ventriculus may remain confined to the left ventral hepatic peritoneal cavity.

The pericardial cavity is similar to that of mammals although the parietal pericardium is continuous with the peritoneal partitions of the coelom. In mammals, a diaphragm separates these cavities.

The pleural cavity has areas of fibrous strands connecting the parietal pleura to the visceral pleura, obliterating the potential space. In the fowl, there is an extensive region that has few delicate strands connecting the two pleura along the dorsolateral aspect of the lung. The lung can collapse inward if the pleural cavity is penetrated along the dorsolateral border.

EFFUSIONS

Effusions can accumulate within any of the cavities. Chronic hepatic disease can result in the formation of a transudate or modified transudate within the perihepatic cavities. Sustained portal hypertension secondary to hepatic fibrosis is suspected to be a common mechanism in pet birds. Hypoproteinemia due to reduced albumin synthesis may also contribute; however, severe hypoproteinemia alone rarely results in ascites, as most birds generally die before the fluid develops. The prominent accumulation of a modified transudate ascitic fluid in poultry is believed to be due to portal hypertension from right-ventricular failure or right–ventricular failure secondary to pulmonary hypertension.

Effusions into the peritoneal cavity are generally the result of inflammatory or malignant diseases. Exudative effusions are more cellular, with a specific gravity greater than 1.020 and total protein greater than 3.0 g/dl. Malignant effusions are not uncommonly associated with hemorrhage or evidence of hemorrhage (histiocytic erythrophagocytosis or cytoplasmic iron-pigment accumulation). Occasionally neoplastic cells may exfoliate into the fluid.

A variety of inflammatory and toxic heart diseases can result in pericardial fluid accumulation. Hemopericardium has been associated with cardiac rupture due to myocardial infarction and dissecting aortic aneurysms, some associated with mycobacterial aoritis.

INFLAMMATORY DISEASE

Many of the inflammatory processes involving the pleural/peritoneum will generally result in the production of a protein-rich exudate with fibrin, desquamated mesothelial cells, and inflammatory cells. This is in contrast with air-sac inflammation that typically forms a dry purulent exudate.

Infectious Disease

Viral Disease. Avian viral serositis is an uncommon viral infection of neonatal and juvenile psittacines in which the causative agent is eastern equine encephalomyelitis (EEE) virus. EEE virus is an alphavirus in the Togaviridae family that uses a mosquito vector. This infection results in a fibrinous epicarditis and the development of abundant coelomic effusion. The ascitic fluid is typically pale yellow with the specific gravity greater than 1.017 and a low cellularity (Fig. 13.1). The serositis involves all serosal surfaces and is characterized by a protein-rich exudate with proliferative and desquamated mesothelial cells, fibrin, and inflammatory cells (Fig. 13.2). Other common gross lesions include hepatomegaly and pulmonary edema/congestion.

The histologic lesions of avian viral serositis are similar to psittacine proventricular dilatation disease with perivascular lymphoplasmacytic accumulations and lymphocytic plasmacytic infiltrates in myenteric ganglia and nerves of crop, proventriculus, ventriculus, and duodenum. Lymphoplasmacytic infiltrates are also seen in the pericardial ganglia, cardiac conduction fibers, and as perivascular foci in brain and spinal cord. Avian viral serositis infection also leads to bursal lymphoid necrosis,

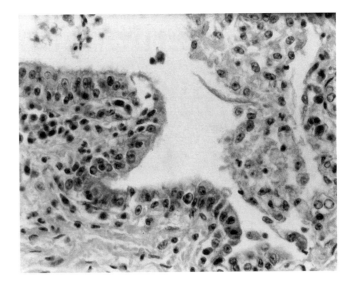

13.2.   Mild serositis with proliferation of mesothelial cells and slight mononuclear cell infiltrate.

hepatocellular necrosis, a heterophilic splenitis, and the prominent serositis.

Polyomavirus infections in both budgerigars and the large psittacines can be associated with the development of hydropericardium and ascites. Viral damage to the vascular endothelium as well as hypoproteinemia associated with liver damage may lead to the serositis, subcutaneous edema, and widespread ecchymotic and petechial hemorrhages (Fig. 13.3). The serositis and pericardial effusion are of low cellularity. A heterophilic serositis can suggest a secondary bacterial or fungal infection. The most consistent lesions of polyomavirus include hepatic necrosis, membranous glomerulopathy, variable karyomegaly of the liver and kidney, and large clear to basophilic intranuclear inclusion bodies of the splenic periarteriolar sheaths.

Herpesvirus (Pacheco's disease virus) will produce multifocal serosal and mesenteric petechiation (Fig. 13.4). The hemorrhages may be secondary to the severe hepatic

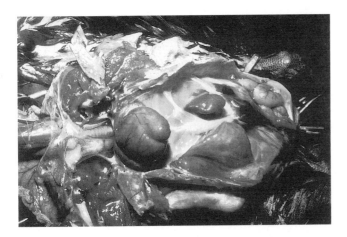

13.1.   Peritoneal fluid and opaque serosal foci of a bird with probable avian serositis virus infection.

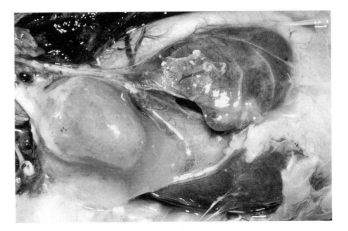

13.3.   Severe serositis and pericardial effusion associated with polyomavirus infection.

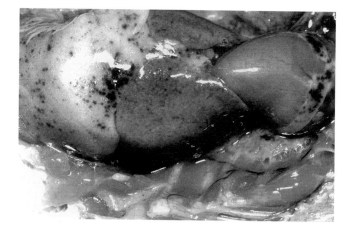

13.4. Mesenteric and serosal petechiae and ecchymoses due to herpesvirus (Pacheco's disease) infection.

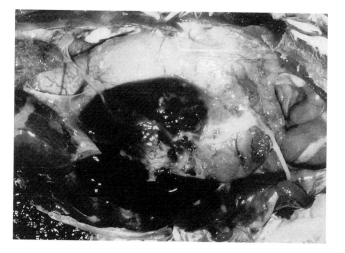

13.6. Salmonella-induced peritonitis. Note the fibrin and purulent material on the serosal surfaces and in the mesentery.

necrosis or viral proliferation in the endothelial cells of blood vessels. The defining lesions of Pacheco's disease virus are hepatic acute diffuse or multifocal necrosis with mixed inflammation, necrotic foci in periarterial lymphatic sheaths of the white pulp or in the red pulp of the spleen, syncytial cells, and eosinophilic intranuclear inclusions.

Uncommon lesions in systemic poxvirus infections of passerines have included air sacculitis, pneumonia, peritonitis, and heart and liver necrosis. The peritonitis is a proliferative lesion characterized by increased size and number of serosal cells, some of which contain cytoplasmic vacuoles and granular eosinophilic inclusions. The diagnosis of poxvirus rests on demonstration of the characteristic intracytoplasmic inclusion bodies generally in proliferative epithelium of the skin or mucosa.

Bacterial Disease. Bacterial peritonitis is an uncommon presentation in pet birds. Most cases of bacterial peritonitis are secondary to a gastroenteritis or perforation of the gastrointestinal tract (Fig. 13.5). The lesions and inflam-

matory cells are generally dependent on the pathogenicity of the bacteria and the chronicity of the disease (Fig. 13.6). In acute to subacute lesions, there will be heterophilic infiltrates, edema, and fibrin deposition (Fig. 13.7). Mycobacterium is the most frequently reported isolate, although this most likely reflects the systemic nature of the infection and ease of recognizing the acid-fast positive bacteria (Fig. 13.8). The inflammation is typically granulomatous, with macrophages, multinucleated giant cells, and scattered nodules of lymphocytes and plasma cells.

Chlamydophila psittaci. The acute lesions of *Chlamydophila psittaci* are of a fibrinous peritoneal exudate, air sacculitis, hepatitis, pericarditis, myocarditis, bronchopneumonia, catarrhal enteritis, nephrosis, and splenitis.

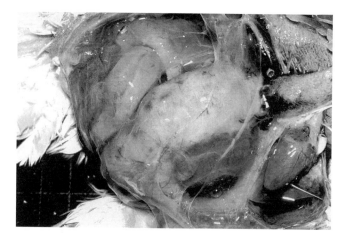

13.5. Bacterial peritonitis. The serosal surfaces are thickened, and there is fibrin and gelatinous fluid accumulation.

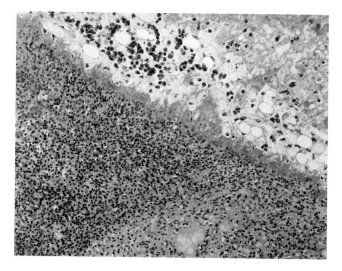

13.7. Bacterial peritonitis with large areas of necrosis, pleocellular inflammation, and fibrin deposition.

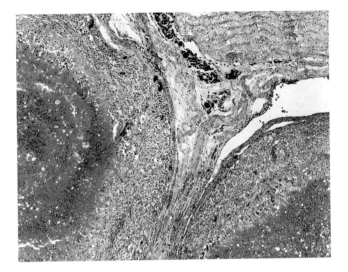

13.8. *Chronic mycobacterial peritonitis with formation of large granulomas.*

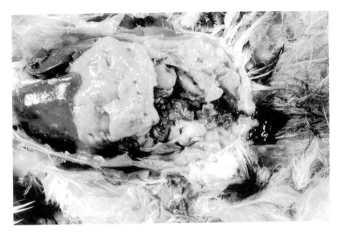

13.10. *Chronic mycotic infection with peritonitis. Large amounts of thickened yellow-white exudate are present.*

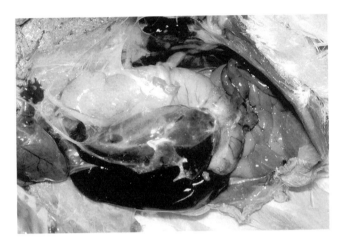

13.9. *Tenacious, slightly opaque, peritoneal exudate seen in* Chlamydophila *infection.*

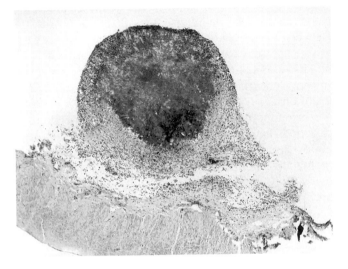

13.11. *Typical serosal mycetoma with a necrotic core surrounded by an inflammatory reaction.*

Fibrin exudation characterizes the peritoneal and epicardial lesions (Fig. 13.9). The single most consistent histologic lesion of this zoonotic disease is a systemic histiocytic inflammation.

Fungal Disease. Fungal peritonitis usually represents an extension of a fungal air sacculitis or pneumonia or, less likely, a gastrointestinal perforation and a mixed infection with bacteria. With an acute infection the mesentery, pericardium, or serosa will be thickened with edema, scattered heterophils, and fibrin deposition. The more chronic lesions contain large amounts of yellow-white caseous exudate (Fig. 13.10). Histologically they are pyogranulomatous to granulomatous lesions with a thick proliferation of epithelioid macrophages, degenerate heterophils, multinucleated giant cells, smaller numbers of lymphocytes and plasma cells, and mats of fungal hyphae. Mycetomas may form with central cores of necrosis (Fig. 13.11).

Protozoal Disease. A serous and fibrinous serositis has been associated with toxoplasma infection of canaries (Serinus canaria) and other small passerine cage birds. Disseminated massive hemorrhage and pulmonary necrosis with intra- and extracellular organisms, a heterophilic interstitial pneumonia, acute hepatitis, splenitis, nephritis, and necrotic nonsuppurative myocarditis characterize the acute phase (see the relevant chapters). Birds surviving the initial infection may develop ocular atrophy. Toxoplasma gondii cysts can be found in the brain and eye, with a nonsuppurative chorioretinitis and meningoencephalitis.

NONINFECTIOUS DISEASE

Egg Yolk Peritonitis

The peritonitis associated with the presence of egg yolk material can range in severity from nonclinical to life threatening. The yolk material (proteins and fats), which in small amounts can be gradually resorbed, generally elicits a mild histiocytic response along the serosa of the intestines and oviduct. Large amounts of yolk material and the presence of bacteria can result in severe adhesions between the loops of intestines and variable organ dysfunction.

Acute egg yolk peritonitis histologically is characterized by large amounts of slightly refractile amphophilic to basophilic, variably sized protein globules deposited on the serosal surfaces (Fig. 13.12). There may be some hemorrhage as well as mild heterophilic inflammation (Fig. 13.13). Egg yolk peritonitis may occur from trauma, salpingitis, rupture of the oviduct, neoplasia, ovarian cystic hyperplasia, and ectopic ovulation due to reverse peristalsis of the oviduct. Most birds with egg yolk peritonitis present in respiratory distress with a distended, fluid-filled abdomen.

Visceral Gout

Visceral gout is the deposition of urates on serosal surfaces. The common sites are the epicardium, pericardium, and serosal surfaces of the proventriculus/ventriculus and liver. Grossly these deposits are gray-white and of variable shape (Fig. 13.14). Histologically many cases are peracute, although there may be heterophilic infiltrates subtending the deposits. These heterophils are generally degenerative or necrotic and are associated with edema and mild hemorrhage/congestion. The urates appear as faint basophilic feathery material on the serosa. Formalin fixation will dissolve most of the crystals, but a negative image can be recognized in most cases with obvious gross lesions (Fig. 13.15). Severe renal lesions are typically associated with visceral gout.

Hemorrhage

Trauma, neoplastic rupture, and toxic exposure (anticoagulant rodenticides) can result in hemorrhage into the

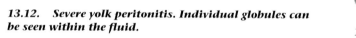

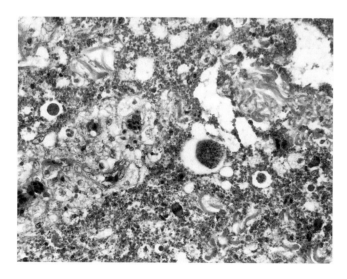

13.12. Severe yolk peritonitis. Individual globules can be seen within the fluid.

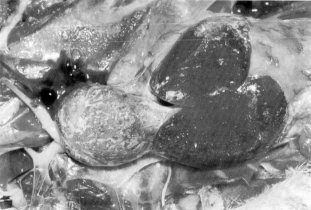

13.14.   Visceral/serosal urate deposition. The reaction must be differentiated from infection.

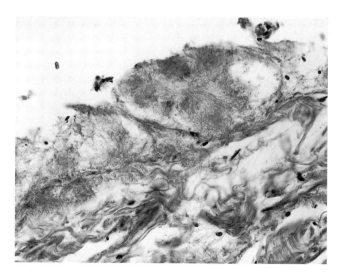

13.13.   Detail of exudate in yolk peritonitis. Basophilic globules of varying sizes characterize the reaction.

13.15.   Detail of serosal crystalline urate deposition.

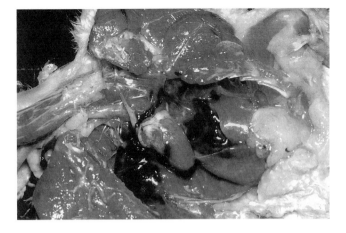

13.16.   *Marked hemorrhage within the peritoneal cavity.*

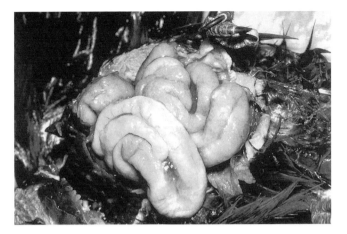

13.17.   *Serosal lymphosarcoma. Markedly thickened and opaque intestinal serosa is seen.*

coelomic cavities (Fig. 13.16). The amount and duration of the hemorrhage will determine the lesions. In all but peracute lesions, there will be an influx of macrophages that exhibit erythrophagocytosis and cytoplasmic hemosiderin pigment accumulation.

Avocado Toxin

Although the toxic principle is unknown, a number of psittacines, passerines, and ratites have died after ingesting avocado fruit. The majority of cases have few gross or histologic lesions. Hydropericardium due to myocardial damage is recognized in some cases. The fluid is described as clear and light tan, with a low specific gravity (less than 1.014). Degeneration and necrosis of myocytes, a marked infiltration of heterophils, and rare early fibroplasia characterize the cardiac lesions. Other lesions include mild nephrosis and pulmonary congestion, edema, and hemorrhage.

NEOPLASTIC DISEASE

The tumors described of the pleural/peritoneum are of systemic and local metastases. These include lymphosarcoma, ovarian/oviductal carcinomas, pancreatic carcinomas, and gastric carcinomas.

Lymphosarcoma (malignant lymphoma) is a common neoplasm of psittacines and passerines. To date, there has been no evidence of a viral link to the tumor formation in pet birds. This neoplasia develops in primary and secondary lymphoid tissues and spreads to other tissues. Diffuse to nodular involvement is characteristic. The liver is most commonly involved, followed by involvement of the spleen and kidneys. These organs will appear enlarged and pale. Serosal infiltration of neoplastic lymphoid cells leads to thickening and opacity of the involved organs (Fig. 13.17). The neoplastic lymphocytes typically have scant to moderate amounts of amphophilic to eosinophilic cytoplasm and a central nucleus with a reticulated to coarse chromatin (Fig. 13.18).

Both oviductal and ovarian tumors can implant widely throughout the coelomic cavity (chapter 6). Carcinomas

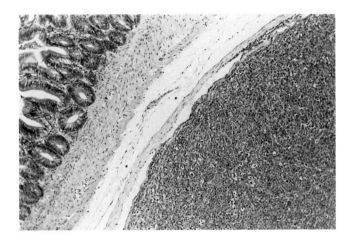

13.18.   *Histologic appearance of serosal lymphosarcoma.*

of the oviduct can appear as columnar epithelial cells forming tubular structures closely resembling cells of normal glands except for their orientation or as nodules composed of cuboidal cells that form definitive tubules to solid sheets. The cells are large and basophilic, with vesicular nuclei and numerous mitotic figures.

Pancreatic adenocarcinomas are rare tumors that may implant on the serosal surfaces and metastasize to the liver or lung. Grossly the typical lesion is of a diffusely enlarged, white, nodular, and firm pancreas. They are most common in the cockatiel and may completely envelope the intestines. Histologically the tumors are comprised of irregular glandular and tubular structures embedded in variable amounts of fibrous connective tissue stroma. The cells are tightly packed columnar cells with large vesicular nuclei, prominent nucleoli, and scant apical cytoplasm.

Primary, malignant gastric neoplasms are seen in psittacine birds (chapter 3), and carcinomas/adenocarcinomas of the proventriculus are more frequently reported than those of the ventriculus. Gastric tumors may appear grossly as a thickening at the junction of proventriculus and ventriculus that presents as a flat or slightly raised subserosal or serosal lesion. Late in the disease, there may be implants or extension to the serosa of ventriculus, intestine, pancreas, and lungs.

ADDITIONAL READING

Bezuidenhout AJ. 1988. Ascites and the anatomy of the peritoneal sacs of broilers. Onderstepoort J Vet Res 1:23–25.

Burger WP, Naude TW, Van Rensburg IB, et al. 1994. Cardiomyopathy in ostriches (Struthio camelus) due to avocado (Persea americana var. guatemalensis) intoxication. J S Afr Vet Assoc 3:113–118.

Campbell TW, Turner O. 1999. Carcinoma of the ventriculus with metastasis to the lungs in a sulphur-crested cockatoo (Cacatua galerita). J Avian Med Surg 13:265–268.

Chalmers GA. 1986. Neoplasms in two racing pigeons. Avian Dis 30:241–244.

Coleman CW. 1995. Lymphoid neoplasia in pet birds: A review. J Avian Med Surg 9:3–7.

Fitzgerald SD, Reed WM, Fulton RM. 1995. Development and application of an immunohistochemical staining technique to detect avian polyomaviral antigen in tissue sections. J Vet Diagn Invest 7:444–450.

Fredrickson TN. 1987. Ovarian tumors of the hen. Environ Health Perspect 73:35–51.

Fudge AM. 1997. What is your diagnosis? J Avian Med Surg 11:279–281.

Goodchild WM. 1970. Differentiation of the body cavities and air sacs of Gallus domesticus post mortem and their location in vivo. Br Poult Sci 11:209–215.

Graham DL, Calnek BW. 1987. Papovavirus infection in hand-fed parrots: Virus isolation and pathology. Avian Dis 31:398–410.

Graham DL. 1993. Special presentation a color atlas of avian chlamydiosis. Semin Avian Exotic Pet Med 2:184–189.

Gravendyck M, Balks E, Schröder-Gravendyck A-S, et al. 1998. Quantification of the herpesvirus content in various tissues and organs, and associated post mortem lesions of psittacine birds which died during an epornitic of Pacheco's parrot disease (PPD). Avian Pathol 27:478.

Gregory CR, Latimer KS, Niagro FD, et al. 1997. Investigations of eastern equine encephalomyelitis virus as the causative agent of psittacine proventricular dilatation syndrome. J Avian Med Surg 11:187–193.

Hargis AM, Stauber E, Casteel S, Eitner D. 1989. Avocado (Persea americana) intoxication in caged birds. J Am Vet Med Assoc 194:64–66.

Harcourt-Brown NH, Gough RE, Drury SE, Higgins RJ. 1998. Serositis in two black-capped conures (Pyrrhura rupicola): A possible viral cause. J Avian Med Surg 12:178–183.

Kajigaya H, Kamemura M, Tanahara N, et al. 1987. The influence of celomic membranes and a tunnel between celomic cavities on cancer metastasis in poultry. Avian Dis 31:176–186.

Kennedy FA, Sattler-Augustin S, Mahler JR, Jansson PC. 1996. Oropharyngeal and cloacal papillomas in two macaws (Ara spp.) with neoplasia. J. Avian Med Surg 10:89–95.

Leach MW, Paul-Murphy J, Lowenstine LJ. 1986. Three cases of gastric neoplasia in psittacines. Avian Dis 33:204–210.

Levy S. 1993. Avocado toxicity: Some considerations. J Assoc Avian Vet 7:160.

Marsh AE, Denver M, Hill FI, et al. 2000. Detection of Sarcocystis neurona in the brain of a Grant's zebra (Equus burchelli bohmi). J Zoo Wildl Med 31:82–86.

O'Toole D, Haven T, Driscoll M, Nunamaker C. 1992. An outbreak of Pacheco's disease in an aviary of psittacines. J Vet Diagn Invest 4:203–205.

Parenti E, Cerruti-Sola S, Turilli C, et al. 1986. Spontaneous toxoplasmosis in canaries (Serinus canaria) and other small passerine cage birds. Avian Pathol 15:183–197.

Ramis A, Tarres J, Fondevila D, Ferrer L. 1996. Immunocytochemical study of the pathogenesis of Pacheco's parrot disease in budgerigars. Vet Microbiol 52:49–61.

Ritchey JW, Degernes LA, Brown TT. 1997. Exocrine pancreatic insufficiency in a yellow-naped Amazon (Amazona ochrocephala) with pancreatic adenocarcinoma. Vet Pathol 34:55–57.

Ritchie BW, Niagro FD, Latimer KS, et al. 1991. Avian polyomavirus: An overview. J Assoc Avian Vet 5:147–153.

Shropshire CM, Stauber E, Arai M. 1992. Evaluation of selected plants for acute toxicosis in budgerigars. J Am Vet Med Assoc 200:936–939.

Stauber E, Papageorges M, Sande R, Ward L. 1990. Polyostotic hyperostosis associated with oviductal tumor in a cockatiel. J Am Vet Med Assoc 196:939–940.

Stoica G, Russo E, Hoffman JR. 1989. Abdominal tumor in a military macaw. Lab Anim 23:17–20.

Straub J, Pees M, Krautwald-Junghanns ME. 2001. Diagnosis of pericardial effusion in birds by ultrasound. Vet Rec 21:149:86–88

Williams SM, Fulton RM, Render JA, et al. 2001. Ocular and encephalic toxoplasmosis in canaries. Avian Dis 45:262–267.

Index